Pediatric Brain and Spine
An Atlas of MRI and Spectroscopy

Ketonen · Hiwatashi · Sidhu · Westesson

L. M. Ketonen
A. Hiwatashi
R. Sidhu
P.-L. Westesson

Pediatric Brain and Spine

An Atlas of MRI and Spectroscopy

With 1427 Figures

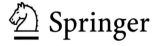 Springer

ISBN 3-540-21340-6
Springer Berlin Heidelberg New York

Library of Congress Control Number: 2004111251

Springer is a part of Springer Science + Business Media

springeronline.com

© Springer-Verlag Berlin Heidelberg 2005
Printed in Germany

Editor: Dr. Ute Heilmann, Heidelberg
Desk editor: Dörthe Mennecke-Bühler, Heidelberg
Production editor: Bernd Wieland, Heidelberg
Cover design: F. Steinen, ᵉStudio Calamar, Spain
Reproduction and Typesetting: AM-productions, Wiesloch
Printing and bookbinding: Stürtz AG, Würzburg

21/3150 – 5 4 3 2 1 0
Printed on acid-free paper

Preface

This is an atlas on contemporary MR imaging of the pediatric central nervous system. We have concentrated on brain imaging, but have an extensive chapter on the spine and a smaller chapter on the head and neck.

The book starts with a chapter on the normal myelinization and normal variance. We are including chapters on malformations, inherited conditions, infection, tumors, trauma, vascular abnormalities, and spine abnormalities. The last chapter of the book is a miscellaneous chapter that includes all those cases that did not fit well in other categories. The chapter on trauma and brain damage includes an extensive section on CNS manifestations of nonaccidental pediatric trauma. There is an also an exciting chapter on fetal MR imaging describing some of the more common abnormalities seen in prenatal imaging. We have intentionally avoided discussing some of the ethical aspects of fetal imaging.

Cases in this book range from those commonly seen in clinical practice to many exceedingly rare conditions. The book format has allowed us to illustrate these unusual cases generously, and in many we have been able to include MR proton spectroscopy and diffusion images. We included a few CT images when they were an essential part of the diagnosis, classic presentations or showed the abnormalities the best. It was not our intention to publish a textbook, but rather an atlas-type book on pediatric neuro-MR imaging. We have concentrated on multiple high-quality images, which will allow the clinician to identify an unknown case relatively quickly by simply comparing the images of his patient with the images in the book. A short discussion is associated with each case, but for more detailed and in-depth information we refer to existing textbooks.

The book is a collaboration between four authors and three collaborators all with different backgrounds, training from different parts of the world and with different clinical experiences. Dr. Leena Ketonen is the lead author and has a long-term interest in pediatric neuro-imaging. During her 20-year career in neuroradiology she has continuously gathered interesting cases. When Dr. Ketonen moved from Massachusetts General Hospital in Boston to the University of Rochester it was quite obvious, looking into her new office, that she had a very extensive collection of such cases. She would have needed a much larger office than the one we were able to offer her just to store her enormous teaching file. Seeing her phenomenal collection of cases and pairing that with our positive experience writing our previous book, *Diffusion-Weighted MR Imaging of the Brain*, it was obvious that we had both an idea and the material for another neuro-imaging book. We decided on the topic of pediatric neuro-imaging with Dr. Ketonen as the lead author. We started out with the intention of having ten cases per chapter, but it soon became obvious that the number of cases would double for many of the chapters. The book is based mainly on Dr. Ketonen's collected cases, backed up by the University of Rochester's teaching file, started many years ago by Dr. Numaguchi. We have incorporated cases of fetal MR imaging (Chap. 11) that we borrowed from Dr. Susan Blaser of the Children's Hospital in Toronto.

Dr. Akio Hiwatashi has been instrumental in correcting, manipulating and formatting the images for this book. Dr. Ravinder Sidhu has been the lead person for looking up background information and making sure we have the most appropriate and up-to-date references. Dr. Westesson has been the leader of the project and has kept it moving forward while writing the head and neck chapter. The contribution of Susan Blaser has been instrumental. Her outstanding collection of prenatal MR cases constitutes the bulk of Chap. 11. In addition we have enjoyed the help of Drs Lawrence Buadu and Sudhir Kathuria for the chapters on miscellaneous conditions and nonaccidental trauma (child abuse).

Our experience from working with Springer on our earlier book was totally positive from the beginning to the end. The printing, editing and image quality along with the layout of the book were first quality and the publisher proved to be able to produce this quality work in a short period of time. This experience has been repeated with this second project. It should be mentioned that we started this book in December of 2003 after the RSNA and it was published less than one year later, which is a remarkable accomplishment thinking of how many high-quality images were included. We would like to thank the editors at Springer, Dr. Heilmann and Mrs. Dörthe Mennecke-

Bühler, our graphic designer at the University of Rochester, Margaret Kowaluk, and our secretaries, Belinda De Libero and Jeanette Griebel. Special thanks go to our families for sacrificing the time and energy that we invested in this project.

Rochester, New York
October 2004

Authors and Collaborators

Susan Blaser, MD
Associate Professor of Neuroradiology
The Hospital for Sick Children
Division of Neuroradiology
and Department of Medical Imaging
The University of Toronto
Toronto, Ontario, Canada
susan.blaser@sickkids.ca

Lawrence Buadu, MD, PhD
Fellow, Division of Diagnostic
and Interventional Neuroradiology
Department of Radiology
University of Rochester School of Medicine
and Dentistry
Rochester, New York, USA
lbuadu@comcast.net

Akio Hiwatashi, MD
Fellow, Division of Diagnostic
and Interventional Neuroradiology
Department of Radiology
University of Rochester School of Medicine
and Dentistry
Rochester, New York, USA
akio_hiwatashi@urmc.rochester.edu

Sudhir Kathuria, MD
Fellow, Division of Diagnostic
and Interventional Neuroradiology
Department of Radiology
University of Rochester School of Medicine
and Dentistry
Rochester, New York, USA
sudhir_kathuria@urmc.rochester.edu

Leena M. Ketonen, MD, PhD
Professor of Radiology
Director, Pediatric Neuroimaging
Division of Diagnostic
and Interventional Neuroradiology
Department of Radiology
University of Rochester School of Medicine
and Dentistry
Rochester, New York, USA
Leena.Ketonen@DI.MDACC.TMC.edu

Ravinder Sidhu, MD
Visiting Assistant Professor
Division of Diagnostic
and Interventional Neuroradiology
Department of Radiology
University of Rochester School of Medicine
and Dentistry
Rochester, New York, USA
ravinder_sidhu@urmc.rochester.edu

Per-Lennart Westesson, MD, PhD, DDS
Professor of Radiology
Director, Division of Diagnostic
and Interventional Neuroradiology
Department of Radiology
and Professor of Clinical Dentistry
University of Rochester School of Medicine
and Dentistry
Rochester, New York, USA

Professor of Oral Diagnostic Sciences
State University of New York at Buffalo
Buffalo, New York, USA

Associate Professor of Oral Radiology
University of Lund
Lund, Sweden

perlennart_westesson@urmc.rochester.edu

Contents

**1 Normal Brain Myelination
and Normal Variants** 1

Introduction 1
**Chronological Imaging Atlas
of Normal Myelination** 2
**Cavum Septi Pellucidi, Cavum Vergae
and Cavum Velum Interpositum** 11
  Cavum Septi Pellucidi and Vergae 11
  Cavum Velum Interpositum 12
Ventriculus Terminalis 14

2 Congenital Brain Malformations 17

Introduction 17
Corpus Callosum Agenesis/Dysgenesis 19
  Completely Absent Corpus Callosum 19
  Near Complete Agenesis of Corpus callosum . 20
Pericallosal Lipoma 22
  Curvilinear Lipoma 22
  Nodular Midline ("Callosal") Lipoma 23
Hydranencephaly 25
  Case 1. Hydranencephaly
    with Increasing Head Size. 25
  Case 2. Hydranencephaly
    with Increasing Head Size. 26
  Case 3. Hydranencephaly
    with Microcephaly. 27
Cephalocele and Meningocele 28
  Occipital Encephalocele 28
  Parietal Cephalocele 29
  Parietal Cephalocele 30
  Skull Base Encephalocele 31
  Parietal Meningocele 32
  Spinal Lipomeningocele 33
Micrencephaly with Lissencephaly 34
Generalized Cortical Dysplasia 35
Schizencephaly 37
  Open Lip Schizencephaly (Type II) 37
  Unilateral Closed Lip Schizencephaly (Type I) 38

Lissencephaly 39
Gray Matter Heterotopia 40
  Subependymal Nodular Heterotopia 40
  Focal Subcortical Heterotopia
    with Agenesis of Corpus Callosum 41
  Focal Subcortical Heterotopia 43
  Band Heterotopia ("Double Cortex") 44
Holoprosencephaly 45
  Septo-Optic Dysplasia in a Teenager. 45
  Septo-Optic Dysplasia. 46
  Alobar Holoprosencephaly 47
  Semilobar Holoprosencephaly 48
  Semilobar Holoprosencephaly
    with Pierre-Robin Syndrome 49
Chiari Malformations 51
  Chiari I Malformation
    with Low but Rounded Tonsils 51
  Unilateral Chiari I Malformation
    with Pointed Tonsils 52
  Chiari II (Arnold-Chiari) Malformation . . . 53
  Chiari II and Meningomyelocele
    in a Newborn. 54
  Chiari III and Occipital Encephalocele 55
  Chiari III and Spina Bifida 56
Dandy-Walker Syndromes 58
  Dandy-Walker Variant
    with Enlargement of Fourth Ventricle . . . 58
  Dandy-Walker Variant
    with No Separate Fourth Ventricle 59
  Dandy-Walker Variant
    with Elevation of Torcula 60
Joubert's Syndrome 61
Rhombencephalosynapsis 63
**Cloverleaf Skull Syndrome
  (Kleeblattschädel Anomaly)** 64
Hemimegalencephaly 66

**3   Inherited Neurological Diseases
and Disorders of Myelin** 69

Introduction 69
Hereditary Myelin Disorders 70
  Krabbe's Disease
    (Globoid Cell Leukodystrophy) 70
  Mucopolysaccharidoses (MPS) 73
  Zellweger Syndrome 78
  Adrenoleukodystrophy 79
  Neuronal Ceroid Lipofuscinosis (NCL). . . . 80
  Mitochondrial Disorders 83
  Cerebellar Degeneration Associated
    with Coenzyme Q10 Deficiency. 90
  Hallervorden-Spatz Disease 91
**Defects in Genes Encoding
  the Myelin Proteins** 93
  Pelizaeus-Merzbacher Disease 93
  p10 p9 Translocation. 95
  18q Syndrome 97
**Disorders in Amino Acid
  and Organic Acid Metabolism** 98
  Phenylketonuria (PKU) 98
  Propionic Acidemia 100
  Maple Syrup Urine Disease (MSUD) 101
  Galactosemia 102
  Late-Onset Type of Ornithine
    Transcarbamylase (OTCD) Deficiency
    with a Recent Occipital Infarct 104
Miscellaneous 106
  Multiple Sclerosis (MS) 106
  Acute Disseminated Encephalomyelitis
    (ADEM). 110
  Perisylvian Syndrome 112
  Merosin-Deficient Congenital
    Muscular Dystrophy (CMD). 114
  Vanishing White Matter (VWM) Disease . . 115
  Megalencephalic Leukoencephalopathy
    with Subcortical Cysts (MLC)
    and Normal Development 117
  Delayed Myelination 119
  Autoimmune Polyglandular Syndrome
    (APS) 121
  Osmotic Myelinolysis
    (Extrapontine Myelinolysis). 123

4   Infection 125

Introduction 125
Meningitis and Complications of Meningitis . . 127
  Acute Pyogenic Meningitis 127
  Subacute Pyogenic Meningitis
    with Hydrocephalus 128
  Suppurative Meningitis with Subdural
    Effusions and Cortical Ischemia 128
  Suppurative Meningitis and Brain Infarct . . 130
  Meningitis with Multiple Infarcts. 131
  Candida Meningitis 132
Brain Abscess. 133
Empyema 135
  Subdural Empyema with Cortical
    and Meningeal Involvement. 135
  Subdural Empyema 136
  Epidural Empyema 137
Septic Emboli 138
Nocardiosis 139
Citrobacter Infections 141
  Citrobacter Meningitis and Cerebritis 141
  Chronic Citrobacter Cerebritis 142
Herpes Simplex Virus Encephalitis. 143
  Neonatal Herpes Simplex
    Virus Encephalitis Type 2 143
  Neonatal Herpes Simplex
    Virus Encephalitis Type 2 144
  Herpes Simplex Virus Encephalitis Type 1. . 147
Congenital Cytomegalovirus Infection 149
Cytomegalovirus Encephalitis 151
Viral Encephalitis (Influenza Encephalopathy) . 152
**Congenital Human Immunodeficiency Virus
  (HIV) Infection.** 153
Cysticercosis 157
  Intraventricular Cysticercosis. 157
  Subarachnoid Cysticercosis 157
  Parenchymal Cysticercosis 158
  Calcified Cysticercosis 159
Tuberculosis 160
  Tubercular Meningitis 160
  Intracranial Tuberculoma 160
Tuberculous Abscesses 161
**Limbic Encephalitis
  (Paraneoplastic Limbic Encephalitis)** 162
Acute Cerebellitis 164
Rasmussen's Encephalitis 165

5 Posterior Fossa Tumors 167

Introduction 167
  Diffusion-Weighted Imaging (DW imaging) 167
  MR Spectroscopy. 167
Medulloblastoma 169
  Solid Medulloblastoma 169
  Hemorrhagic/Necrotic Medulloblastoma . . 170
  Medulloblastoma with CSF Seeding 172
Cerebellar Pilocytic Astrocytoma 173
  Mostly Solid Cerebellar Pilocytic
    Astrocytoma 173
  Cystic Cerebellar Pilocytic Astrocytoma
    with Mural Nodule 175
Ependymoma 176
Brain Stem Glioma 178
Epidermoid Tumor 180
Arachnoid Cyst. 181
Von Hippel-Lindau Disease (VHL) 182
Acute Lymphoblastic Leukemia
  (Precursor B) 184
Chordoma 185

6 Supratentorial Brain Tumors 187

Introduction 187
  DW Imaging 188
  MR Spectroscopy. 188
Glioblastoma Multiforme (GBM). 189
Juvenile Pilocytic Astrocytoma (JPA) 191
Mixed Pleomorphic Xanthoastrocytoma
  (PXA) and Ganglioglioma 192
Oligodendroglioma 194
Ependymoma 197
Choroid plexus papillomas 199
  Choroid Plexus Papilloma in the Trigone . . 199
  Choroid Plexus Papilloma at the Foramen
    of Monro 201
Gliomatosis Cerebri 202
Ganglioglioma 203
Central Neurocytoma 206
Dysembryoplastic Neuroepithelial Tumor
  (DNET) 208
Germinoma of the Pineal Region 208
Pineal Teratoma 210
Pineoblastoma. 211
Pineal Embryonal Carcinoma 212
Primitive Neuroectodermal Tumor (PNET) . . 214
Atypical Teratoid Rhabdoid Tumor 215
Esthesioneuroblastoma 217

Trigeminal Neurofibroma 218
Eosinophilic Granuloma 220
Craniopharyngioma. 220
Pituitary Adenoma 222
  Pituitary Macroadenoma 222
  Pituitary Microadenoma (Prolactinoma) . . 224
Subependymal Giant Cell Astrocytoma (SEGA) 225
Atypical Meningioma 226
Congenital Brain Tumors 229
  Congenital Teratoma 229
  Congenital Glioblastoma Multiforme 230
Orbital Juvenile Pilocytic Astrocytoma (JPA) . . 230
Optic Pathway Glioma 232
Hypothalamic Hamartoma
  (Hamartoma of Tuber Cinereum) 233

7 Brain Damage. 235

Introduction 235
Nonaccidental Trauma 236
  Scalp Injury (Subgaleal Hemorrhage) 236
  Skull Fracture 237
  Subdural Hemorrhage. 238
  Subarachnoid Hemorrhage 239
  Parenchymal Hemorrhage and Ischemia . . 240
  Diffuse Axonal Injury 241
  Hypoxic Ischemic Injury 242
  Infarct. 243
  Atrophy 244
  Venous Sinus Thrombosis. 245
  Thalamic Infarcts in a
    Shaken Infant Syndrome 245
Epidural and Subdural Hematoma 247
  Epidural Hematoma (EDH) 247
  Subdural Hematoma (SDH) 249
Contusion 251
Diffuse Axonal Injury (DAI) 252
  DAI in Corpus Callosum and Parenchyma . 252
  Hemorrhagic Contusion with DAI 254
  Multiple Areas of DAI in Corpus Callosum . 255
  DAI with Excitotoxic Mechanism. 256
Periventricular Leukomalacia (PVL),
  Preterm Hypoxic Ischemic
  Encephalopathy (HIE) 258
  Periventricular Leukomalacia
    with White Matter Aplasia 258
  Periventricular Leukomalacia
    with Thin Corpus Callosum. 259
  Unilateral PVL 260
  Periventricular Leukomalacia with
    Dystrophic Parenchymal Calcification . . 260

Hypoxic Ischemic Encephalopathy (HIE) 263
   Hypoxic Ischemic Encephalopathy
      with Infarcts 263
   Hypoxic Ischemic Encephalopathy
      with Brain Edema 263
   Hypoxic Ischemic Encephalopathy
      Post-Surgery 263
   Hypoxic Ischemic Encephalopathy
      with Seizures 265
Hypoxic Encephalopathy in Near-Drowning . . 267
Multicystic Encephalomalacia 268
Status Epilepticus and Postictal Stage 270
   Status Epilepticus with Partially
      Reversible Tissue Changes. 270
   Status Epilepticus with Permanent
      Tissue Damage 272
Cortical Laminar Necrosis 275
Cyclosporin-Induced Encephalopathy 277
Pontine and Extrapontine Myelinolysis
   in the Setting of Rapid Correction
   of Hyponatremia 278
Cephalhematoma 280
   CT Scan of Cephalhematoma 280
   MR Imaging of Cephalhematoma 281
   Cephalhematoma and
      Hypoxic-Ischemic Insult 283

8 Vascular Disorders 287

Introduction 287
Childhood Cerebrovascular Diseases
   with Infarct 288
   Dissection 288
   Sickle Cell Hemoglobinopathy with Infarct . 292
   Herpesvirus Infections of the CNS
      and Vascular Thrombosis 296
   CNS Vasculitis and Infarct 298
Wiskott-Aldrich Syndrome (WAS),
   Vasculitis and Infarct 301
Arteriovenous Malformations (AVMs) 302
Cavernous Malformation 306
   Solitary Intrinsic Parenchymal Lesion 306
   Solitary Exophytic Cavernous
      Malformation. 307
   Solitary Cavernous Malformation
      with Developmental Venous Anomaly . . 308
   Multiple Cavernous Malformations 309
   Cavernous Malformation Simulating
      Neoplasm with Major Bleed 311
Developmental Venous Anomaly 312
Capillary Telangiectasia 314

Sinovenous Thrombosis 315
   Transverse Sinus Thrombosis
      Extending Into Superior Sagittal,
      Sigmoid and Jugular Sinus 315
   Evolution of Transverse Sinus Thrombosis . 316
Sturge-Weber (SWS) Syndrome and Lack
   of Flow Through the Superior Sagittal
   Sinus Simulating Chronic Superior
   Sagittal Sinus Thrombosis 318
Iatrogenic Sinus Thrombosis in an
   Infant Treated with Extracorporeal
   Membrane Oxygenation (ECMO) 320
Intracranial Aneurysm 322
   Berry Aneurysm 322
   Fusiform Aneurysm 323
   Berry Aneurysm with Significant
      Vasospasm 324
Hemolytic Uremic Syndrome (HUS) 326
Intracerebral Hematoma 327
Moyamoya Disease 329
   Bilateral Moyamoya Disease 329
   Bilateral Moyamoya Disease
      with a Major Infarct 330
   Unilateral Moyamoya (Variant) 330
   Sickle cell Disease Leading
      to Moyamoya Disease 330
Vein of Galen Malformation 332

9 Head and Neck 335

Introduction 335
Multinodular Goiter 335
Thyroglossal Duct Cyst 337
Tornwaldt Cyst 339
Cystic Hygroma in Neck of Newborn 340
Neurofibromatosis 342
   Plexiform Neurofibromatosis of the Neck . . 342
   Neurofibromatosis of the Orbit 343
Kikuchi Disease 344
Dermoid 346
Schwannoma of the Tongue 348
Pleomorphic Adenoma of the Nose. 349
Rhabdomyosarcoma 350
Acinic Cell Carcinoma of the Parotid Gland . . 352
Anophthalmos 354
Wolf-Hirschhorn Syndrome 356
Retinopathy of Prematurity 357
Hemangioma 358
   Hemangioma of the Parotid Gland 358
   Hemangioma of the Face and Orbit 359
Langerhans Cell Histiocytosis 360

Osteosarcoma of the Cranium 362
Fibrous Dysplasia 364
Bilateral Coronoid Hyperplasia
   of the Mandible Causing Trismus 365
Dental Radicular Cyst 367
Mastoiditis with Sigmoid Sinus Thrombosis . . 368
Arteriovenous Fistula of Vertebral Artery . . . 369

10 Spine 371

Introduction 371
Chiari I Malformation 372
Tethered Cord with Lipoma 373
   Case 1 373
   Case 2 374
Ventriculus Terminalis
   of the Conus Medullaris 375
Diastematomyelia 376
   Separate Thecal Sacs 376
   Single Thecal Sac 376
Dermal Sinus Tract 378
Spinal Lipomas 380
   Case 1. Intra- and Extramedullary Lipomas . 380
   Case 2. Extramedullary Cervical Lipoma
      with Cord Compression 381
   Case 3. Intradural, Extramedullary Lipoma
      at the Conus 382
Caudal Regression Syndrome 383
Congenital Spinal Scoliosis,
   Kyphosis and Kyphoscoliosis 384
   Lumbar Hemivertebra 384
   Thoracic Hemivertebra 386
   Kyphosis 387
Arthrogryposis (Larsen's Syndrome) 388
Mucopolysaccharidoses (MPS) 388
   Hurler/Scheie Syndrome (MPS Type I H/S) . 388
   Morquio's Syndrome (MPS Type IV-A) . . . 390
Spinal Cord Astrocytoma 391
Intraspinal Ependymoma 394
   Holocord Ependymoma 394
   Conus Ependymoma 395
Neurofibromatosis Type 1 (NF-1) 396
Neurofibromatosis Type 2 (NF-2) 398
Neurofibroma 400
Metastatic Disease from CNS Primary Tumor . 402
   Intradural, Extramedullary Metastases
      (Drop Metastases) 402
   Intramedullary Metastases 403
Neuroblastoma 404
Ganglioneuroma 406

Ependymoblastoma 407
Meningioma 408
Meningeal Sarcoma 410
Rhabdomyosarcoma 411
   Primary Rhabdomyosarcoma 411
   Metastatic Rhabdomyosarcoma 412
Teratoma 413
Sacrococcygeal Teratoma 414
Osteochondroma 415
Hemangioma 417
Spinal Trauma 418
   Ligament Injury and Subluxation
      with Acute Cord Edema 418
   Myelomalacia 419
Brachial Plexus Trauma 421
   Nerve Root Avulsion from Accident 421
   Obstetric Brachial Plexus Injury 422
   Blunt Trauma to the Brachial Plexus 423
Epidural Hematoma 425
Spine Fractures 426
   Lumbar Spine Burst Fracture 427
   Lumbar Spine Compression Fracture 428
Spondylolisthesis 430
   Case 1. Spondylolisthesis
      With Spinal Canal Narrowing 430
   Case 2. Spondylolisthesis
      Without Spinal Canal Narrowing 430
Acute Disseminated Encephalomyelitis
   (ADEM) 432
   ADEM of Thoracic Cord 432
   ADEM of Cervical Cord 433
Epidural Abscess 434
Subacute Combined Degeneration
   of Spinal Cord (B12 Deficiency) 435

11 Fetal Imaging 437

Introduction 437
Normal MR Images of Fetus 438
   Normal Fetus 438
   Parasagittal Images of Normal Development 439
Anencephaly 440
Holoprosencephaly 441
   Alobar Holoprosencephaly 441
Alobar Holoprosencephaly 442
Septo-Optic Dysplasia 443
Aplasia of the Corpus Callosum 444
Dandy-Walker Malformation 445
Fetal Hydrops 446
Fetal Sacrococcygeal Teratoma 448

12 Miscellaneous 449

Introduction 449
Neurofibromatosis 451
   Neurofibromatosis 1
      and Bilateral Optic Nerve
      and Chiasm Glioma 451
   Neurofibromatosis 1
      and Unilateral Optic Nerve Glioma 452
   Neurofibromatosis 1 and "Hamartomas":
      Myelin Vacuolization in
      Supratentorial Area 452
   Neurofibromatosis 1 and "Hamartomas":
      Myelin Vacuolization in Cerebellum
      and Pons 453
   Neurofibromatosis 1 and
      Plexiform Neurofibroma of the Skin . . . 454
Sturge-Weber Syndrome 456
   Classic Sturge-Weber Syndrome 456
   Leptomeningeal Angioma
      and Prominent Choroid Plexus 457
   Classic Sturge-Weber Syndrome with
      Hemiatrophy and Calvarial Changes . . . 458
Tuberous Sclerosis 460
   Tuberous Sclerosis and Subependymal
      Nodules and Cortical Tubers 460
   Tuberous Sclerosis and Radial Bands
      and Cortical Tubers 461
   Tuberous Sclerosis
      and Parenchymal Calcification 462
   Tuberous Sclerosis and Cortical
      Dysplasia-Mimicking Lesion 463
   Tuberous Sclerosis and Giant Cell
      Astrocytoma, Subependymal
      and Subcortical Tubers 463
   Tuberous Sclerosis and Low-Grade Glioma . 465

Mesial Temporal Sclerosis 467
   Bilateral Mesial Temporal Sclerosis 467
   Hippocampus, Fornix and Mamillary
      Body Involvement in a Patient
      with Mesial Temporal Sclerosis 468
   Unilateral Mesial Temporal Sclerosis 469
Pituitary-Hypothalamic Axis Anomalies . . . 470
   Absent Pituitary Gland 470
   Ectopic Posterior Pituitary Gland 471
   Thickening of the Pituitary Stalk 472
Posterior Reversible Encephalopathy
  Syndrome (PRES) 474
Arachnoid Cyst 476
   Arachnoid Cyst with Enlargement
      of the Calvaria 476
   Arachnoid Cyst with Midline Cyst 477
   Arachnoid Cyst with Calvarial Remodeling . 478
   Arachnoid Cyst in the Posterior Fossa . . . 478
Dermoid Cyst (Ectodermal Inclusion Cyst) . . . 480
Neuroepithelial (Ependymal) Cyst 481
Temporal Lobe Cysts
  and Fetal Alcohol Syndrome 483
Lenticulostriate Vasculopathy 485
Craniosynostosis 487

Subject Index 489

Normal Brain Myelination and Normal Variants

Introduction

Normal brain myelination is a process that begins during the fifth fetal month and continues in the postnatal brain. It has important implications in normal brain development. The organized order of myelination emphasizes the role of imaging examinations of developmentally delayed children who often show no structural brain alterations despite suspicion of brain maturation delay. During the first months of life, the myelination process follows well-defined steps. Even the appearance of the normal fetal brain follows predictable steps. The timing of the appearance of the different sulci in the fetal brain is available using MR imaging. It is considered to be a good marker of fetal brain maturation. In general, in the postnatal brain the myelination progresses from caudal to cephalad and from dorsal to ventral. Therefore the occipital lobes myelinate before the frontal lobes and the dorsal brainstem does so before the ventral brainstem. The myelination progresses more rapidly in the functional areas used early in life. The myelination progresses rapidly during the two first years of life and slows markedly after that. MR imaging studies suggest that white matter myelination can be considered as an indicator of functional brain maturation. Myelination also progresses differently in compact (corpus callosum, internal capsule, cerebral peduncle) than in non-compact (peripheral white matter and corona radiata) white matter. Although myelination is initially greater in compact white matter, the change in myelination may be greater in non-compact white matter during the first few years of infancy.

From the imaging point of view, brain maturation can be followed in both T1- and T2-weighted images, although it occurs at different rates in T1 and T2 images. The newborn T1-weighted image is grossly similar to the adult T2-weighted image in that white matter has lower signal intensity than gray matter. The overall appearance of the newborn brain on the T2-weighted image is grossly similar to that of the adult on the T1-weighted image in that the white matter has higher signal intensity than the gray matter. The brain myelination reaches the adult appearance at the age of 2 years. The only area that can still exhibit a persistent T2 hyperintensity on MR images at about 2 years of age (and well beyond that) is considered to be the peritrigonal region, the so-called terminal zone. However, a persistent T2 hyperintensity has been noted in the frontotemporal subcortical regions beyond that age in normal children suggesting, that the so-called terminal zones are subcortical areas rather than the peritrigonal area. The terminal zones do not stain for myelin until the fourth decade of life. Persistent T2 hyperintensity may be seen until the second decade in these areas. Complete myelination takes place by about age 3 years in the subcortical regions. It is important to differentiate the terminal areas from white matter injury, such as periventricular leukomalacia.

Diffusion images and ADC maps give the same information: in both the signal intensity is proportional to water diffusion only. On DW images of the neonatal brain there is marked contrast between the hyperintense gray matter and the hypointense white matter. This contrast is more marked in premature neonates than in term neonates. The ventrolateral thalami of the newborn stand out on DW image and should not be misinterpreted as pathological restricted diffusion in the neonatal brain. It becomes progressively less hyperintense until the age of 4 months when it is isointense to the rest of the gray matter. As the brain matures, the contrast between the gray and white matter diminishes.

Suggested Reading

1. Carmody DP, Dunn SM, Boddie-Willis AS, DeMarco JK, Lewis M (2004) A quantitative measure of myelination development in infants, using MR images. Neuroradiology 8 Jul (Epub ahead of print) DOI: 10.1007/s00234-004-1241-z
2. McGraw P, Liang L, Provenzale JM (2002) Evaluation of normal age-related changes in anisotropy during infancy and childhood as shown by diffusion tensor imaging. AJR Am J Roentgenol 6:1515–1522
3. Parazzini C, Baldoli C, Scotti G, Triulzi F (2002) Terminal zones of myelination: MR evaluation of children aged 20–40 months. AJNR Am J Neuroradiol 10:1669–1673

Chronological Imaging Atlas of Normal Myelination

Figures 1.1 to 1.8 illustrate the process of normal myelination starting with a fetus aged 28 weeks and ending with a normal pattern in a 7-year-old. We have included MR spectroscopy for all cases available.

Figure 1.1

28 gestational week fetus (courtesy Susan Blazer, M.D.)

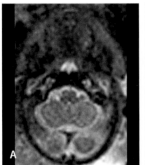

T2-weighted image.
Medulla

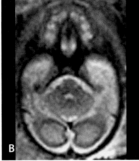

T2-weighted image.
Pons

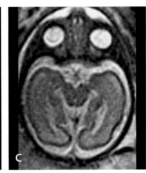

T2-weighted image.
Midbrain

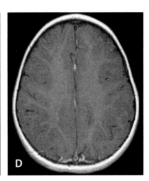

T2-weighted image.
Basal ganglia

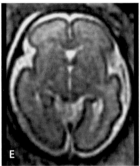

T2-weighted image.
Sylvian fissure level

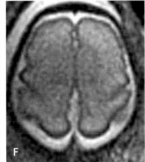

T2-weighted image.
Centrum semiovale

Figure 1.2

17-day-old male

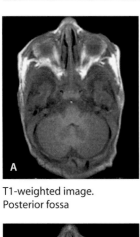

T1-weighted image.
Posterior fossa

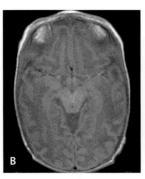

T1-weighted image.
Suprasellar cistern

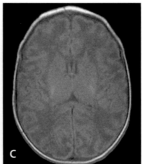

T1-weighted image.
Basal ganglia

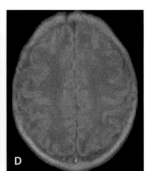

T1-weighted image.
Centrum semiovale

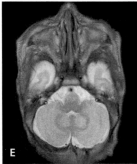

T2-weighted image.
Posterior fossa

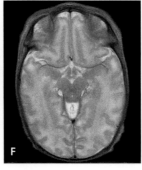

T2-weighted image.
Suprasellar cistern

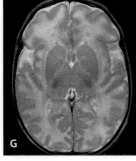

T2-weighted image.
Basal ganglia

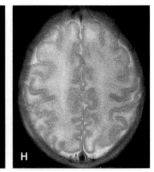

T2-weighted image.
Centrum semiovale

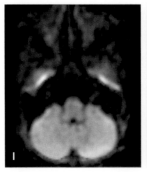

DW image.
Posterior fossa

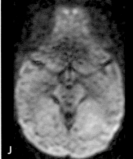

DW image.
Suprasellar cistern

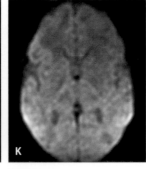

DW image.
Basal ganglia

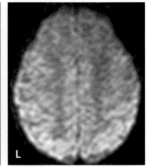

DW image.
Centrum semiovale

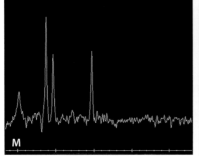

MR spectroscopy. TE=144 ms

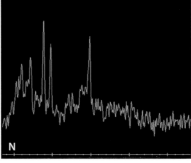

MR spectroscopy. TE=35 ms

Figure 1.3

4-month-old female

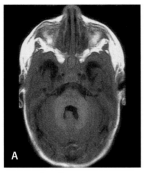

T1-weighted image.
Posterior fossa

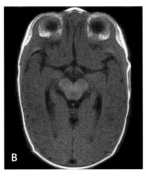

T1-weighted image.
Suprasellar cistern

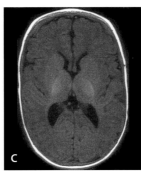

T1-weighted image.
Basal ganglia

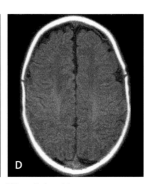

T1-weighted image.
Centrum semiovale

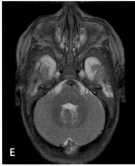

T2-weighted image.
Posterior fossa

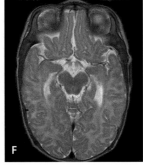

T2-weighted image.
Suprasellar cistern

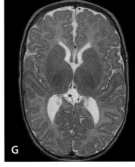

T2-weighted image.
Basal ganglia

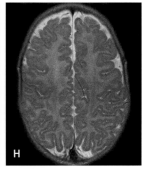

T2-weighted image.
Centrum semiovale

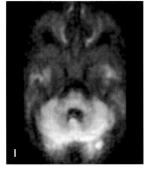

DW image.
Posterior fossa

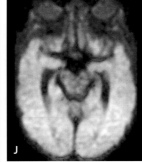

DW image.
Suprasellar cistern

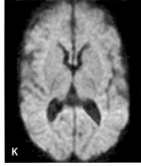

DW image.
Basal ganglia

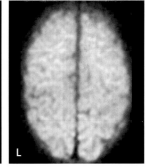

DW image.
Centrum semiovale

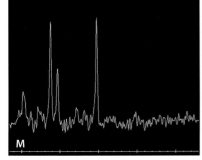

MR spectroscopy. TE=144 ms

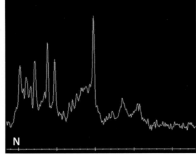

MR spectroscopy. TE=35 ms

Figure 1.4

6-month-old male

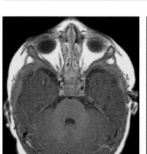

T1-weighted image.
Posterior fossa

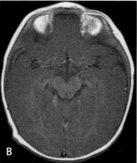

T1-weighted image.
Suprasellar cistern

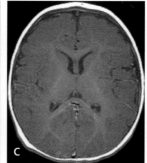

T1-weighted image.
Basal ganglia

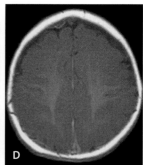

T1-weighted image.
Centrum semiovale

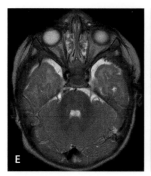

T2-weighted image.
Posterior fossa

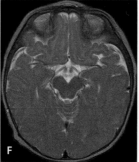

T2-weighted image.
Suprasellar cistern

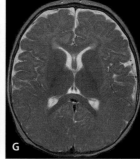

T2-weighted image.
Basal ganglia

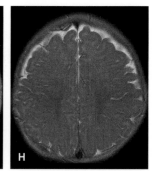

T2-weighted image.
Centrum semiovale

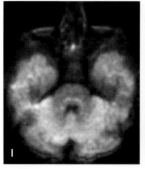

DW image.
Posterior fossa

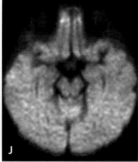

DW image.
Suprasellar cistern

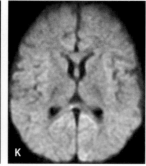

DW image.
Basal ganglia

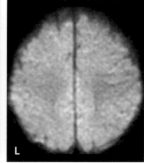

DW image.
Centrum semiovale

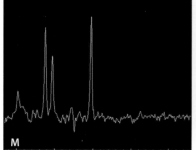

MR spectroscopy. TE=144 ms

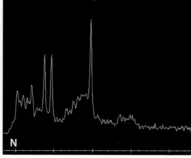

MR spectroscopy. TE=35 ms

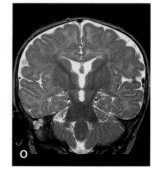

Coronal T2-weighted image

Figure 1.5

10-month-old male

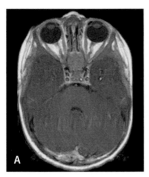

Contrast-enhanced
T1-weighted image.
Posterior fossa

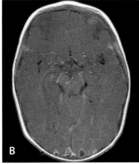

Contrast-enhanced
T1-weighted image.
Suprasellar cistern

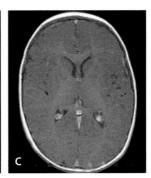

Contrast-enhanced
T1-weighted image.
Basal ganglia

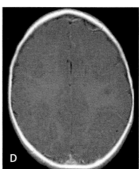

Contrast-enhanced
T1-weighted image.
Centrum semiovale

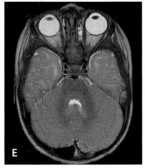

T2-weighted image.
Posterior fossa

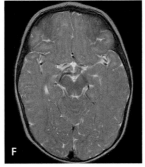

T2-weighted image.
Suprasellar cistern

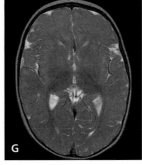

T2-weighted image.
Basal ganglia

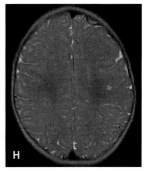

T2-weighted image.
Centrum semiovale

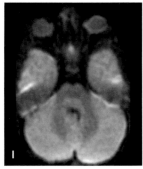

DW image.
Posterior fossa

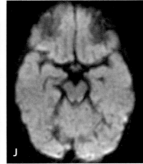

DW image.
Suprasellar cistern

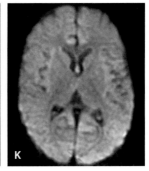

DW image.
Basal ganglia

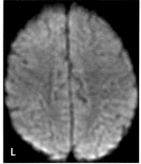

DW image.
Centrum semiovale

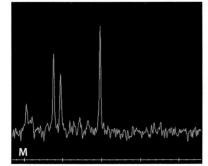

MR spectroscopy. TE=144 ms

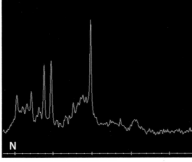

MR spectroscopy. TE=35 ms

Figure 1.6
13-month-old male

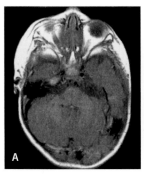

T1-weighted image.
Posterior fossa

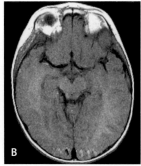

T1-weighted image.
Suprasellar cistern

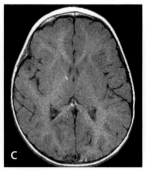

T1-weighted image.
Basal ganglia

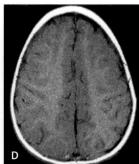

T1-weighted image.
Centrum semiovale

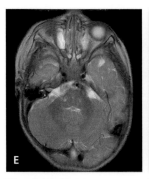

T2-weighted image.
Posterior fossa

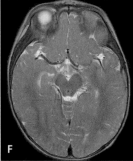

T2-weighted image.
Suprasellar cistern

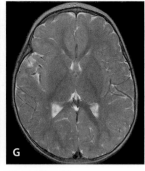

T2-weighted image.
Basal ganglia

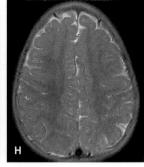

T2-weighted image.
Centrum semiovale

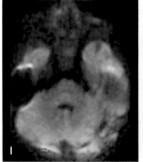

DW image.
Posterior fossa

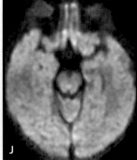

DW image.
Suprasellar cistern

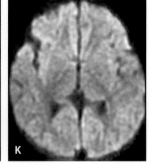

DW image.
Basal ganglia

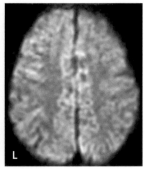

DW image.
Centrum semiovale

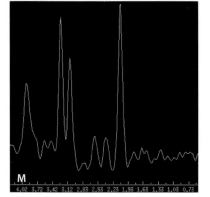

MR spectroscopy. TE=144 ms

Figure 1.7

25-month-old female

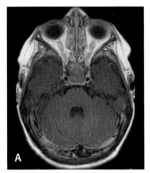

Contrast-enhanced
T1-weighted image.
Posterior fossa

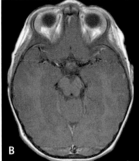

Contrast-enhanced
T1-weighted image.
Suprasellar cistern

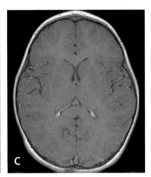

Contrast-enhanced
T1-weighted image.
Basal ganglia

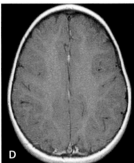

Contrast-enhanced
T1-weighted image.
Centrum semiovale

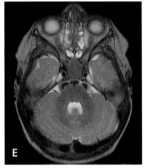

T2-weighted image.
Posterior fossa

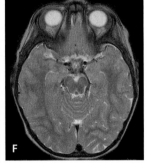

T2-weighted image.
Suprasellar cistern

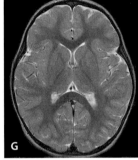

T2-weighted image.
Basal ganglia

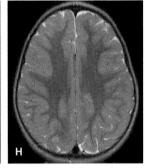

T2-weighted image.
Centrum semiovale

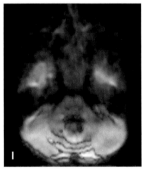

DW image.
Posterior fossa

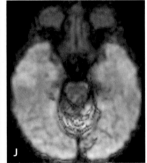

DW image.
Suprasellar cistern

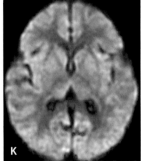

DW image.
Basal ganglia

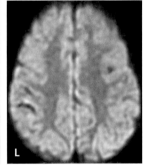

DW image.
Centrum semiovale

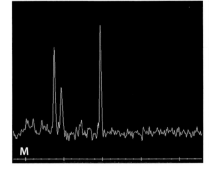

MR spectroscopy. TE=144 ms

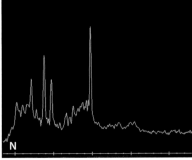

MR spectroscopy. TE=35 ms

Figure 1.8

7-year-old male

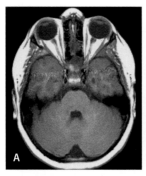

T1-weighted image.
Posterior fossa

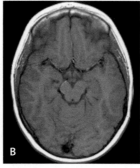

T1-weighted image.
Suprasellar cistern

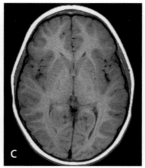

T1-weighted image.
Basal ganglia

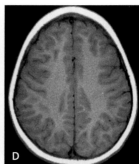

T1-weighted image.
Centrum semiovale

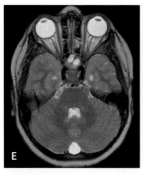

T2-weighted image.
Posterior fossa

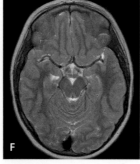

T2-weighted image.
Suprasellar cistern

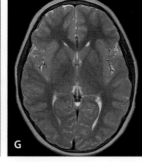

T2-weighted image.
Basal ganglia

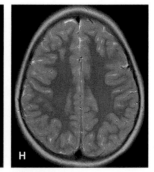

T2-weighted image.
Centrum semiovale

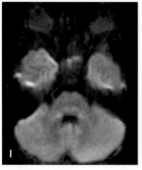

DW image.
Posterior fossa

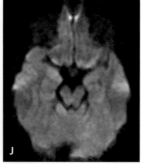

DW image.
Suprasellar cistern

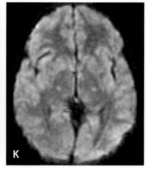

DW image.
Basal ganglia

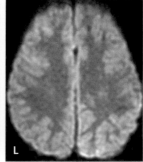

DW image.
Centrum semiovale

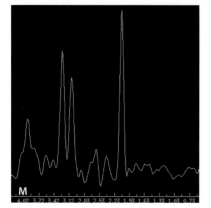

MR spectroscopy. TE=144 ms

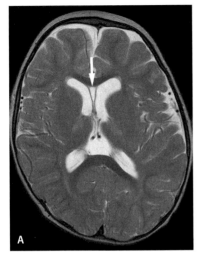 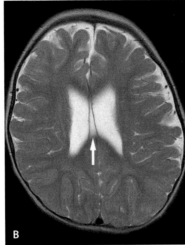 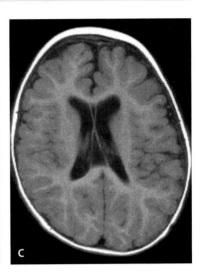

Figure 1.9

Cavum septi pellucidi and vergae

Cavum Septi Pellucidi, Cavum Vergae and Cavum Velum Interpositum

Cavum Septi Pellucidi and Vergae

Clinical Presentation

A 21-month-old male with developmental delay.

Images (Fig. 1.9)

A. T2-weighted image shows cavum septi pellucidi between the frontal horns (*arrow*).
B. T2-weighted image shows cavum vergae between the bodies of the lateral ventricles (*arrow*)
C. T1 FLAIR image. The CSF in the cavum follows CSF signal in all sequences

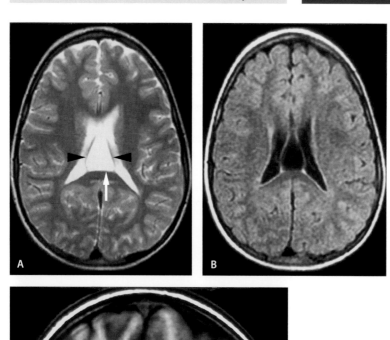

Figure 1.10

Cavum velum interpositum

Cavum Velum Interpositum

Clinical Presentation

A 6-year-old female with headaches. Cavum is considered as an incidental finding.

Images (Fig. 1.10)

A. T2-weighted image shows a triangular CSF space (*arrow*) between and below the fornices (*arrowheads*) with its apex pointed anteriorly

B. FLAIR image reveals the signal intensity of the CSF inside the cavum to be near isointense to the ventricle CSF. This is due to different velocities of the CSF

C. Coronal SPGR image confirms the location of the cavum

Discussion

Cavum septi pellucidi is a CSF collection between the two leaves of the septum pellucidum posterior to the genu of the corpus callosum and anterior to the foramina of Monro. It is present in most fetuses and in 80% of term infants up to the age of 3 months. Although until recently it was considered an incidental finding, cavum septi pellucidi is more commonly seen in pugilists and after a head trauma. Recently it has also been associated with schizophrenia. The increased prevalence of cavum septi pellucidi, cavum vergae and corpus callosum dysgenesis in schizophrenics supports the concept that abnormal development of the brain may play an important role in this disorder. These structures are closely related developmentally to the limbic system, which has been implicated in the etiology of schizophrenia. The portion of the cavum septi pellucidi extending posterior to the fornices is known as the cavum vergae. It is rarely seen without cavum septi pellucidi. The cavum vergae is bordered posteriorly by the splenium of the corpus callosum, and superiorly by the body of the corpus callosum. Although it usually is an incidental finding, it may become very large and cause compression upon the foramina of Monro leading to hydrocephalus.

Cavum veli interpositum is produced by an infolding of pia matter between the roof of the third ventricle and forniceal fibers. This CSF space between the pial layers is known as the cistern of the velum interpositum and it contains the posterior medial choroidal arteries and the internal cerebral veins. On MR images and CT scan it appears as a triangular CSF space with its apex pointed anteriorly. When the cistern is very large it is called the cavum. The cavum lies below the fornices and above the internal cerebral veins. It should not be confused with an arachnoid cyst or an epidermoid tumor that can be present is this region.

Suggested Reading

Chen CY, Chen FH, Lee CC, Lee KW, Hsiao HS (1998) Sonographic characteristics of the cavum velum interpositum. AJNR Am J Neuroradiol 19:1631–1635

Degreef G, Lantos G, Bogerts B, Ashtari M, Lieberman J (1992) Abnormalities of the septum pellucidum on MR scans in first-episode schizophrenic patients AJNR Am J Neuroradiol 13:835–840

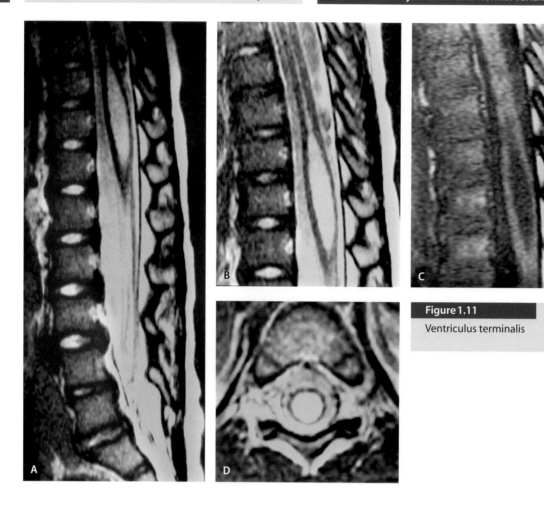

Figure 1.11

Ventriculus terminalis

Ventriculus Terminalis

Clinical Presentation

A 2-year-old girl was examined because of walking difficulties and suspicion of tethered cord.

Images (Fig. 1.11)

A. Sagittal T2-weighted image of the lumbosacral spine reveals normal location of the conus. It shows a large cystic dilatation in the conus
B. Sagittal T2-weighted magnified image of the conus shows again a smooth cystic dilatation that is hyperintense on T2-weighted image
C. On T1-weighted image the cyst follows the CSF signal
D. Axial T2-weighted image shows the central location of the ventriculus terminalis

Discussion

The final stage of development of the distal spinal cord begins at about 38 days of gestation. In this process the central lumen of the caudal neural tube decreases in size and the segment formed includes the conus, filum terminale and ventriculus terminalis. Thus the ventriculus terminalis is a cavity situated at the conus medullaris enclosed by ependymal tissue and normally present as a virtual cavity or as a mere ependymal residue. In rare cases, and almost exclusively in children, the ventriculus terminalis may be wide enough to be visualized by imaging studies, such as MR imaging. It represents a transient finding in young children. On rare occasions, a cystic dilatation of the central conus medullaris may be seen and this is probably the result of a persistent ventriculus terminalis. Cystic dilatation is usually described in children in association with a tethered cord. However, an asymptomatic, localized dilatation of the ventriculus terminalis is considered a normal developmental phenomenon that can be seen on imaging.

Suggested Reading

Celli P, D'Andrea G, Trillo G, Roperto R, Acqui M, Ferrante L (2002) Cyst of the medullary conus: malformative persistence of terminal ventricle or compressive dilatation? Neurosurg Rev 1/2:103–106

Coleman LT, Zimmerman RA, Rorke LB (1995) Ventriculus terminalis of the conus medullaris: MR findings in children. AJNR Am J Neuroradiol 7:1421–1426

Congenital Brain Malformations

Introduction

In the past brain malformations were the domain of the neuropathologist, but with advanced neuroimaging these conditions can also be studied in great detail in the living patient. Knowledge of normal brain development is the basis for understanding malformations. Imaging of congenital brain malformations is important to understand etiologies, to guide therapy and genetic counseling, and to evaluate prognosis.

Congenital brain pathology is clinically suspected when there is a prior abnormal prenatal ultrasound or an abnormal physical examination after birth. There is an especially high index of suspicion in infants with dysmorphic features or macrocephaly, but also premature infants belong to the high-risk group. Screening of these patients is appropriate as well as infants with an abnormal neurological examination or low APGAR scores.

Congenital brain anomalies can be classified according to the stage of central nervous system development when the gestational disturbance occurred. Van der Knaap and Valk have developed a classification system based on the MR imaging appearance and timing of the embryological failure. Their classification is based on Volpe's classification for congenital malformations of the brain that is based on the chronology of normal development and is based on four major categories (Table 2.1).

Anencephaly is the most common congenital malformation in human fetuses. This malformation is in most cases incompatible with life. Cephaloceles are significantly less frequent than anencephaly. They are also less common than meningomyelocele. There are strong geographic differences in the distribution of the various types of cephaloceles.

Table 2.1. Classification of congenital brain anomalies

Gestational age	Stage/etiology	Malformation
3–4 weeks	Dorsal induction	Anencephaly Cephalocele Chiari II
5–8 weeks	Ventral induction	Porencephalies Septo-optic dysplasia Pituitary maldevelopment Posterior fossa malformations
2–5 months	Neuronal proliferation	Microcephaly Megalencephaly Hemimegalencephaly Neurocutaneous syndromes
2–5 months	Neuronal migration	Schizencephaly Lissencephaly Heterotopias Polymicrogyria
6 months to postnatal and adult		Maturation and dysmyelinating disorders Metabolic disorders Toxic effects Encephaloclastic disorders

During ventral induction, a series of events lead to the formation of two separate cerebral hemispheres. Disturbances in development during this period lead to a spectrum of porencephalies, such as alobar and semilobar holoprosencephaly. The incidence of holoprosencephaly is approximately 1 per 13,000 live births. Most cases are sporadic, but mothers with diabetes, toxoplasmosis, syphilis, rubella and alcoholism have an increased risk for holoprosencephaly. Holoprosencephaly is also associated with chromosomal anomalies such as trisomies 13 and 15. Dandy-Walker syndrome is another disorder of ventral induction.

Disorders of neuronal proliferation, differentiation and histogenesis include micrencephaly, which refers to a small but normally developed brain. Macrencephaly is an abnormally large but otherwise normally developed brain. This is usually a familiar finding. Other rare causes for a large head include leukodystrophies such as Alexander's and Canavan's disease. Hemimegalencephaly is characterized by unilateral hemispherical enlargement. Clinically these children have intractable seizures, hemiplegia and severe developmental delay. Disorders of histogenesis are a large group of malformations including phakomatoses, congenital neoplastic lesions, and vascular malformations.

Despite the good visualization of posterior fossa anomalies by MRI, a great deal of confusion persists regarding the terminology and nosology of these lesions. Various classifications regarding the posterior fossa cyst or cyst-like CSF collections have been reported. There is substantial variation in the literature concerning the precise timing of the various events in human brain development. However, most authorities agree about the relative sequence. The flocculi of the cerebellum and the entire vermis are known as paleocerebellum and the remainder of the cerebellar hemispheres is referred to as the neocerebellum. Dysgenesis of the paleocerebellum includes Dandy-Walker malformation and variant, Joubert's syndrome, vermian aplasia-hypoplasia and rhombencephalosynapsis. Dysgenesis of the neocerebellum includes cerebellar hemispheric aplasia-hypoplasia and cerebellar dysplasia. Cysts or cyst-like malformations are commonly seen in the cerebellum and they include mega cisterna magna, Blake's pouch, arachnoid, and epidermoid and neuroepithelial cysts.

During neuronal proliferation the vast majority of neurons and a large number of glial cells are generated in the subventricular location or germinal matrix. During this phase the cells differentiate into specific cell lines with various functions. This phase is followed by the neuronal migration phase. Congenital disorders as a result of abnormal proliferation, differentiation and histogenesis that first manifest during this time include diffuse lesions such as phakomatoses or focal findings such as aqueductal stenosis. Neuronal migration is the time between the third and fifth gestational month when neurons migrate from their site of origin in the subventricular region to their final destination within the cortex. During the migration, as the cerebral hemispheres enlarge, the distance to be moved from the subventricular zone to the cortex increases. The migrating cells move along specialized radial glial fibers that span from the ventricle surface to the pia of the developing hemisphere. The sulcation is a complex process and it coincides with a maximal increase in the volume of the cerebral cortex. This leads to a large cortical surface area that is necessary to accommodate an increasing number of migrating neurons without an increase in cerebral volume. Disorders of neuronal migration include various forms of schizencephaly, lissencephalies, various gray matter heterotopias, polymicrogyria and dysgenesis of the corpus callosum. The process of development does not end with morphological development and neuronal migration. There is still a long process of myelination and maturation ahead with further cell differentiation. This process can also be interrupted in various stages.

Suggested Reading

Ball WS Jr (1997) Pediatric neuroradiology. Lippincott Williams and Wilkins, Philadelphia

Barkovich JA (2000) Pediatric neuroimaging, 3rd edn. Lippincott Williams Wilkins, Philadelphia

Patel S, Barkovich AJ (2002) Analysis and classification of cerebellar malformations. AJNR Am J Neuroradiol 23:1074–1087

Van der Knaap MS, Valk J (1988) Classification of congenital abnormalities of the CNS. AJNR Am J Neuroradiol 9:315–326

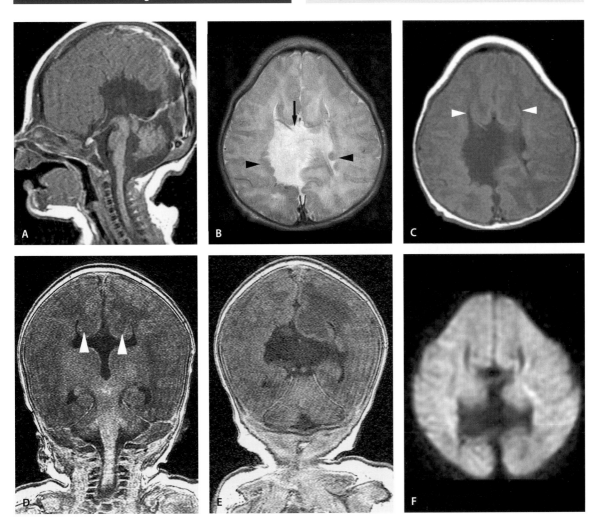

Figure 2.1
Completely absent corpus callosum

Corpus Callosum Agenesis/Dysgenesis

Completely Absent Corpus Callosum

Clinical Presentation

A 2-day-old girl with suspicion of brain anomalies in fetal ultrasound.

Images (Fig. 2.1)

A. Sagittal T1-weighted image shows absence of the corpus callosum. Sulci radiate to the third ventricle because of the lack of formation of the cingulate gyrus/sulcus

B. T2-weighted image shows agenesis of corpus callosum. Subependymal nodular heterotopia is also noted (*arrowheads*). A high-riding third ventricle opens into an interhemispheric cyst (*arrow*). The lateral ventricles are widely apart and the frontal horns are pointed

C. T1-weighted image shows agenesis of corpus callosum and the midline cyst. The fontal horns are
wide apart (*arrowheads*) because if the high-riding third ventricle. Subependymal nodular heterotopia is also noted. Note the pointed forehead in
this patient with metopic suture closure seen on
CT

D. Coronal SPGR image reveals the typical "Viking
helmet" or "moose head" configuration of the ventricles and high-riding third ventricle. Probst bundles are longitudinally oriented white matter
tracts that parallel the insides of the lateral ventricles (*arrowheads*). Hippocampi are vertically oriented

E. Coronal SPGR image through the large midline
cyst

F. DW image shows agenesis of corpus callosum

Near Complete Agenesis of Corpus callosum

Clinical Presentation

A 3-year-old male with developmental delay, walking
difficulties and speech delay.

Images (Fig. 2.2)

A. Sagittal T1-weighted image shows near complete
absence of corpus callosum and cingulate gyrus,
only a small rostrum is present (*arrow*). Prominent massa intermedia is seen (*arrowhead*). Sulci
radiate to the third ventricle because of lack of the
cingulate gyrus

B. Coronal SPGR image shows the typical "Viking
helmet" configuration of the ventricles. There is
absent falx anteriorly with mild interdigitation of
gyri

C. Coronal SPGR image more posteriorly shows
high-riding third ventricle

Discussion

The corpus callosum may be partially formed (dys-
genic) or completely absent (agenic) or hypoplastic
(completely present, but thin). Complete agenesis of
the corpus callosum results from an insult that occurs
before the initial induction of the structure at
8 weeks, and it is highly associated with other CNS
anomalies such as Chiari II malformation, Dandy-

Walker malformation, lipoma, abnormalities of neuronal migration and organization, dysraphic anomalies, encephaloceles, Aicardi's syndrome, cerebellar
anomalies, septo-optic dysplasia, ocular anomalies,
other midline facial anomalies and congenital heart
disease. Corpus callosum dysgenesis is often associated with midline lipoma.

The development of the corpus callosum takes
place between the 12th and 20th week of gestation.
When the corpus callosum is hypoplastic, it is the
posterior portion that is nearly always affected. The
corpus callosum is a midline commissural fiber tract
that develops from the commissural plate in the dorsal aspect of the lamina terminalis. When the corpus
callosum is absent, the connections that would normally cross the midline instead turn in the interhemispheric fissure and run parallel to the fissure in
the medial walls of the lateral ventricle to form the
longitudinal callosal bundles of Probst.

MR imaging is the modality of choice. The presence of parallel lateral ventricles, without the normal
convergence of bodies, radial orientation of interhemispheric gyri, colpocephaly, and longitudinal
white matter tracts at the superomedial aspect of lateral ventricle (bundles of Probst, non-crossed callosal fibers) are suggestive of corpus callosum anomalies. Development of the limbic system and corpus
callosum are intimately related and the rudimentary
fornix lies inferior and medial to the longitudinal callosal bundle. Typically there is a high-riding third
ventricle opening into the interhemispheric fissure or
an interhemispheric cyst.

Diffusion tensor MR imaging is useful in the evaluation of white matter configuration in callosal dysgenesis. Clinically, patients with isolated corpus callosum dysgenesis may be asymptomatic; if it is associated with a syndrome, the symptoms are usually de-
termined by the associated syndrome.

Suggested Reading

Doffe L, Adamsbaum C, Rolland Y, Robain O, Ponsot G, Kalifa G
(1996) Corpus callosum agenesis and parasagittal interhemispheric cyst. J Radiol 77:427–430
Lee SK, Mori S, Kim DJ, Kim SY, Kim SY, Kim DI (2004) Diffusion tensor MR imaging visualizes the altered hemispheric fibre connection in callosal dysgenesis. AJNR Am J Neuroradiol 25:25–28
Rubinstein D, Youngman V, Hise JH, Damiano TR (1994) Partial development of the corpus callosum. AJNR Am J Neuroradiol 15:869–875

Figure 2.2

Figure 2.2

Near complete agenesis of corpus callosum

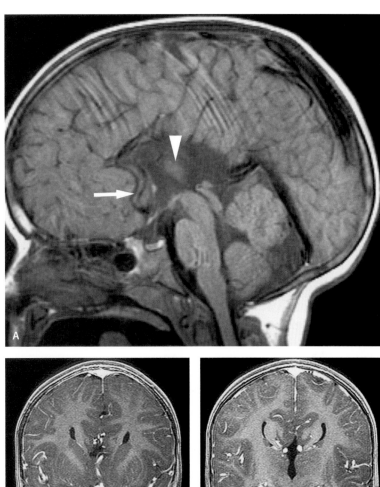

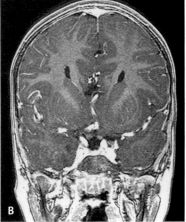

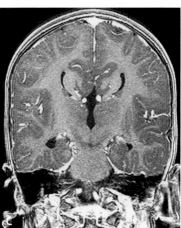

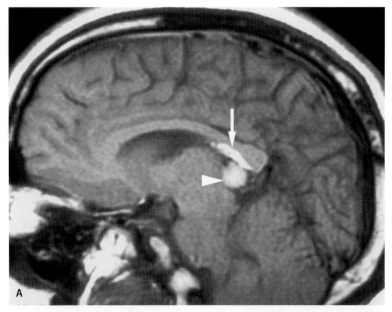

Figure 2.3

Curvilinear lipoma

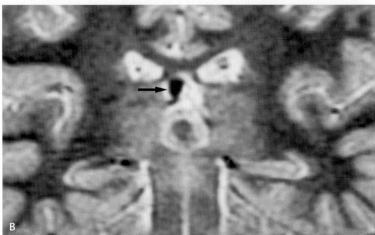

Pericallosal Lipoma

Curvilinear Lipoma

Clinical Presentation

An asymptomatic 17-year-old male who had a CT scan because of head trauma was noted to have a large pineal gland and pericallosal lipoma. Both lesions have been stable in annual examinations.

Images (Fig. 2.3)

A. Sagittal T1-weighted image with contrast enhancement demonstrates a curvilinear pericallosal lipoma (*arrow*). A large enhancing pineal gland (*arrowhead*) is also seen
B. The lipoma (*arrow*) is of low signal on coronal T2-weighted image

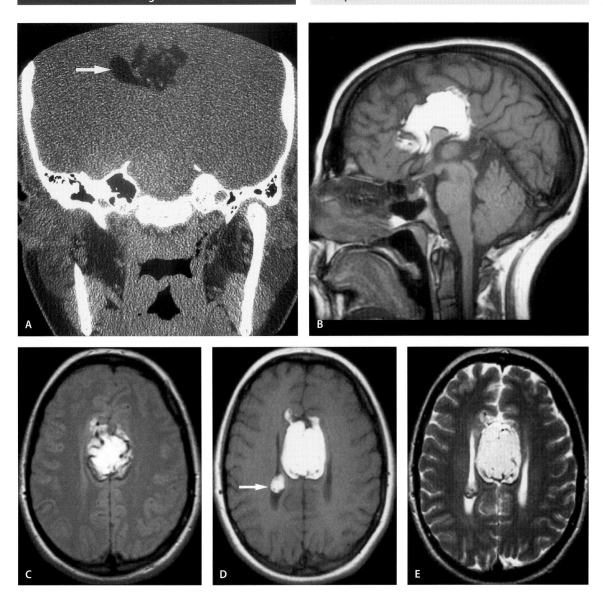

Figure 2.4

Nodular midline ("callosal") lipoma

Nodular Midline ("Callosal") Lipoma

Clinical Presentation

A 20-year-old female had MR scan as seizure work-up. She is mildly developmentally delayed.

Images (Fig. 2.4)

A. Coronal CT scan demonstrates a fat-attenuation mass in the region of corpus callosum (*arrow*)
B. Sagittal T1-weighted image reveals a hyperintense mass above the frontal horns of the lateral ventricles. Note the absence of corpus callosum and cingulate gyrus

C. Proton density image shows a hyperintense mass with several flow voids consistent with pericallosal arteries

D. T1-weighted image confirms the fatty nature of the midline mass lesion. Note the fatty choroid plexus (*arrow*) and absent corpus callosum seen as widely separated and parallel lateral ventricles

E. T2-weighted image. Thin rim of calcification is seen in both midline lipoma and choroid plexus

Discussion

Pericallosal lipoma ("lipoma of the corpus callosum") is a rare anomaly of the CNS that is found in 1 of 2,500 to 1 of 25,000 autopsies. This anomaly is frequently associated with anomalies of the corpus callosum, especially the absence of corpus callosum. The pericallosal lipoma can be considered as a congenital malformation resulting from abnormal persistence and mal differentiation of the meninx primitiva during the development of arachnoid cisterns. When the meninx primitiva persists, instead of being absorbed, it differentiates into lipomatous tissue. Lipoma may develop in any of the cerebral cisterns, but they are most frequent in the area of the corpus callosum. They may be seen in the quadrigeminal/ambient cistern as well.

Two types pericallosal lipoma have been described based on MR imaging findings. One is tubulonodular type and the other is a curvilinear type. The former is usually anterior and often associated with extensive callosal and facial anomalies. The second type is a thin and elongated sliver of fat located more posteriorly. The former is more common. Intracranial lipomas are often associated with vascular anomalies including that of an aneurysm. This could be explained by the fact that both share the same malformation origin, i.e. persistence and abnormal differentiation of the primitive meninx. There may be other explanations as well. When abnormal vasculature is imaged with the time-of-flight technique, it may be obscured by the intrinsic hyperintensity of the lipoma with this technique, but it is revealed by phase-contrast MR angiography. CT angiography may also be useful since the lipoma appears as a low-density lesion contrasted with high-density contrast material in the vessels.

Interhemispheric lipomas are associated with seizures in about half of the patients. The tubulonodular type of lipoma is more often associated with clinical anomalies and symptoms than the curvilinear type. When other associated anomalies such as neuronal migration and gyration anomalies are present, they may be more symptomatic than the lipoma itself.

Suggested Reading

Ickowitz V, Eurin D, Rypens F, et al (2001) Prenatal diagnosis and postnatal follow-up of pericallosal lipoma: report of seven new cases. AJNR Am J Neuroradiol 22:767–772

Truwit CL, Barkovich AJ (1990) Pathogenesis of intracranial lipoma: an MR study in 42 patients. AJR Am J Roentgenol 4:855–864

Figure 2.5

Case 1. Hydranencephaly with increasing head size

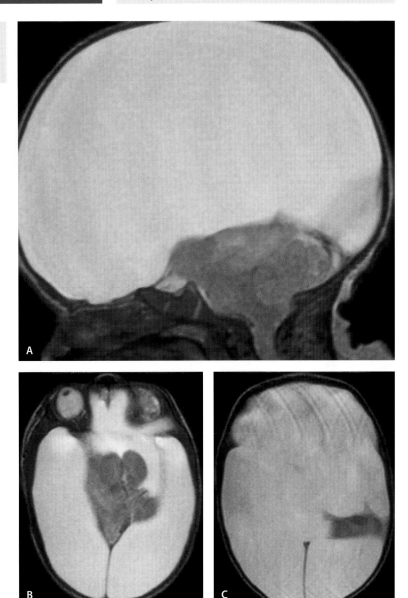

Hydranencephaly

Case 1. Hydranencephaly with Increasing Head Size

Clinical Presentation

A 1-month-old male with increasing head circumference and failure to thrive.

Images (Fig. 2.5)

A. Sagittal T2-weighted image demonstrates fluid
   filling most of the cranium in the expected location of the cerebral hemispheres. Only the cerebellum and part of the thalami are present
B. Axial T2-weighted image shows the brainstem and
   cerebellum to be present
C. Axial T2-weighted image through the expected
   hemispheres shows a portion of residual temporal
   lobe on the left

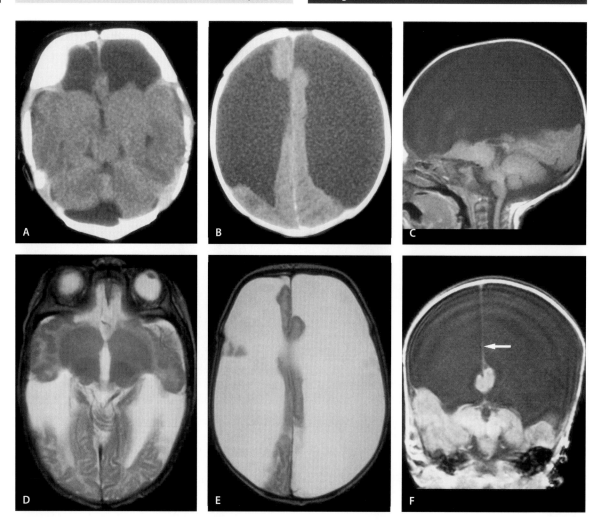

Figure 2.6

Case 2. Hydranencephaly with increasing head size

Case 2. Hydranencephaly with Increasing Head Size

Clinical Presentation

A 5-week-old male with abnormal fetal ultrasound and increasing head circumference presents for MRI for evaluation of "hydrocephalus".

Images (Fig. 2.6)

A. Noncontrast CT through the temporal lobes reveals normal-appearing lower temporal lobes with abnormal CSF collection frontally

B. CT image reveals that CSF replaces the hemispheric brain tissue with a thin residual midline and occipital lobe brain

C. Sagittal T1-weighted image shows that the areas supplied by posterior cerebral artery are preserved

Figure 2.7
Case 3. Hydranencephaly with microcephaly

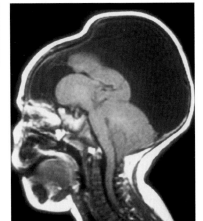 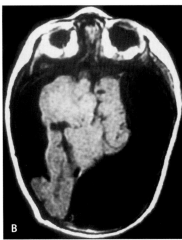

D. T2-weighted image shows normal lower medial temporal and occipital lobes. The thalami are not fused

E. T2-weighted image shows that CSF occupies most of the space normally filled with brain

F. Coronal SPGR image shows also that areas supplied by the posterior cerebral artery are preserved. The falx (*arrow*) is partially normal

Case 3. Hydranencephaly with Microcephaly

Clinical Presentation

An 8-months-old female with microcephaly has "irregular" head and failure to thrive.

Images (Fig. 2.7)

A. Sagittal T1-weighted image shows portions of frontal lobes, midbrain and cerebellum to be present

B. Axial T1-weighted image shows only portions of temporal lobe and midbrain to be present. Most of the cranium is filled with fluid

Discussion

Anencephaly is the most common congenital malformation in human fetuses. This malformation is in most cases incompatible with life. It is a globally destructive process of the CNS that is characterized total or near total absence of cerebral hemispheres but intact calvaria and meninges. The cerebral hemispheres are replaced with a thin sac filled with CSF and necrotic residua. Involvement of the brain suggests intrauterine ischemia and infarctions. Internal carotid arteries are believed to be occluded after the normal development of the hemispheres. Hydranencephaly has also been described in association with herpes simplex, CMV and toxoplasma infections. Some parts of the brain may be preserved; these include the orbital surface of frontal lobes and inferior, medial aspects of the temporal and occipital lobes. These are areas supplied by the posterior cerebral arteries. The basal ganglia and thalami are typically preserved and they are not fused. The posterior fossa is morphologically normal. It is sometimes a diagnostic problem to separate hydranencephaly from severe hydrocephalus, since the cortical mantle may be very thin and compressed against the calvaria. Hydrocephalic children have usually macrocephaly, whereas children with hydranencephaly are usually normocephalic. This distinction is important, since hydrocephalic children may benefit from shunting, Alobar holoprosencephaly may also simulate hydranencephaly, but infants with the former always present with midline cleft anomalies with no formation of falx.

Suggested Reading

McAbee GN, Chan A, Erde EL (2000) Prolonged survival with hydranencephaly: report of two patients and literature review. Pediatr Neurol 1:80–84

Poe LB, Coleman L (1989) MR of hydranencephaly. AJNR Am J Neuroradiol 1 [5 Suppl]:S61

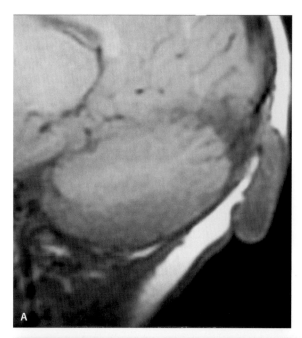

Figure 2.8
Occipital encephalocele

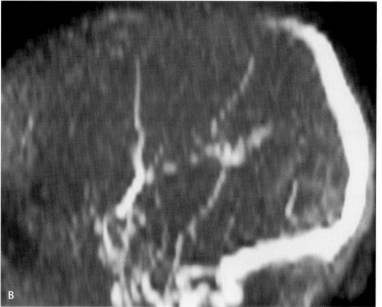

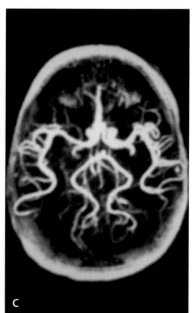

Cephalocele and Meningocele

Occipital Encephalocele

Clinical Presentation

A 5-month-old asymptomatic girl noted to have a "lump" in her occiput.

Images (Fig. 2.8)

A. Sagittal T1-weighted image reveals a defect in the occipital bone through which herniate a dysplastic portion of brain, CSF and meninges

B. Sagittal MR venography (2D TOF) reveals a patent superior sagittal sinus at normal location

C. MR angiography (3D TOF) of the circle of Willis shows patency and normal location of the arteries

Figure 2.9

Parietal cephalocele

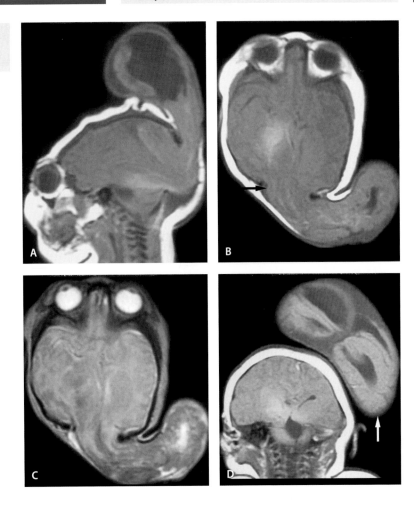

Parietal Cephalocele

Clinical Presentation

A 1-day-old female with cephalocele presents for MRI before surgery to verify the contents of the sac.

Images (Fig. 2.9)

A. Sagittal T1-weighted image shows a large midline bony defect through which brain, meninges and CSF herniate, most likely also ventricles

B. Axial T1-weighted image confirms the large bone defect (*arrow*) with herniating brain tissue

C. T2-weighted image better outlines the herniating brain tissue and CSF

D. Coronal T1-weighted image shows the contents of the herniating cephalocele (*arrow*)

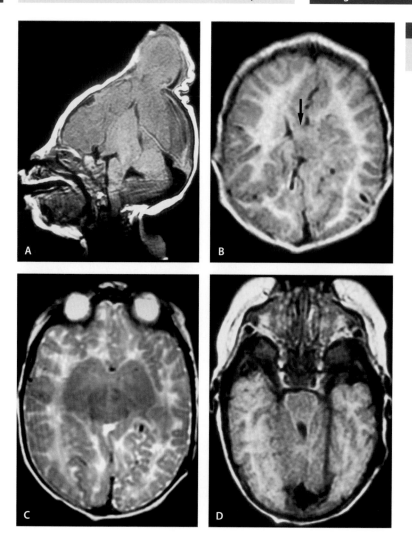

Figure 2.10

Parietal cephalocele

Parietal Cephalocele

Clinical Presentation

A 1-day-old with cephalocele presents for MRI before surgical planning.

Images (Fig. 2.10)

A. Sagittal midline section reveals at the posterior fontanelle region a large bone defect through which brain tissue herniates
B. FLAIR image shows irregular cortical and subcortical brain tissue at the midline (*arrow*)
C. T2-weighted image through the basal ganglia level shows fused thalami and patent venous sinuses
D. FLAIR image shows narrow upper pons and wide incisura of tentorium

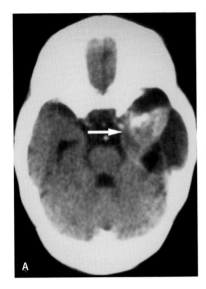
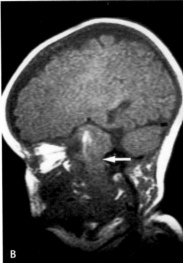
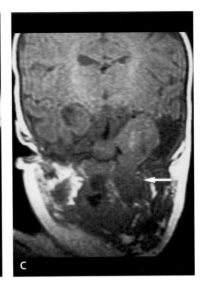

Figure 2.11

Skull base encephalocele

Skull Base Encephalocele

Clinical Presentation

A 5-month-old female with neck and parapharyngeal mass that during later surgery proved to be brain tissue with hamartomatous areas.

Images (Fig. 2.11)

A. Contrast-enhanced CT scan shows abnormal-appearing soft tissue in the left middle cranial fossa (*arrow*) surrounded by a large CSF space. Heterogeneous enhancement is seen in the medial temporal lobe

B. Sagittal T1-weighted image reveals dumbbell shaped brain tissue (*arrow*) herniating inferiorly from the cranial cavity to the oropharynx

C. Coronal T1-weighted image shows the herniating brain tissue in the oropharynx (*arrow*), left to the clivus. The signal is heterogeneous corresponding to the hamartomatous changes seen in pathology. A large CSF space is seen lateral to this abnormal brain tissue within the cranium. A normal hippocampus is not identified in this side

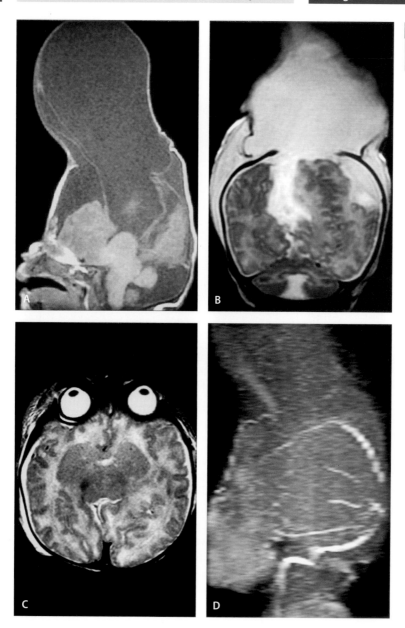

Figure 2.12

Parietal meningocele

Parietal Meningocele

Clinical Presentation

A 1-day-old female with a parietal "mass" presents for imaging evaluation of the contents of the cephalocele before surgery.

Images (Fig. 2.12)

A. Sagittal T1-weighted image shows a large parietal bony defect and CSF-containing sac that is in direct continuation with the intracranial CSF space and ventricles. Note the hypoplastic cerebellum with a large retrocerebellar CSF space consistent with Dandy-Walker variant

B. Coronal T2-weighted image shows monoventriculia and communication of the ventricular system with this extracranial CSF collection

C. Axial T2-weighted image shows nonfused thalami

D. Sagittal MR venography (2D phasecontrast) reveals a patent superior sagittal sinus that has a normal location

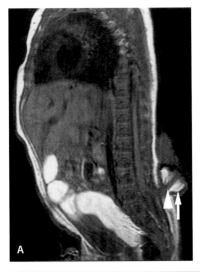
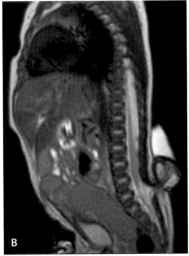
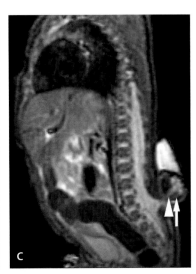

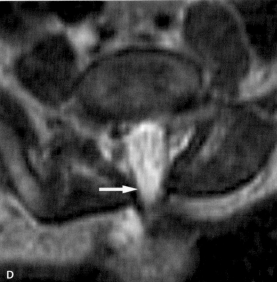

Figure 2.13

Spinal lipomeningocele

Spinal Lipomeningocele

Clinical Presentation

A 1-day-old female with a soft lumbar midline "mass" presents for imaging evaluation of the spinal axis and the lumbar mass. At surgery no neural elements were found in the sac. No other anomalies were found in the spinal canal or brain.

Images (Fig. 2.13)

A. Sagittal T1-weighted image shows midline lipomeningocele and tethered cord. The sac contains a thick fibrous band (*arrowhead*), fat (*arrow*) and fluid

B. Sagittal T2-weighted image demonstrates the bright signal fluid and intermediate signal fat

C. On sagittal STIR image the fat is very dark (*arrow*) and the fluid component very bright. The fibrous band (*arrowhead*) is well contrasted by the dark fat

D. Axial T2-weighted image shows the connection of the lipomeningocele with the spinal canal (*arrow*)

Discussion

Anomalies resulting from disturbance of primary neurulation are the most common and also the most severe congenital malformations. As a general rule the earlier the developmental arrest occurs the most severe is the resulting malformation. Anencephaly is the most common congenital malformation in the human fetus. Time-wise it occurs around the fourth week of gestation. The malformation is incompatible with life and most fetuses are stillborn. The remainder die within a few days of birth. Many of the dysraphic anomalies, such as anencephaly, exencephaly and craniorachischisis, are not compatible with life. From a neuroimaging standpoint more important are lesions that are compatible with life such as cephalocele, meningocele and myelomeningocele. The term cephalocele refers to a situation where intracranial contents herniate through a congenital defect in the skull and dura. Cephaloceles are classified by their contents and by the location of the cranial defect through which the herniation occurs. The herniating neural tissue that is usually covered by skin may include meninges, brain parenchyma, ventricles and vascular structures.

Cephaloceles are significantly less common than anencephaly. There are strong geographic differences in the distribution of the various subtypes of cephaloceles. Occipital cephaloceles are most common among the white population in Europe and North America while sincipital cephalocele is most frequent in South East Asia and Russia. There is also sex distribution among the cephaloceles: occipital cephalocele are more frequent in females, whereas parietal and sincipital cephaloceles are more frequent in males. The size of the occipital cephalocele varies from a tiny occipital mass to a large cephalocele containing most of the brain tissue. The cephalocele can appear as a broad-based or pedunculated mass attached to the brain tissue by a narrow pedicle. The lesion is usually covered with dura and skin. In addition to the primary bone defect at the site of the cephalocele, there is usually enlargement of the foramen magnum and agenesis of the arch of C1. CT and MR imaging are helpful in evaluating the contents of the sac. MR venography is an important means of visualizing the venous sinuses, especially the superior sagittal and transverse sinuses which is important prior to surgical intervention.

Parietal cephaloceles are rare compared to occipital ones. They also may vary in size, shape and content. They are usually located near the anterior or posterior fontanelle rather than along the sagittal suture. Sincipital cephaloceles are relatively rare in Europe and North America, but frequent in South East Asia. Sincipital cephaloceles usually appear as an external mass along the nose and orbital margin. Small nasoethmoidal and nasofrontal cephaloceles may even go undetected.

Skull base cephalocele is the rarest type of cephalocele. They are the most difficult to diagnosis because there is no external visible mass. Failure to recognize the existence of skull base cephalocele may lead to misdiagnosis as a pharyngeal soft-tissue mass leading to biopsy or surgical intervention.

Suggested Reading

Larsen CE, Hudgins PA, Hunter SB (1995) Skull-base meningoencephalocele presenting as a unilateral neck mass in a neonate. AJNR Am J Neuroradiol 16:1161–1163
Patterson RJ, Egelhoff JC, Cron KR, Ball WS Jr (1998) Atretic parietal cephaloceles revisited: an enlarging clinical and imaging spectrum? AJNR Am J Neuroradiol 19:791–795

Micrencephaly with Lissencephaly

Clinical Presentation

An 8-month-old female with small head and developmental delay.

Images (Fig. 2.14)

A. Axial T2-weighted image reveals small head with lack of gyration and dilated occipital horns. The extra-axial CSF space is wide
B. Sagittal T1-weighted image shows small head, sloping forehead and small brain with prominent CSF spaces. The gyration is primitive

Discussion

Microcephaly is a descriptive term and means small head size, but otherwise normal brain. It can also be seen in underlying brain hypoplasia or as a consequence of an acquired destructive process. Micrencephaly means small brain. The etiology is heterogeneous and varies from an inherited to an acquired lesion. Micrencephaly is part of many syndromes: Alpert, Cockayne, Menke, and Rubinstein-Taubi. It

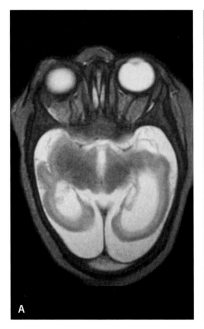
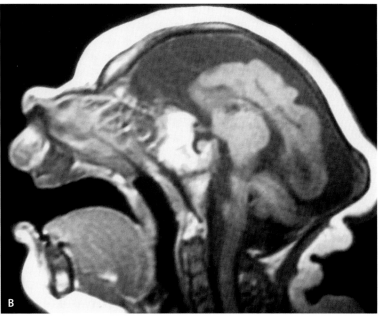

Figure 2.14
Micrencephaly with lissencephaly

results from insult that interferes with normal neuronal proliferation in the fetus between 2 and 4 months of gestation at the time of neuronal proliferation, differentiation and histogenesis. It is part of the fetal alcohol syndrome with many other somatic anomalies. Intrauterine infections, toxic effects and some medications may also lead to micrencephaly. Toxoplasmosis and rubella are often implicated in micrencephaly. It is also part of many chromosomal disorders. Clinically it is associated with various degrees of mental retardation and often seizures.

Suggested Reading

Mishra D, Gupta VK, Nandan D, Behal D (2002) Congenital intrauterine infection like syndrome of microcephaly, intracranial calcification and CNS disease. Indian Pediatr 39:866–869

Riley EP, McGee CL, Sowell ER (2004) Teratogenic effects of alcohol: a decade of brain imaging. Am J Med Genet 15:35–41

Woods CG (2004) Human microcephaly. Curr Opin Neurobiol 14:112–117

Generalized Cortical Dysplasia

Clinical Presentation

A 5-year-boy who was profoundly mentally retarded and suffered from intractable seizures presented for MR imaging. He died at the age of 7 years and the postmortem brain showed generalized cortical dysplasia without any major malformation of the external gyral pattern. The neuropathological examination of cortical dysplasia revealed abnormally thickened cortex with indistinct demarcation of the gray-white matter junction. In many areas, the cortex contained increased numbers of large neurons with disordered cortical lamination. Additionally there were heterotopic neurons scattered throughout the white matter with decreased myelination of the underlying white matter.

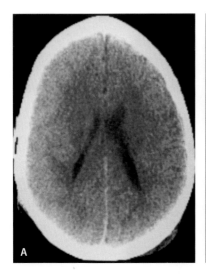 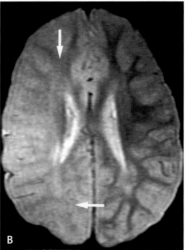 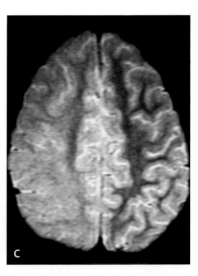

Figure 2.15

Generalized cortical dysplasia

Images (Fig. 2.15)

A. Noncontrast CT reveals normal appearing white-gray interface on the left. The white matter volume is decreased on the right with a poorly visualized gray-white interface

B. T2-weighted image shows a poorly defined gray-white matter border on the right (*arrow*) with an abnormal high signal mainly in the posterior aspect of the hemisphere (*arrow*)

C. T2-weighted image through the centrum semiovale reveals poor demarcation between the gray and white matter with abnormal high signal in the underlying white matter

Discussion

Malformations of cortical development are classified on the basis of imaging features and stages of cortical development. They are grouped by causes of the malformation: abnormal glial and neuronal proliferation, abnormal neuronal migration and abnormal cortical organization. Malformations of cortical development are thought to be an important element of the pathogenesis of epilepsy in over 75% of children undergoing epilepsy surgery. The structural malformation may extend beyond the findings seen on conventional, anatomic MRI. The metabolic alterations in the cortex are not depicted by anatomic imaging, but DW imaging and MR spectroscopy may be sensitive indicators of altered metabolic activity and water diffusion. Malformations in cortical development may collectively be described as neuronal migration disorders, but they represent a heterogeneous group of cortical abnormalities manifested by anomalies of site, thickness and organization of the cortex due to complete or partial failure of the neuroblasts to migrate to their expected location that occurs between 8 and 16 weeks of gestation.

Cortical dysplasia is a pathological disorder of the neocortex that includes an increased number of abnormal neurons within the gray matter in an abnormal cytoarchitectural pattern of cortical lamination. It includes a wide spectrum of gray and white matter abnormalities that range from mild cortical disruption to complete derangement of neocortical lamination with dysmorphic neurons with or without balloon cells. Clinically neuronal migration defects range from those that are incompatible with life to asymptomatic.

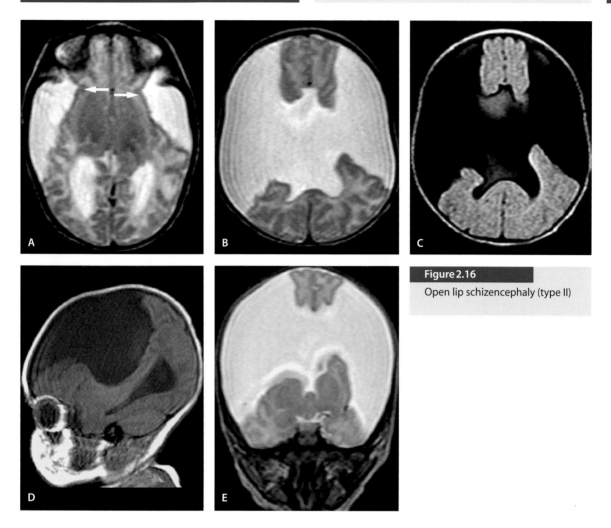

Figure 2.16
Open lip schizencephaly (type II)

Suggested Reading

D'Incerti L (2003) Morphological neuroimaging of malformations of cortical development. Epileptic Disord [Suppl] 2:S59–S66

Fountas KN, King DW, Meador KJ, Lee GP, Smith JR (2004) Epilepsy in cortical dysplasia: factors affecting surgical outcome. Stereotact Funct Neurosurg 1:26–30

Kazee AM, Lapham LW, Torres CF, Wang DD (1991) Generalized cortical dysplasia. Clinical and pathologic aspects. Arch Neurol 8:850–853

Van der Knaap MS, Valk J (1988) Classification of congenital abnormalities of the CNS. AJNR Am J Neuroradiol 1988 2:315–326

Schizencephaly

Open Lip Schizencephaly (Type II)

Clinical Presentation

A 2-year-old male with seizures, spastic quadriparesis and developmental delay presents for MR imaging.

Images (Fig. 2.16)

A. T2-weighted image at the level of the thalami shows dilatation of the sylvian fissures bilaterally (*arrows*). The clefts are lined by cortex

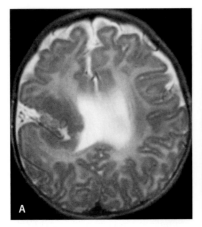 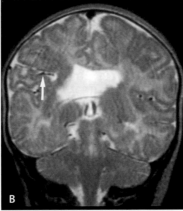

Figure 1.17

Unilateral closed lip
schizencephaly (type I)

B. T2-weighted image at the level of the lateral ventricles shows bilateral open lip schizencephaly lined by cortex

C. FLAIR image confirms the findings in B. The cleft extends from the ventricle surface to convexity

D. Sagittal T1-weighted image shows a large open lip schizencephaly

E. Coronal T2-weighted image also shows bilateral open lip schizencephaly. The thalami are separated. The septum pellucidum is absent, as it is in 80% of cases

Unilateral Closed Lip Schizencephaly (Type I)

Clinical Presentation

A 3-month-old female with abnormal ultrasound and CT scan.

Images (Fig. 2.17)

A. Axial T2-weighted image reveals a right-sided partially open cleft lined by heterotopic gray matter extending to the body of the right lateral ventricle. The septum pellucidum is absent

B. Coronal T2-weighted image shows a thin corpus callosum. The septum pellucidum is absent. Some MCA vessels are seen in the cleft that is outlined on both sides by thick and heterotopic cortex (*arrow*)

Discussion

Schizencephaly is an uncommon congenital disorder of cerebral cortical development, defined as a gray matter-lined cleft extending from the pial surface to the ventricle. It may be close lip or open lip depending upon the thickness of cleavage line of cerebrospinal fluid lined by gray matter. The clefts may be unilateral or bilateral. Patients present with a wide range of neurological symptoms. Unilateral cleft may be asymptomatic. Large bilateral clefts may lead to significant developmental delay, mental retardation and seizures. The condition is often associated with heterotopias and periopercular dysplasias.

CT scanning can demonstrate the cleft as a linear hypodense line extending from the cerebral cortex to the lateral ventricle. In open type, changes of the inner bony vault may be seen due to CSF pulsations. MR imaging is more sensitive than CT scanning in detecting the clefts with gray matter lining as well as in demonstrating other anatomic changes in schizencephaly. Schizencephaly may be inherited or may be a result of an early intrauterine insult, such as exposure to toxins, infection or trauma.

Suggested Reading

Barkovich AJ, Norman D (1988) MR imaging of schizencephaly. AJR Am J Roentgenol 150:1391–1396

Packard AM, Miller VS, Delgado MR (1997) Schizencephaly: correlations of clinical and radiological features. Neurology 48:1426–1434

Figure 2.18

Lissencephaly

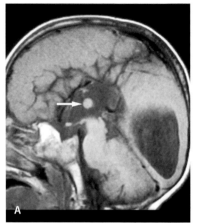
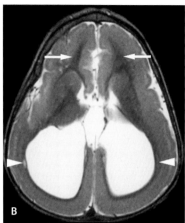

Lissencephaly

Clinical Presentation

X-linked lissencephaly. A 3-year-old male with microcephaly, profound developmental delay and seizures. Patient's mother has seizures and band heterotopia.

Images (Fig. 2.18)

A. Sagittal T1-weighted image reveals only a few medial sulci that abnormally radiate toward the third ventricle because of absence of the cingulate gyrus and corpus callosum. The massa intermedia is prominent (*arrow*)

B. T2-weighted image shows a smooth outer cortical layer with near absent gyri. There is colpocephaly and a high-riding third ventricle due to absent corpus callosum. Shallow Sylvian fissures are present. The frontal horns are small and pointed. Only a small layer of myelinated white matter is seen frontally (*arrows*). The thickened cortex is striated with a thin layer of high signal between cortex and gray matter (*arrowheads*)

Discussion

Lissencephaly, or "smooth brain" in its classic form, belongs to the neuronal migrational disorder group. The syndrome is characterized by no or few cerebral gyri and sulci. Smooth brain can exist also as a consequence of CMV infection or other infectious diseases. Lissencephaly can be divided into two main groups and further into a number of subcategories upon morphology of the brain and associated brain anomalies. The two main groups are: type I (classic form) and type II (cobblestone form). Classic (type I) lissencephaly is seen in chromosome 17-linked lesions (in Miller-Dieker syndrome and in isolated lissencephaly) and in X-linked lissencephaly. X-linked lissencephaly is seen usually in males and subcortical band heterotopia in females. In cobblestone lissencephaly there is an irregular interface between gray and white matter. This lissencephaly is seen in three rare entities: Fukuyama congenital muscular dystrophy, Walker-Warburg syndrome, and muscle-eye-brain disease. On MR and CT imaging, lissencephaly shows an hour-glass or "figure-8" configuration of the brain in axial images because of incomplete or lacking opercularization of the insula. A surface gyral pattern predicts associated chromosomal anomaly (there are various deletions of genes that govern specific stages of neuronal migration). The ventricles are usually mildly enlarged with colpocephaly. The frontal horns are small and anteriorly pointed. The cortex is markedly thickened. The claustrum and extreme capsule are typically absent. The thickened cortex has four layers instead of the normal six layers.

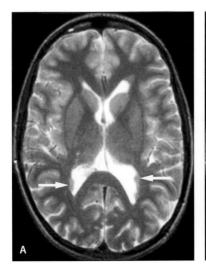 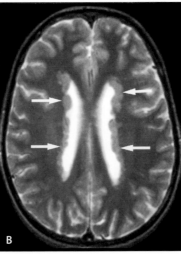

Figure 2.19

Subependymal nodular heterotopia

Suggested Reading

Barkovich AJ (1998) Neuroimaging manifestations and classification of congenital muscular dystrophies. AJNR Am J Neuroradiol 8:1389–1396

Dobyns WB, Truwit CL, Ross ME, et al (1999) Differences in the gyral pattern distinguish chromosome 17-linked and X-linked lissencephaly. Neurology 53:270–277

Pilz DT, Matsumoto N, Minnerath S, et al (1998) LIS1 and XLIS (DCX) mutations cause most classical lissencephaly, but different patterns of malformation. Hum Mol Genet 13:2029–2037

Santavuori P, Valanne L, Autti T, Haltia M, Pihko H, Sainio K (1998) Muscle-eye-brain disease: clinical features, visual evoked potentials and brain imaging in 20 patients. Eur J Paediatr Neurol 1:41–47

Van der Knaap MS, Valk J (1988) Classification of congenital abnormalities of the CNS. AJNR Am J Neuroradiol 2:315–326

Vasconcelos MM, Guedes CR, Domingues RC, Vianna RN, Sotero M, Vieira MM (1999) Walker-Warburg syndrome. Report of two cases. Arq Neuropsiquiatr 3A:672–627

Gray Matter Heterotopia

Subependymal Nodular Heterotopia

Clinical Presentation

A 16-year-old female with seizures.

Images (Fig. 2.19)

A. T2-weighted image reveals round, smooth masses of gray matter that line the occipital horns (*arrows*) and left frontal horn. There are more lesions on the left

B. T2-weighted image reveals multiple round gray matter nodules that bulge into the ventricle (*arrows*)

Focal Subcortical Heterotopia with Agenesis of Corpus Callosum

Clinical Presentation

A 12-year-old female with seizures.

Images (Fig. 2.20)

A. Sagittal T1-weighted image shows absent corpus callosum

B. T2-weighted image reveals an irregular mass of heterotopic gray matter in the left frontal lobe (*arrow*). The left lateral ventricle is deformed. No falx is seen anteriorly

C. T2-weighted image through the parietal region shows heterotopic gray matter (*arrow*)

D. T1-weighted image at the same level as C demonstrates well the gray/white matter differentiation and heterotopic gray matter

E. Coronal SPGR image shows typical "Viking helmet" appearance of the ventricles. There is a lipoma (*arrow*) between the left frontal horn and heterotopic gray matter

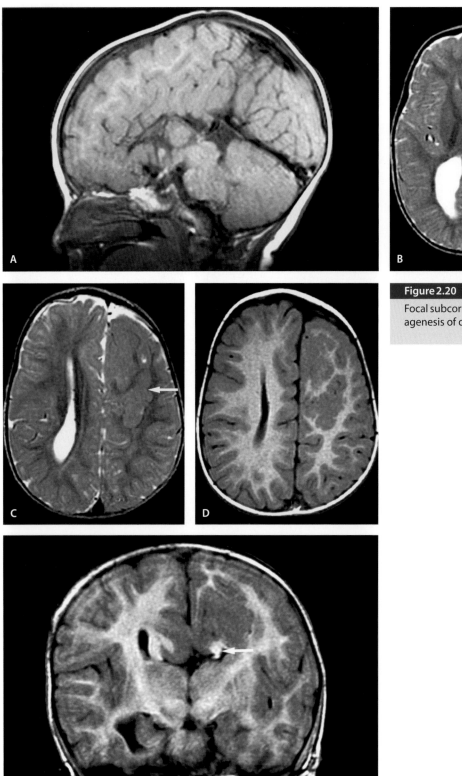

Figure 2.20

Focal subcortical heterotopia with agenesis of corpus callosum

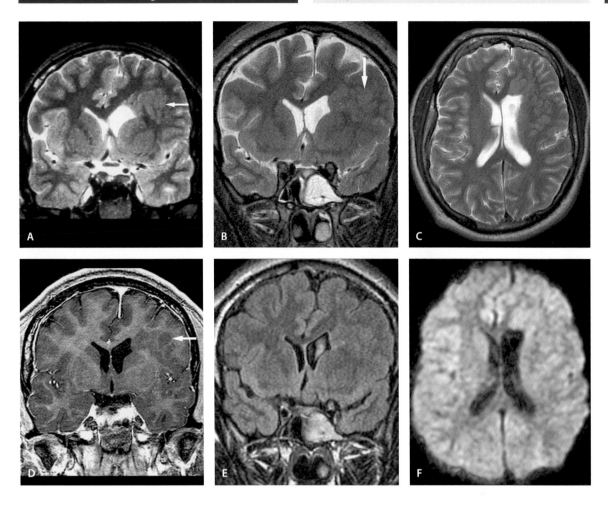

Figure 2.21

Focal subcortical heterotopia

Focal Subcortical Heterotopia

Clinical Presentation

A 15-year-old male with history of intractable seizures since age 10 years.

Images (Fig. 2.21)

A. Coronal T2-weighted image at the age of 15 years reveals clusters of gray matter inside the frontal lobe white matter (*arrow*). The left frontal horn is deformed

B. Coronal T2-weighted image several years later shows features that are identical to those shown in A. Clusters of gray matter nodules (*arrow*) are again seen on the left

C. Axial T2-weighted image shows a tumor-like collection of gray matter nodules adjacent the left frontal horn that is deformed

D. Coronal SPGR image separates well the gray and white matter with left frontal heterotopia (*arrow*)

E. The heterotopic gray matter is isointense to cortical gray matter on FLAIR image

F. No diffusion abnormality is seen on DW image

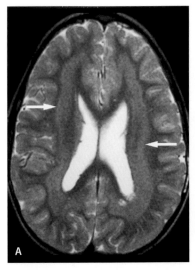 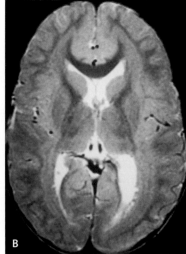 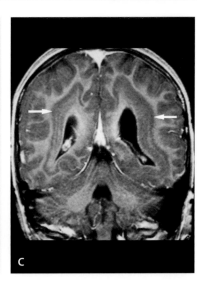

Figure 2.22

Band heterotopia ("double cortex")

Band Heterotopia ("Double Cortex")

Clinical presentation

A 6-year-old male with intractable seizures.

Images (Fig. 2.22)

A. Axial T2-weighted image demonstrates a symmetric subcortical band of tissue isointense to gray matter (*arrows*). The subcortical white matter appears normal
B. On axial proton density image the band of tissue remains isointense to gray matter
C. On coronal SPGR image the gray matter band follows smoothly the cortical gray matter (arrows)

Discussion

Heterotopia refers to collections of neurons and glia in abnormal locations secondary to arrest of migration of neurons. Heterotopia can be subependymal, focal subcortical, or band-formed, parallel to the ventricular wall (double cortex). Heterotopia is isodense with cortical gray matter on all imaging sequences and does not enhance after gadolinium administration. Fluorodeoxyglucose positron emission tomographic study demonstrates glucose uptake similar to that of cortex. MR spectroscopy may show reduced N-acetyl aspartate levels as neurons are dysfunctional in heterotopia

Subependymal Heterotopia Subependymal heterotopia is the most common type of heterotopia. The nodules are smooth, ovoid, with the long axis typically parallel to the ventricular wall. It can be differentiated from subependymal hamartomas in tuberous sclerosis which are irregular and show enhancement.

Focal Heterotopia Focal heterotopia produces variable motor and intellectual impairment, depending on the size and location of the lesion. The foci of focal heterotopia may coexist with other malformations such as schizencephaly, micrencephaly, polymicrogyria, dysgenesis of corpus callosum or absence of septum pellucidum.

Band Heterotopia/Double Cortex Band heterotopia/double cortex is predominantly seen in females (90%). On imaging, band heterotopia is seen as bands of gray matter between the lateral ventricle and cerebral cortex, separated from both by a layer of white matter. Band heterotopia may be complete, surrounded by white matter, or partial. The frontal lobes are more commonly involved.

Suggested Reading

Barkovich AJ (2000) Morphologic characteristics of subcortical heterotopia: MR imaging study. AJNR Am J Neuroradiol 21:290–295

Hayden SA, Davis KA, Stears JC, Cole M (1987) MR imaging of heterotopic gray matter. J Comput Assist Tomogr 11:878–879

Widjaja E, Griffiths PD, Wilkinson ID (2003) Proton MR spectroscopy of polymicrogyria and heterotopia. AJNR Am J Neuroradiol 24:2077–2081

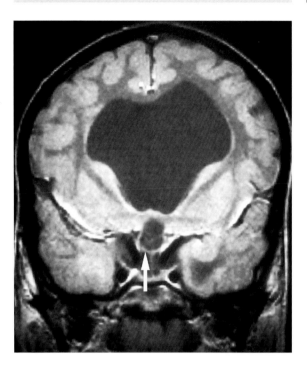

Figure 2.23

Septo-optic dysplasia in a teenager

Holoprosencephaly

Septo-Optic Dysplasia in a Teenager

Clinical Presentation

A 13-year-old girl with mild developmental delay and visual symptoms.

Images (Fig. 2.23)

A. Coronal proton density image shows absent septum pellucidum with squared-off appearance of frontal horns with inferior pointing. Optic nerves and chiasm are small (*arrow*)

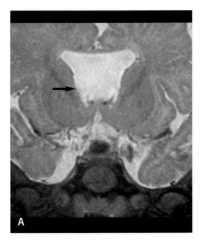 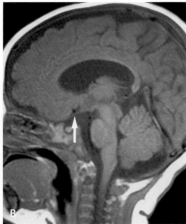 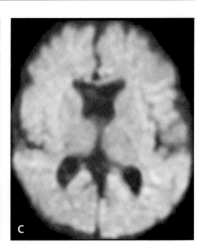

Figure 2.24

Septo-optic dysplasia

Septo-Optic Dysplasia

Clinical Presentation

A 6-month-old female with optic disc hypoplasia and nystagmus.

Images (Fig. 2.24)

A. Coronal T2-weighted image shows box-like frontal horns with inferior pointing (*arrow*). The septum pellucidum is absent
B. Sagittal T1-weighted image shows small optic nerve (*arrow*). The corpus callosum is thin
C. DW image shows no signal abnormality, but the septum is seen to be absent

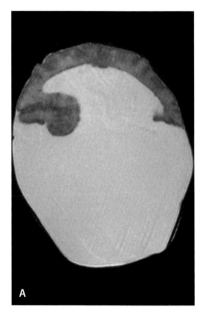 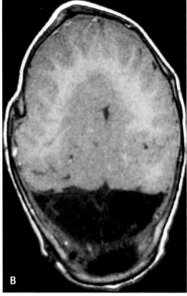 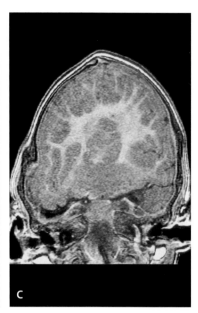

Figure 2.25

Alobar holoprosencephaly

Alobar Holoprosencephaly

Clinical Presentation

An 18-month-old girl, a former 34-week premature baby diagnosed with hydrocephalus or ventricular abnormality in utero. She has facial dysmorphism with hypotelorism.

Images (Fig. 2.25)

A. Axial T2-weighted image demonstrates a central monoventricle with minimal residual frontal brain tissue
B. Axial T1-weighted image reveals fused midline structures
C. Coronal SPGR image confirms the presence of fused midline structures and thalami. Abnormal cortical gyration is present

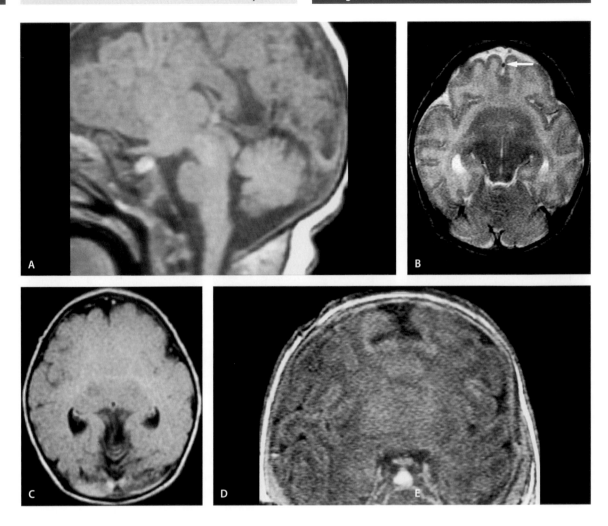

Figure 2.26

Semilobar holoprosencephaly

Semilobar Holoprosencephaly

Clinical Presentation

A 6-day-old female with abnormal prenatal ultrasound image.

Images (Fig. 2.26)

A. Sagittal T1-weighted image shows no normal CSF space in the midline above the aqueduct. However, a rudimentary third ventricle is seen

B. Axial T2-weighted image shows a rudimentary interhemispheric fissure with an azygos anterior cerebral artery (*arrow*). The thalami are fused. No third ventricle is visualized

C. Axial FLAIR confirms the absent midline structures and fused thalami

D. Coronal SPGR image reveals rudimentary interhemispheric fissure and fused frontal lobes. Normal-appearing optic chiasm and pituitary gland are present

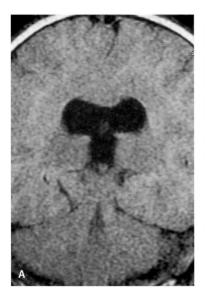
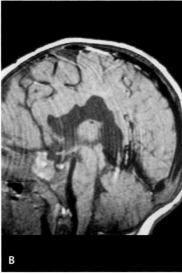
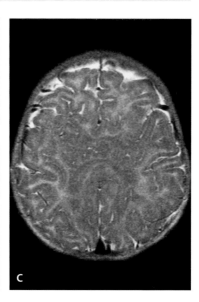

Figure 2.27

Semilobar holoprosencephaly with Pierre-Robin syndrome

Semilobar Holoprosencephaly with Pierre-Robin Syndrome

Clinical Presentation

A 10-month-old girl with developmental delay and Pierre-Robin syndrome.

Images (Fig. 2.27)

A. Coronal FLAIR image shows absent interhemispheric fissure and fusion of the gray and white matter across the midline. The septum pellucidum is absent. Deep sulci with decreased white matter volume are seen
B. Sagittal T1-weighted image reveals that body of the corpus callosum buckled superiorly with normal genu and splenium
C. Axial T2-weighted image confirms the absence of interhemispheric fissure in the middle and fusion of the gray and white matter across the midline

Discussion

Holoprosencephaly is a midline malformation of the anterior brain, skull and face resulting from the failure of the embryonic prosencephalon to undergo segmentation and cleavage into two separate cerebral hemispheres. Holoprosencephaly is of three subtypes: alobar, semilobar and lobar holoprosencephaly. Also the absence of the septum pellucidum with septo-optic dysplasia (De Morsier syndrome; absent septum, small optic nerves) develops at the same stage and can be considered as a mild form of holoprosencephaly.

Alobar Holoprosencephaly Alobar holoprosencephaly is the most severe form. Affected fetuses are often spontaneously aborted. On imaging, the brain is small and the hemispheres are completely fused as one entity. The basal ganglia and thalami are also fused. The ventricular system is seen as a single cavity and is in continuity with a large dorsal cyst.

Semilobar Holoprosencephaly Semilobar holoprosencephaly is less severe with less reduction in brain volume. The interhemispheric fissure is partially fused, but the thalami are partially separated. A single ventricle is present but indication of development of the third ventricle is seen.

Lobar Holoprosencephaly In lobar holoprosencephaly, the brain is generally of normal volume and shows almost complete separation into two hemispheres. The falx is often dysplastic anteriorly but otherwise normal. The ventricular system is well defined but may be dysmorphic. The septum pellucidum is absent. The corpus callosum is absent or dysmorphic.

Suggested Reading

Castillo M, Bouldin TW, Scatliff JH, Suzuli K (1993) Radiologic-pathologic correlation. Alobar holoprosencephaly. ANJR Neuroradiol 14:1151–1156

Simon EM, Barkovich AJ (2001) Holoprosencephaly: new concepts. Magn Reson Imaging Clin North Am 9:149–164

Thomas NA, Cherian A, Sridhar S (2002) Holoprosencephaly. Postgrad Med 49:173–174

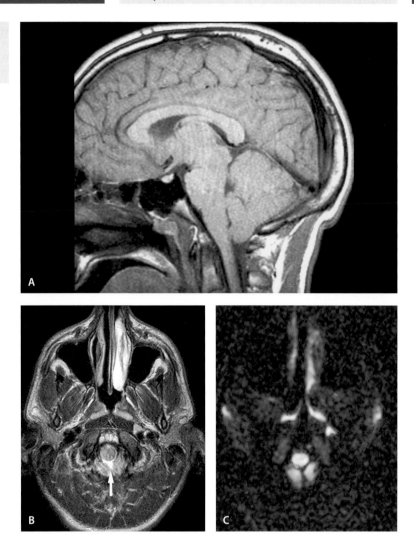

Chiari Malformations

Chiari I Malformation with Low but Rounded Tonsils

Clinical Presentation

A 15-year-old male with headache and neck pain. Suboccipital craniectomy relieved the symptoms.

Images (Fig. 2.28)

A. Sagittal T1-weighted image shows low-lying tonsils (6 mm below the foramen magnum)
B. Axial T2-weighted image shows crowding at the foramen magnum with no CSF around the tonsils (*arrow*)
C. DW image shows normal signal intensity in the medulla and low-lying tonsils

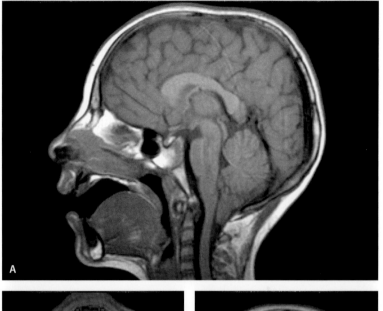

Figure 2.29

Unilateral Chiari I malformation with pointed tonsils

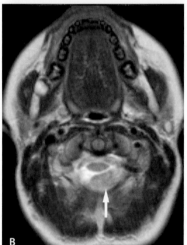

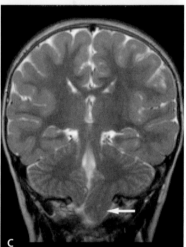

Unilateral Chiari I Malformation with Pointed Tonsils

Clinical Presentation

A 7-year-old girl with Noonan syndrome (synonym: Turner-like syndrome, Turner's phenotype with normal karyotype) presents with neck pain.

Images (Fig. 2.29)

A. Sagittal T1-weighted image reveals descent of the pointed tonsil through the foramen magnum and absence of CSF within the cisterna magna. The fourth ventricle locates normally
B. Axial T2-weighted image shows the large left tonsil in the upper cervical canal behind the cord (*arrow*)
C. Coronal T2-weighted image confirms the low position of the left tonsil and vertically oriented sulci (*arrow*)

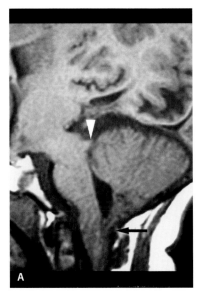 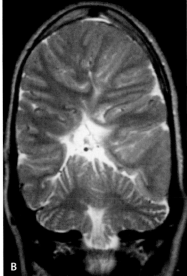 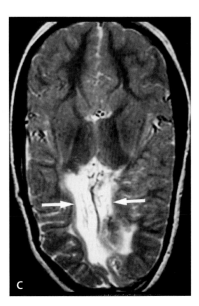

Figure 2.30

Chiari II (Arnold-Chiari) malformation

Chiari II (Arnold-Chiari) Malformation

Clinical Presentation

A 6-year-old girl with history of meningomyelocele repair as a newborn. She presents for cranial MR evaluation and ventricle size assessment.

Images (Fig. 2.30)

A. Sagittal T1-weighted image demonstrates small posterior fossa, low-lying fourth ventricle, descent of the cerebellar vermis through the foramen magnum (*arrow*) and tectal beaking (*arrowhead*)
B. Coronal T2-weighted image shows absence of the falx with interdigitation of the paramedian gyri
C. Axial T2-weighted image through the brain shows shunted hydrocephalus with vertically oriented ventricles (*arrows*). The absence of the falx is apparent. There is corpus callosum hypoplasia posteriorly and the lateral ventricles are medially located and separated only by a straight sinus. The white matter volume is reduced posteriorly

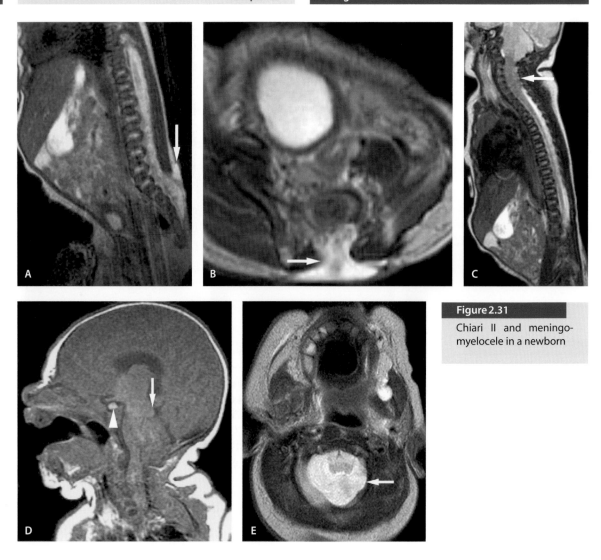

Figure 2.31

Chiari II and meningo-myelocele in a newborn

Chiari II and Meningomyelocele in a Newborn

Clinical Presentation

A 1-day-old baby girl with meningomyelocele presents for cranial MR evaluation.

Images (Fig. 2.31)

A. Sagittal T2-weighted image through the lower spinal canal shows spinal dysraphism and meningomyelocele (*arrow*). The cord is tethered and ends at neural placode (non-neurulated neural tissue)
B. Axial T2-weighted image shows better the midline dysraphism and contents of the sac (*arrow*)

C. Sagittal T2-weighted image shows the low-lying vermis and tonsils (*arrow*) are seen down at T1 level
D. Sagittal T1-weighted image through the brain shows better the small posterior fossa, low tonsils and vermis, small fourth ventricle and tectal beaking (*arrow*). The corpus callosum is difficult to visualize at this age. Note the normal bright signal of newborn pituitary gland (*arrowhead*)
E. Axial T2-weighted image above the foramen magnum shows a wide foramen and cerebellar hemisphere "wrapping around" the medulla (*arrow*)

Figure 2.32

Chiari III and occipital encephalocele

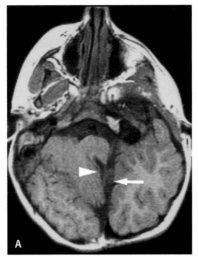
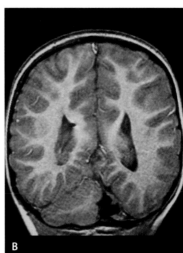

Chiari III and Occipital Encephalocele

Clinical Presentation

A 3-year-old girl who had occipital encephalocele resection as a newborn. MR imaging has shown findings of Chiari II malformation. She presents because of increasing gait difficulties over the past 2 months.

Images (Fig. 2.32)

A. Axial T1-weighted image shows absent left cerebellar hemisphere (*arrow*) and hypoplastic right cerebellar hemisphere. The fourth ventricle is low lying. The right cerebellar hemisphere "wraps around" the brainstem (arrowhead)

B. Coronal SPGR image shows small posterior fossa and absent left cerebellar hemisphere

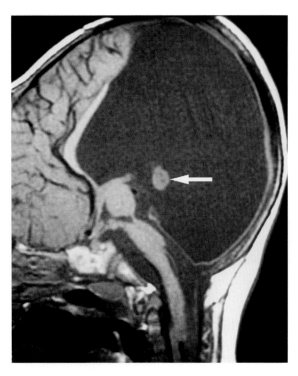

Figure 2.33
Chiari III and spina bifida

Chiari III and Spina Bifida

Clinical Presentation

An 11-month-old girl with spina bifida and choking spells.

Images (Fig. 2.33)

A. Sagittal T1-weighted image shows hypoplastic cerebellar hemisphere (*arrow*), small brainstem and a large posterior CSF space. There is also a prominent CSF space anterior to the pons. Corpus callosum is thin and splenium absent

Discussion

The Chiari malformations (I–IV) are a group of disorders involving mainly the posterior fossa. Chiari type I malformation is the most common cerebellar abnormality identified on MRI. It may not be related to the other two, however, Types II and III are likely related to each other. Chiari type IV malformation is a severe cerebellar hypoplasia without displacement of brain through the foramen magnum. Although Chiari described type IV malformation, it is likely not a distinct entity and probably represents a variation of cerebellar hypoplasia. The normal position of the cerebellar tonsils varies according to the age of the patient. In a newborn the cerebellar tonsils locate slightly inferiorly to the foramen magnum. In adults the tonsils usually locate about the foramen magnum. Cerebellar tonsils that located <3 mm below the foramen magnum may be considered normal and this can be called benign tonsillar ectopia. Tonsils that are 3–6 mm below the foramen magnum are indeterminate and their significance needs to be correlated with a clinical symptomatology.

Tonsils more than 6 mm below the foramen magnum are considered definitely abnormal and compatible with Chiari type I malformation. They are usually pointed (peg-like) rather than rounded with vertically oriented sulci. The Chiari I malformation is more common in females. The symptoms include headaches, neck pain, and progressive ataxia and gait abnormalities. Some patients have hydrocephalus. Dilatation of the central spinal canal (hydromyelia) is found in 20–80% of patients. The foramen magnum looks "crowded" with small/absent CSF spaces.

The Chiari type II malformation (synonym: Arnold-Chiari malformation) is a complex set of anomalies involving cerebellum, brain and spinal cord. Virtually all patients present with meningomyelocele at birth. After repair of the meningomyelocele, most patients will develop hydrocephalus and require CSF shunting. Although this spinal dysraphism may involve any part of the canal, it is most common in the lumbar region. When the meningomyelocele involves the craniocervical junction it may be considered a Chiari III malformation. Intracranially most Chiari malformations may be traced to the presence of a small posterior fossa. The cerebellum "wraps" around the medulla and "towers" upwards. The foramen magnum is wide and the tentorial incisura is hypoplastic and this results in a scalloped appearance of the posterior surface of the clivus and petrosal bones making the internal auditory canals short.

All these findings are related to mesodermal dysplasia. In this syndrome, the cerebellar tonsils and inferior vermis herniate inferiorly through the foramen magnum. The fourth ventricle is small and elongated and herniates often down to the upper cervical canal. A "normal" sized fourth ventricle in Chiari II patients is most likely enlarged and abnormal. The upper medulla kinks at the attachment with a dentate ligament; this is called a "cervicomedullary kink" and is best seen in a sagittal image. The dorsal midbrain in these patients demonstrates fusion of the superior and inferior colliculi making the tectum appear beaked. The midbrain is heart-shaped. The brain stem nuclei are disorganized. The cerebellum towers superiorly via the wide tentorial incisura. The corpus callosum may be hypoplastic or absent. In these cases the white matter of the forceps major is deficient resulting in dilatation of the atria and occipital horns of the lateral ventricles (colpocephaly). Gray matter heterotopias are uncommon but may be present. The falx cerebri may be hypoplastic, absent or fenestrated and this leads to midline interdigitation of gyri. The third ventricle is small and the massa intermedia of the thalami appear enlarged in mid-sagittal images. The ventricles are pointed anteriorly and hydrocephalus is common.

The Chiari type III malformation includes the Chiari II anomalies in addition to cervical spina bifida and high cervical or low occipital meningoencephalocele. The encephalocele usually involves the cerebellum and upper cervical spinal cord but may also include part of the brain. Thus the herniated tissue may contain brain, CSF and commonly venous structures. The contents of herniated the sac are composed of disorganized, non-functioning brain, which may be safely resected. MR venography is useful before the surgery to verify the location of the draining sinuses.

Suggested Reading

Castillo M, Quencer RM, Dominguez R (1992) Chiari III malformation: imaging features. AJNR Am J Neuroradiol 13:1609–1616

Patel S, Barkovich AJ (2002) Analysis and classification of cerebellar malformations. AJNR Am J Neuroradiol 23:1074–1087

Tortori-Donati P, Rossi A, Biancheri R, Cama A (2001) Magnetic resonance imaging of spinal dysraphism. Top Magn Reson Imaging 6:375–409

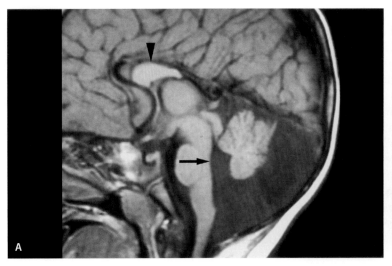
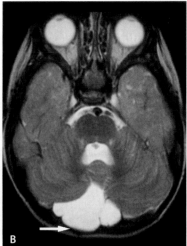

Figure 2.34

Dandy-Walker variant with enlargement of fourth ventricle

Dandy-Walker Syndromes

Dandy-Walker Variant with Enlargement of Fourth Ventricle

Clinical Presentation

A 3-year-old female with macrocephaly, ataxia and developmental delay.

Images (Fig. 2.34)

A. Sagittal T1-weighted image shows vermian hypoplasia. A large retrocerebellar cyst communicates with an enlarged fourth ventricle (*arrow*). Mild cerebellar hypoplasia is present. Torcular is below the lambdoid confluence. Note the corpus callosum dysgenesis (*arrowhead*): the posterior part is absent and the gyri radiate into the posterior third ventricle

B. T2-weighted image better reveals the cerebellar hemisphere and vermian hypoplasia, retrocerebellar cyst and scalloped occipital bone (*arrow*). Falx cerebelli is present

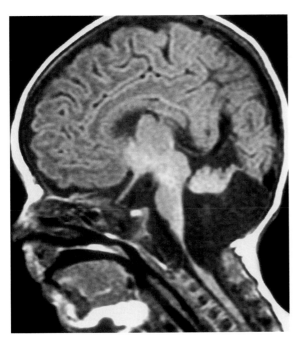

Dandy-Walker Variant with No Separate Fourth Ventricle

Clinical Presentation

A 6-day-old female with swallowing difficulties and abnormal head ultrasound image is referred for MRI scan.

Images (Fig. 2.35)

A. Sagittal T1-weighted image reveals a large posterior fossa fluid collection that extends to the upper spinal canal. The foramen magnum is enlarged. There is hypoplasia of the inferior vermis of the cerebellum. Superior vermis present in the midline. There is significant decrease in the AP dimension of the medulla

Figure 2.35

Dandy-Walker variant with no separate fourth ventricle

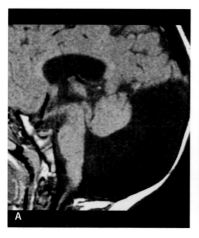 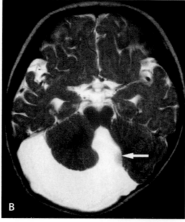 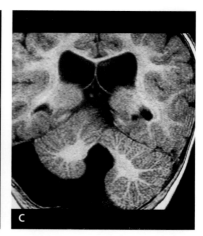

Figure 2.36

Dandy-Walker variant with elevation of torcula

Dandy-Walker Variant with Elevation of Torcula

Clinical Presentation

A 10-month-old male who had an abnormal prenatal ultrasound image.

Images (Fig. 2.36)

A. Sagittal T1-weighted image demonstrates a large posterior fossa cyst that communicates with the fourth ventricle elevating the cerebellar vermis and torcular Herophili
B. Axial T2-weighted image shows a large CSF-intensity fluid collection that expands the posterior fossa on the right and communicates in the midline with the fourth ventricle (*arrow*)
C. Coronal SPGR image shows asymmetry of the cerebellar hemispheres; the right cerebellar hemisphere is hypoplastic

Discussion

Dandy-Walker syndromes (DWS) result in partial or complete vermian aplasia and a large posterior fossa cyst that displaces the cerebellum and replaces the fourth ventricle. There is upward displacement of the transverse sinuses, tentorium and torcular Herophili. It is considered that mega cisterna magna and DWS may represent a continuum of developmental anomalies of the posterior fossa, which therefore form a spectrum of the same syndrome complex. DWS may be caused by maldevelopment of the outlet foramina of Magendie and Luschka of the fourth ventricle with resultant cystic ventricular dilatation and displacement of the adjacent cerebellum. DWS is associated with a number of genetic syndromes including Aicardi's syndrome, neurocutaneous melanosis, coarctation of the aorta, cardiac defects, hemangiomas, and Warburg's syndrome. The multitude of CNS anomalies coexist with DWS and Dandy-Walker variant, the most common of which are dysgenesis of the corpus callosum, gray matter heterotopias and polymicrogyria.

The Dandy-Walker variant, the most common form of this anomaly demonstrates partial dysgenesis of the vermis and remnant fourth ventricle that communicates with retrocerebellar cyst.

The classic clinical presentation of DWS is macrocephaly, developmental delay and seizures. All three are usually present only in a minority of patients. The majority of DWS patients present with hydrocephalus; most patients with Dandy-Walker variant have normal-size ventricles.

Suggested Reading

Altman NR, Naidich TP, Braffman BH (1992) Posterior fossa malformations. AJNR Am J Neuroradiol 13:691–724
Frieden IJ, Reese V, Cohen D (1996) PHACE syndrome. The association of posterior fossa brain malformations, hemangiomas, arterial anomalies, coarctation of the aorta and cardiac defects, and eye abnormalities. Arch Dermatol 132:307–311

Joubert's Syndrome

Clinical Presentation

New onset of seizures in a developmentally delayed female known to have quadrigeminal cistern mass since the age of 13 years when she was diagnosed with cerebellar malformation. Clinically and radiologically this patient is best categorized as Joubert's syndrome, although radiological features of Dandy-Walker syndrome (posterior fossa cyst) and rhombencephalosynapsis (partially fused cerebellar hemispheres) are also present.

Images (Fig. 2.37)

A. Sagittal T1-weighted image shows severe hypoplasia of the vermis with direct communication between the fourth ventricle and the extracerebellar CSF space. A thickened and horizontally oriented superior cerebellar peduncle is seen (*arrow*) caused by reorganization of normally decussating axons. A histologically proven hyperintense quadrigeminal plate cistern dermoid tumor is seen
B. Sagittal T2-weighted image confirms the findings seen in A
C. T1-weighted image shows the slender cerebellar peduncles (*arrows*) that result in the molar tooth configuration
D. T2-weighted image demonstrates disorganized cerebellar hemispheres (*arrows*) with element of midline fusion as seen in rhombencephalosynapsis

E. Coronal SPGR image with contrast enhancement shows the close contact of the cerebellar hemispheres in the midline (*arrow*) due to the absent vermis
F. DW image demonstrates slightly higher signal in the cerebellum (*arrow*)
G. On ADC map, the cerebellum shows a slightly lower signal intensity than the cerebrum

Discussion

Joubert's syndrome is a rare condition representing one of the developmental defects of the cerebellar vermis associated with episodic hyperpnea, and apnea, abnormal eye movements, and mental retardation. Associated findings may include unsegmented midbrain tectum, occipital meningoencephalocele, callosal dysgenesis, chorioretinal coloboma, sacral dermal sinus, polydactyly, and cystic kidney disease. The clinical presentation of these patients is very heterogeneous. No specific chromosome locus has been identified.

MR imaging findings are characteristic. The most consistent radiological changes of the syndrome are complete absence of the vermis which results in a "bat-wing" and "triangular" fourth ventricle. The characteristic appearance of the midbrain, with enlarged superior cerebellar peduncles with absence of their decussation has been called the "molar tooth sign". A cleft is seen between the two cerebellar hemispheres. Dysgenesis of the corpus callosum is often present. Encephalomeningocele and delayed myelination of the cerebral white matter may also be seen. There is some controversy concerning the definition of this syndrome and whether the diagnosis is made by combination of radiological and clinical findings or based on radiological or clinical findings alone.

Suggested Reading

Maria BL, Boltshauser E, Palmer SC, Tran TX (1999) Clinical features and revised diagnostic criteria in Joubert's syndrome. J Child Neurol 14:583–590
McGraw P (2003) The molar tooth sign. Radiology 229:671–672
Sener RN (1995) MR imaging of Joubert's syndrome. Comput Med Imaging Graph 19:481–486

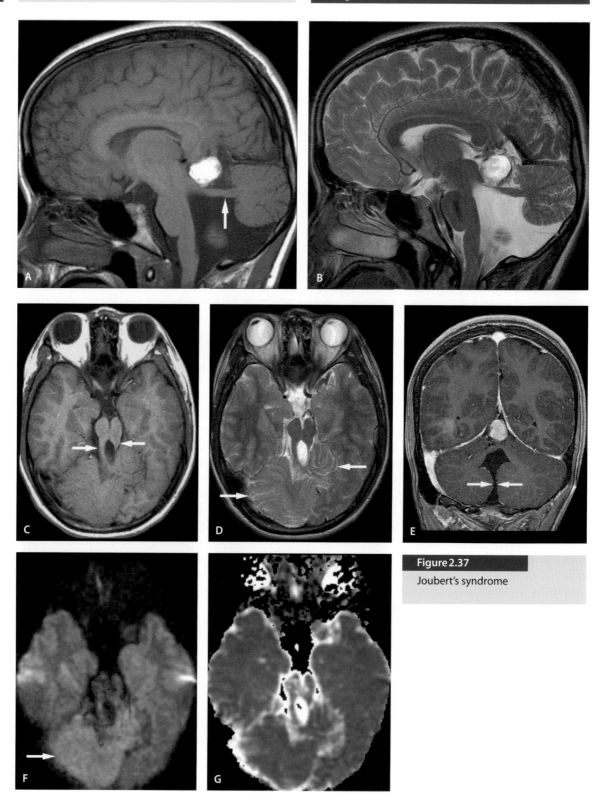

Figure 2.37

Joubert's syndrome

Figure 3.38

Rhombencephalosynapsis

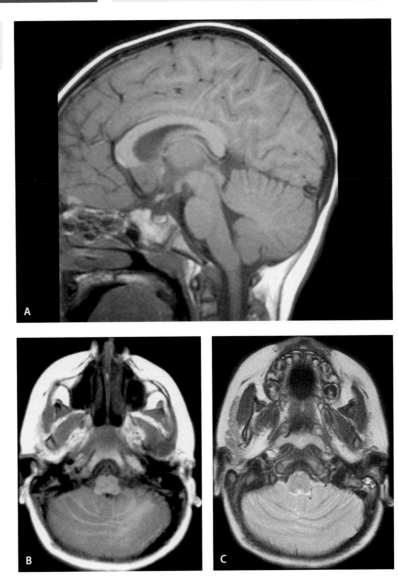

Rhombencephalosynapsis

Clinical Presentation

A 3-year-old female with delay in motor development and falls.

Images (Fig. 2.38)

A. Sagittal T1-weighted image shows a small fourth ventricle in the normal location
B. Axial T1-weighted image demonstrates fused cerebellar hemispheres with absent vermis
C. Axial T2-weighted image confirms the T1 findings: fused cerebellar hemispheres and absent vermis

Discussion

Rhombencephalosynapsis is a rare congenital malformation of the posterior fossa consisting of vermian agenesis or severe hypogenesis, fusion of the cerebellar hemispheres, and apposition or fusion of the dentate nuclei. Associated anomalies include hydrocephalus, fusion of the inferior colliculi, deficiency or absence of septum pellucidum, and hypoplasia of the anterior commissure.

MR imaging features of rhombencephalosynapsis are characteristic. A diamond-shaped fourth ventricle, instead of the normal crescent shape, is seen on axial sections. This abnormal configuration of the fourth ventricle indicates vermian hypogenesis or agenesis, since fusion or apposition of the dentate nuclei and middle cerebellar peduncles can be seen behind a pointed fourth ventricle.

Suggested Reading

Altman NR, Naidich TP, Braffman BH (1992) Posterior fossa malformations. AJNR Am J Neuroradiol 13:691–724

Utsunomiya H, Takano K, Ogasawara T, Hashimoto T, Fukushima T, Okaza M (1998) Rhombencephalosynapsis: cerebellar embryogenesis. AJNR Am J Neuroradiol 19:547–549

Cloverleaf Skull Syndrome (Kleeblattschädel Anomaly)

Clinical Presentation

A 1-day-old female with brain anomaly in the prenatal ultrasound image.

Images (Fig. 2.39)

A. Sagittal T1-weighted image demonstrates a flat head with hydrocephalus. No well-defined corpus callosum is present. Midbrain and cerebellar structures are dysmorphic
B. T2-weighted image demonstrates enlarged middle cranial fossa bilaterally with enlargement of the temporal horns. The thalami are not fused (*arrows*). Severely exophthalmic eyes are present
C. Proton density image confirms the T2-weighted image findings
D. Coronal SPGR image demonstrates significant hydrocephalus above the foramina of Monro with normal-sized third ventricle (*arrow*)

Discussion

With this syndrome there is a trilobed skull deformity at birth due to intrauterine fusion of the coronal and lambdoid sutures. The head is flat and trilobular in appearance caused by hydrocephalus in combination with congenital closure of the coronal and lambdoid sutures. The patient has a beak-like nose, microphthalmia with proptosis. The patient also has a high forehead with midfacial hypoplasia and downward displacement of the ears. The syndrome is equally common in males and females. Prognosis is poor in severe cases. These cranial abnormalities can be seen as an isolated finding or associated with other localized malformations in spine or extremities, associated with generalized chondrodystrophy or in families with inherited craniosynostosis.

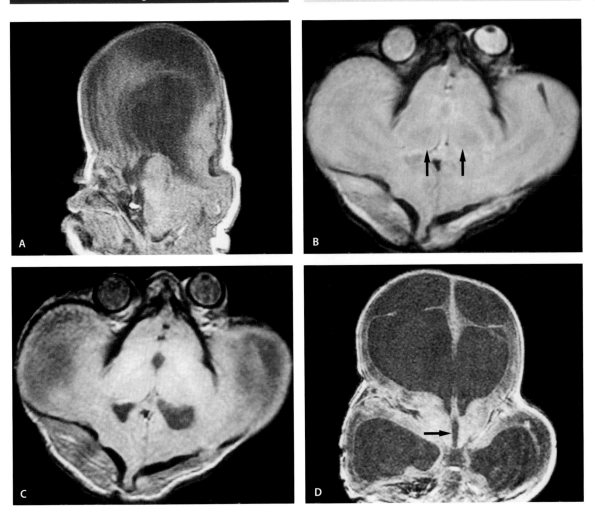

Figure 2.39

Cloverleaf skull syndrome (kleeblattschädel anomaly)

Suggested Reading

Iannaccone G, Gerlini G (1974) The so-called "cloverleaf skull syndrome". A report of three cases with a discussion of its relationships with thanatophoric dwarfism and the craniostenoses. Pediatr Radiol 2:175–184

Lowe LH, Booth TN, Joglar JM, Rollins NK (2000) Midface anomalies in children. Radiographics 20:907–922

Young RS, Pochaczevsky R, Leonidas JC, Wexler IB, Ratner H (1973) Thanatophoric dwarfism and cloverleaf skull. Radiology 106:401–405

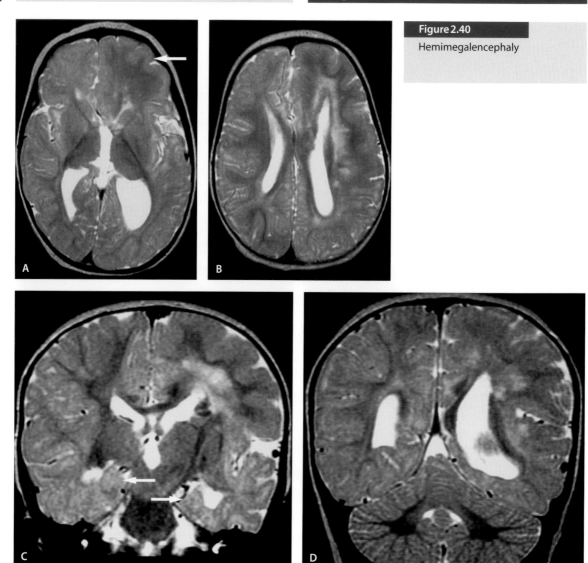

Figure 2.40

Hemimegalencephaly

Hemimegalencephaly

Clinical Presentation

14-month-old male with seizures.

Images (Fig. 2.40)

A. Axial T2-weighted image shows overall enlargement of the left cerebral hemisphere, end especially the posterior aspect. The gyri are broadened on left frontal area as compared to the right hemisphere consistent with pachygyria (*arrow*). The posterior aspect of the left lateral ventricle is abnormally enlarged and the left frontal horn has a straight contour. The corpus callosum is hypoplastic.

B. The hemispheric asymmetry is better seen on the higher T2-weighted image. The left frontal lobe white matter appears abnormally hyperintense around the ventricle. Ventricle asymmetry is again appreciated,

C. Coronal T2-weighted image through the hippocampi reveals poor rotation of the hippocampi that are unusually round (*arrows*). The periventricular white matter hyperintensity and hemispheric asymmetry is again appreciated. The left sylvian fissure is open.

D. Coronal T2-weighted image demonstrates normal posterior fossa structures with ventricular and white matter asymmetry in the supratentorial area.

Discussion

Hemimegalencephaly is a rare disorder of neuronal and glial proliferation. Neuronal migration defects occur in the affected hemisphere with areas or pachygyria, polymicrogyria and heterotopia commonly seen. It is characterized by asymmetry of the hemispheres and cortical dysplasia. It can be isolated or associated with several neurocutaneous syndromes. Infants with this condition present with seizures and severe encephalopathy, although normal Neurologic development has also been described.

MR shows hemispheric hypertrophy with ipsilateral ventricular atrium dilatation, frontal horn straightening, abnormal gyral pattern, and a thick cortex on the enlarged side, an "occipital sign" (displacement of the occipital lobe across the midline), and gliosis in the white matter on affected side.

Chapter 2

Hemimegalencephaly or focal hemimegalencephaly may be confused with low-grade glioma or as a part of ganglioglioma/gangliocytoma spectrum. Features that may be useful in distinguishing focal hemimegalencephaly from tumor are lack of mass effect, lack of edema, and no change on follow-up examinations.

Suggested Reading

Flores-Sarnat L (2002) Hemimegalencephaly: part 1. Genetic, clinical, and imaging aspects. J Child Neurol 17:373–384

Griffiths PD, Gardner SA, Smith M, Rittey C, Powell T (1998) Hemimegalencephaly and focal megalencephaly in tuberous sclerosis complex. AJNR Am J Neuroradiol 19:1935–1938

Yagishita A, Arai N, Tamagawa K, Oda M (1998) Hemimegalencephaly: signal changes suggesting abnormal myelination on MRI. Neuroradiology 40:734–738

Inherited Neurological Diseases and Disorders of Myelin

Introduction

The history of clinical description of genetically inherited white matter diseases is long. More than 100 years ago the pathological description of Pelizaeus-Merzbacher disease started the history of leukodystrophies, followed by a description of metachromatic leukodystrophy and Krabbe disease.

The original term of leukodystrophy has been changed to leukoencephalopathy to better cover the group of diseases. This term better describes the group of diseases that not only include loss of previously formed myelin, but also hypomyelination (delay in normal myelination process) and failure to myelinate at all or failure to maintain normal myelination, such as destruction of myelin. In the past 10 years our understanding of the diseases has increased and simultaneously new leukoencephalopathy syndromes have been defined. In spite of all the genetic, biochemical marker and imaging advances, a significant number of white matter leukoencephalopathy syndromes remain without specific diagnosis. Our prospective has broadened with the new discoveries associated with CNS involvement, such as defects in genes coding for protein that are not typically associated with myelin sheath that can cause myelin disorders.

CT and later MR imaging markedly changed our concept of white matter abnormalities. New imaging techniques such as DW imaging, ADC maps and proton and phosphorus MRS have helped further to characterize the leukoencephalopathies.

MRI imaging has become a routine clinical tool for the evaluation of brain maturation and myelination in young children. The maturation and decrease in brain water content and increase in macromolecules such as myelin reflects signal intensity changes in standard T1- and T2-weighted images. The maturation process can also cause alterations in brain water diffusion that can be seen and analyzed quantitatively with diffusion tensor (DT) imaging. DT imaging characterizes the 3D spatial distribution of water diffusion in each MRI voxel.

The first DT imaging studies in human brain maturation were performed on preterm and term neonates and revealed that the isotropic diffusion coefficient decreases and the diffusion anisotropy increases with increasing gestational age. This technique was later applied to normal brain development in children. From normal brain development the use of DT imaging has been expanded in pathological CNS conditions. DT imaging has been used as an early indicator of white matter demyelination and to monitor the severity of the white matter change before it is seen in conventional MR sequences. Use of more sophisticated techniques will generate new opportunities to provide clinically useful information early in the disease process and detect CNS dysfunction that have been previously been considered beyond the capabilities of routine imaging techniques.

Suggested Reading

Engelbrecht V, Scherer A, Rassek M, Witsack HJ, Modder U (2002) Diffusion-weighted MR imaging in the brain in children: findings in the normal brain and in the brain with white matter diseases. Radiology 222:410–418

Holland BA, Haas DK, Norman D, Brant-Zawadzki M, Newton TH (1986) MRI of normal brain maturation. AJNR Am J Neuroradiol 7:201–208

Kreis R, Hofmann L, Kuhlmann B, Boesch C, Bossi E, Huppi PS (2002) Brain metabolite composition during early human brain development as measured by quantitative in vivo 1H magnetic resonance spectroscopy. Magn Reson Med 48:949–958

Mukherjee P, Miller JH, Shimony JS, et al (2002) Diffusion-tensor MR imaging of gray and white matter development during normal human brain maturation. AJNR Am J Neuroradiol 23:1445–1456

Schneider JF, Il'yasov KA, Boltshauser E, Hennig J, Martin E (2003) Diffusion tensor imaging in cases of adrenoleukodystrophy: preliminary experience as a marker for early demyelination? AJNR Am J Neuroradiol 24:819–824

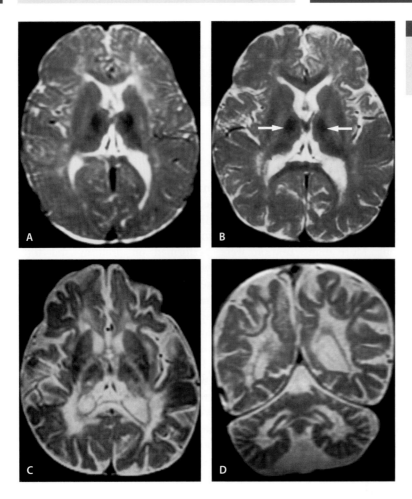

Hereditary Myelin Disorders

Krabbe's Disease
(Globoid Cell Leukodystrophy)

Infantile Type with Progression Over Time and Cerebellar Involvement

Clinical Presentation

A floppy female infant with irritability and hyperacusis. She had also feeding difficulties.

Images (Fig. 3.1)

A. T2-weighted (conventional SE) image at the age of 12 months shows nonspecific hyperintensity around the frontal horns, atria and putamen. Although CT at the age of 11 months did not demonstrate calcification, the globus pallidus low signal can be related to mineral accumulation

B. T2-weighted image at the age of 13 months demonstrates increased low signal in the globus pallidi and thalami (*arrows*). The corpus callosum and frontal white matter myelination have progressed at the same time with increase in hyperintensity at the posterior limb of the internal capsule

C. T2-weighted image at the age of 22 months. There is severe loss of hemispheric white matter with abnormal hyperintensity and deep sulci. An abnormal high signal is seen in both pulvinar regions, the posterior limb of internal capsules and insular cortices. Hyperintensity in the anterior thalamic and lentiform nucleus have progressed with decreased volume of the gray nuclei. At the same time the patient stopped interacting with her environment

D. Coronal T2-weighted image at the age of 32 months. The white matter hyperintensity has progressed significantly and now also the cerebellar white matter is hyperintense. There is diffuse volume loss

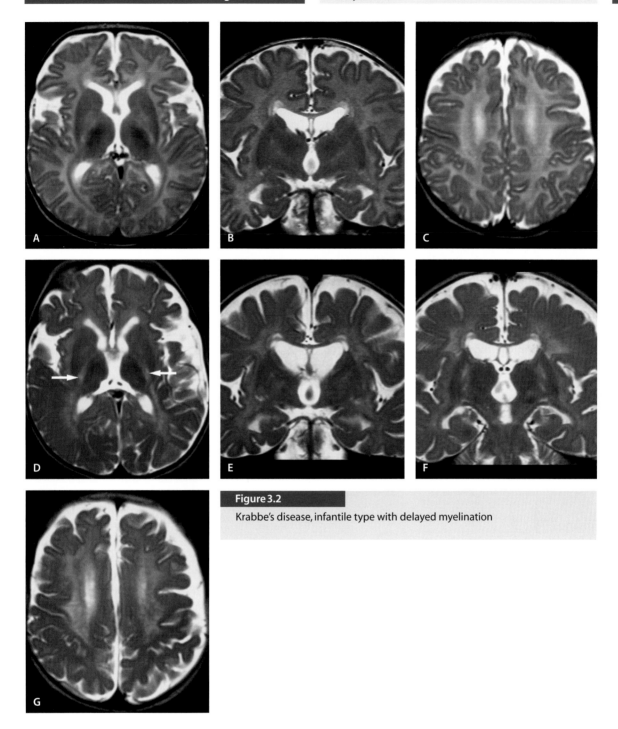

Figure 3.2

Krabbe's disease, infantile type with delayed myelination

Infantile Type with Delayed Myelination

Clinical Presentation

A 3-month-old male with irritability.

Images (Fig. 3.2)

A. Axial T2-weighted image at the age of 3 months shows prominence of sylvian fissures and cortical sulci

B. Coronal T2-weighted image at the age of 3 months reveals mild prominence of cortical CSF spaces

C. Axial T2-weighted image through the centrum semiovale shows nonmyelinated white matter

D. Axial T2-weighted image at the age of 6 months reveals hyperintensity on the posterior limb of internal capsules that normally are myelinated at this age (*arrows*). Abnormal white matter hyperintensity is also seen behind the trigones. Diffuse volume loss has progressed

E. Coronal T2 image at the age of 6 months shows progression of the periventricular white matter hyperintensity. Diffuse atrophy has progressed with dilated ventricles and sulci. Hippocampi are atrophic

F. Coronal T2-weighted image posterior to the image shown in E reveals progression of the periventricular and internal capsule white matter hyperintensity. The diffuse atrophy is well seen by progressive ventricular dilatation

G. At the age of 6 months the global volume loss has progressed. White matter volume has decreased and hyperintensity has also progressed

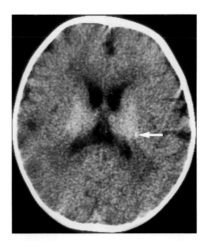

Figure 3.3

Krabbe's disease, infantile type with caudate calcification

Infantile Type with Caudate Calcification

Clinical Presentation

A 6-month-old female infant with irritability, spasticity and blindness

Image (Fig. 3.3)

A. Noncontrast CT scan shows thalamic and caudate body calcification (*arrow*). Mild periventricular hypodensity is seen

Discussion

Krabbe's disease is a neurodegenerative disease characterized by severe destruction of myelin and the presence of globoid bodies in the white matter. The biochemical defect is marked by deficiency of lysosomal enzyme, galactosylceramidase, resulting in accumulation of galactocerebroside. It is an autosomal recessive childhood disorder with the gene localized at chromosome 14. Krabbe's disease is classically divided into three groups: early infantile, late infantile and juvenile forms. Others have simplified the classification into "infantile" and "late onset". The infantile form is the most common subtype and generally presents with progressive irritability, vision loss, hyperacusis and rapid motor or mental decline and death usually occurs by 2 years of age. The late onset type presents after 10 years of age and mimics a peripheral neuropathy.

MR imaging demonstrates diffuse abnormalities of the white matter, which may be difficult to appreciate at the very early stage, when the nonmyelinated white matter is still normally hyperintense on T2-weighted images. CT imaging may be more helpful in the initial stages and shows symmetrically increased attenuation within the basal ganglia, thalami, and centrum semiovale. Progressive cerebral and cerebellar atrophy are seen in the late stage of the disease. Pyramidal tract involvement is the characteristic feature of the disease. In late onset disease, a hyperintense signal may be seen in the white matter, mostly in the posterior regions, with frequent involvement of the splenium of the corpus callosum.

MR spectroscopy reveals prominent peaks from choline-containing areas with high creatine and inositol peaks. The NAA peak is markedly reduced and the choline to NAA ratio is abnormally high. The lactic acid peak may be seen in some cases. This constellation MR spectroscopy finding is seen of extensive demyelination, gliosis, and loss of axons in the involved white matter. The latter two events occur in the later stages of Krabbe's disease.

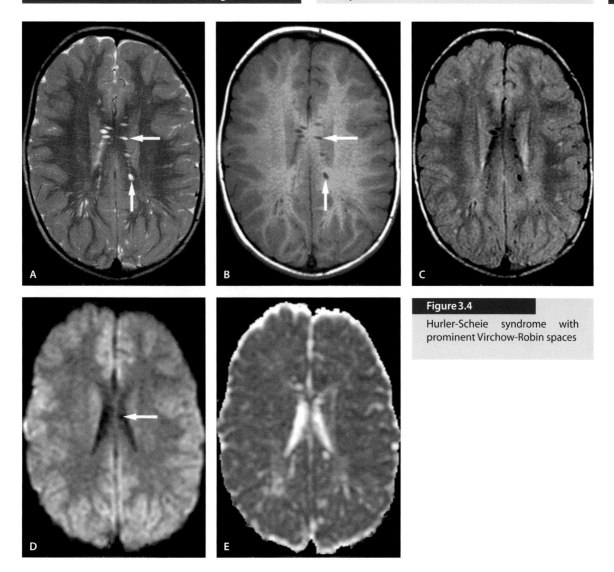

Figure 3.4

Hurler-Scheie syndrome with prominent Virchow-Robin spaces

Suggested Reading

Farina L, Bizzi A, Finocchiro G, et al (2000) MR imaging and proton MR spectroscopy in adult Krabbe disease. AJNR Am J Neuroradiol 21:1478–1482

Farley TJ, Ketonen LM, Bodensteiner JB, Wang DD (1992) Serial MRI and CT findings in infantile Krabbe disease. Pediatr Neurol 6:455–458

Given CA 2nd, Santos CC, Durden DD (2001) Intracranial and spinal MR imaging findings associated with Krabbe's disease. ANJR Am J Neuroradiol 22:1782–1785

Zarifi MK, Tzika AA, Astrakas LG, Poussaint TY, Anthony DC, Darras BT (2001) Magnetic resonance spectroscopy and magnetic resonance imaging findings in Krabbe's disease. J Child Neurol 16:522–526

Mucopolysaccharidoses (MPS)

Hurler-Scheie Syndrome with Prominent Virchow-Robin Spaces (MPS I H/S)

Clinical Presentation

A 5-year-old male with known MPS I presents for MRI with headaches.

Images (Fig. 3.4)

A. T2-weighted image shows characteristic dilated Virchow-Robin perivascular spaces, where mucopolysaccharides accumulate in phagocytic cells. They are characteristically seen in the peritrigonal region and corpus callosum (*arrows*)

B. The dilated perivascular spaces are hypointense on T1-weighted image (*arrows*)

C. The perivascular spaces on the corpus callosum follow the CSF signal on FLAIR image. The peritrigonal perivascular spaces range from low to isointense to CSF

D. The wide perivascular spaces on the corpus callosum are hypointense on DW image (*arrow*)

E. On ADC map the perivascular spaces are hyperintense

Hurler-Scheie Syndrome with Atrophy (MPS I H/S)

Clinical Presentation

A 22-year-old female who presents with cord compression symptoms. She has normal intelligence (see also Chapter 10).

Images (Fig. 3.5)

A. Sagittal T1-weighted image shows dilated ventricles. Note the significantly narrowed upper spinal canal and cord compression. For more details see Chapter 10 (Spine)

B. T2-weighted image shows honeycomb appearance of the thalami (*arrows*). Ventriculomegaly is present with prominent sylvian fissures. Dilated peritrigonal Virchow-Robin spaces are also present. Both frontal lobes show fine network of signal abnormality

C. T2-weighted image. Prominent perivascular spaces are seen throughout the white matter, the frontal lobes being the least involved

D. FLAIR image demonstrates better the thalamic abnormalities

E. FLAIR image shows periventricular white matter hyperintensities

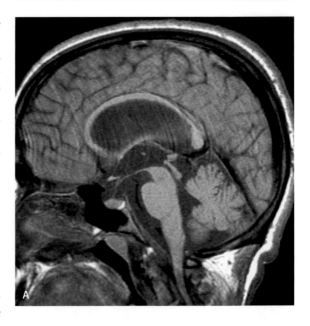

Figure 3.5 A

Hurler-Scheie syndrome with atrophy

F. Contrast-enhanced T1-weighted image fails to demonstrate enhancement in the thalamic cribriform lesions

G. DW image shows hypointensity in the thalami consistent with increased diffusibility

H. The fine white matter changes and prominent perivascular space in the frontoparietal area are difficult to appreciate on DW image

I. On ADC map the thalami show hyperintensity; there is no restricted diffusion

J. Exponential image reveals hypointensity in the thalami, consistent with increased diffusion

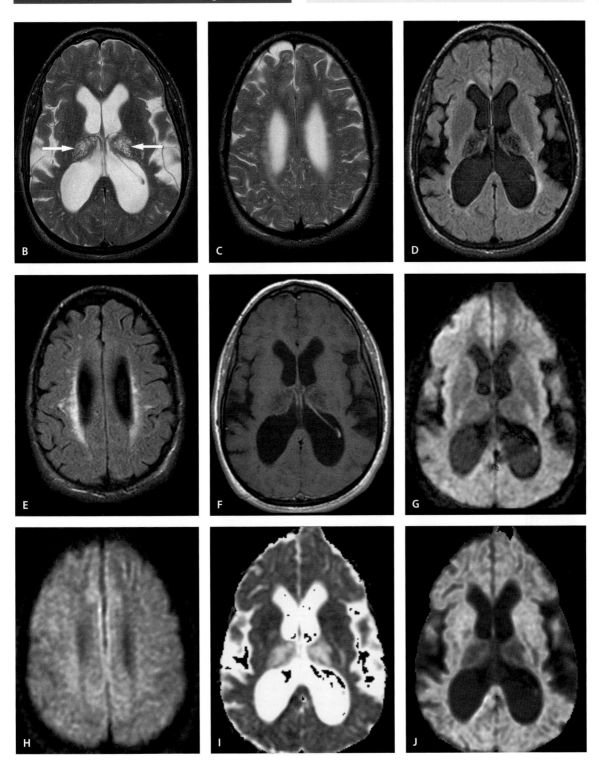

Figure 3.5 B–J

Hurler-Scheie syndrome with atrophy

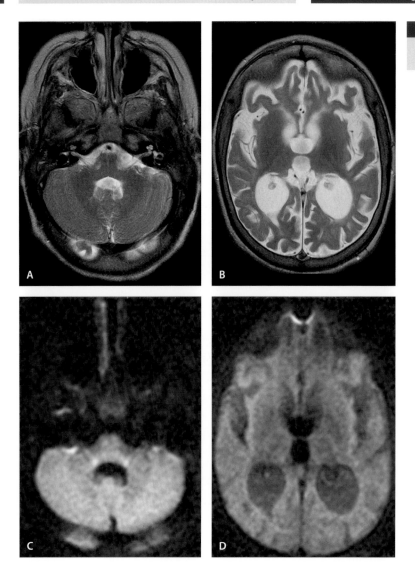

Figure 3.6
Sanfilippo syndrome

Sanfilippo Syndrome (MPS III)

Clinical Presentation

A 6-year-old female with Sanfilippo syndrome has been stable and interacting until 5 months ago, when she experienced a rapid downhill course. Now she is in a vegetative state with posturing.

Images (Fig. 3.6)

A. Axial T2-weighted image through the cerebellum is normal
B. T2 image through the basal ganglia shows lack of myelination in the anterior limb of the internal capsule with poor myelination of the posterior limb. Normal basal ganglia structures are not identified as separate structures. There is diffuse periventricular and subcortical white matter T2 hyperintensity, and also there is low volume of white matter, thin corpus callosum and cortical volume loss with deep gyri
C and D. No abnormality is seen in the DW images

Discussion

MPS are inherited metabolic disorders due to deficiency of lysosomal enzymes involved in the degeneration of glycosaminoglycans. Undegraded glycosaminoglycans accumulate in lysosomes and affect tissue function. MPS have been divided into seven major types. The classification is based on the deficient enzyme responsible for the disease. They share many clinical features, including multiple system involvement, organomegaly, dysostosis multiplex, facial abnormalities ("gargoylism", coarse faces), hearing and vision loss, joint involvement, cardiac involvement and central nervous system involvement. Profound mental retardation may be found in Hurler, Hunter's and Sanfilippo syndromes (MPS types I, II, and III), but normal intellect may be retained in other MPS. All MPS have autosomal recessive inheritance, except of MPS II which is X-linked.

Imaging findings of the brain in the MPS include delayed myelination, atrophy, varying degrees of hydrocephalus, and white matter changes. The white matter and corpus callosum show a cribriform appearance due to dilated perivascular spaces filled with glycosaminoglycans (mucopolysaccharides)

Hurler Syndrome (MPS I)
Hurler syndrome is characterized by deficiency of alpha-iduronidase leading to the storage and massive excretion of dermatan sulfate and heparin sulfate. In addition to the imaging findings of brain parenchyma mentioned above, progressive white matter involvement may be seen in Hurler syndrome. It may be differentiated into three different subtypes based on age at onset and severity of the clinical symptoms. The natural history of white matter abnormalities in patients with MPS is still unclear. It has been suggested that the degree of MR changes in patients with MPS does not always reflect their neurological impairment.

Hurler-Scheie Syndrome (MPS I H/S)
Hurler-Scheie syndrome represents an intermediate variant of the previous MPS type I syndrome with clinical symptoms manifesting between 3 and 8 years of age. Most patients have normal or near-normal intelligence. Cervical spinal cord compression is a typical feature. Most patients survive to adulthood.

Hunter's Syndrome (MPS II)
Hunter's syndrome is due to deficiency of iduronate 2-sulfatase enzyme. These children tend to have severe mental retardation and deafness. Communicating hydrocephalus is common. MR studies typically demonstrate thickened dura, cortical atrophy, and perivascular "pits", seen as low and high signal cystic foci on T1- and T2-weighted images.

Sanfilippo Syndrome (MPS III)
Sanfilippo syndrome (MPS III), is characterized by lysosomal accumulation of the glycosaminoglycan (GAG) heparan sulfate (HS). In humans, the disease manifests in early childhood with severe developmental retardation, and is characterized by a combination of progressive mental deterioration from the third year of life, hepatosplenomegaly and a typical facial appearance (mild 'Hurler' phenotype), leading to death in the second decade. MR imaging shows white matter abnormalities, cortical atrophy and ventricular enlargement, while other findings may include thickening of the diploë, callosal atrophy, and basal ganglia involvement. Cerebellar changes have also been described. Atrophy and abnormal or delayed myelination have been described to precede the onset of overt neurological symptoms.

Sly Disease (MPS VII)
Sly disease is caused by deficiency of beta-glucuronidase enzyme. Progressive hearing loss leading to early deafness is a prominent feature of this disease. On imaging, odontoid hypoplasia is the distinct feature.

Suggested Reading

Barone R, Nigro F, Triulzi F, Masumeci S, Fiumara A, Pavone L (1999) Clinical and neuroradiological follow-up in mucopolysaccharidosis type III (Sanfilippo syndrome). Neuropediatrics 5:270–274

Barone R, Parano E, Trifiletti RR, Fiumara A, Pavone P (2002) White matter changes mimicking a leukodystrophy in a patient with mucopolysaccharidosis: characterization by MRI. J Neurol Sci 195:171–175

Lee C, Dineen TE, Brack M, Kirsch JE, Runge VM (1993) The mucopolysaccharidoses: characterization by cranial MR imaging. AJNR Am J Neuroradiol 14:1285–1292

Parsons VJ, Hughes DG, Wraith JE (1996) Magnetic resonance imaging of the brain, neck and cervical spine in mild Hunter's syndrome (mucopolysaccharidoses type II). Clin Radiol 51:719–723

Zafeiriou DI, Augoustidou-Savvopoulou P, Papadopoulou FA, et al (1998) MRI findings in mild mucopolysaccharidosis II (Hunter's syndrome). Eur J Paediatr Neurol 2:153–156

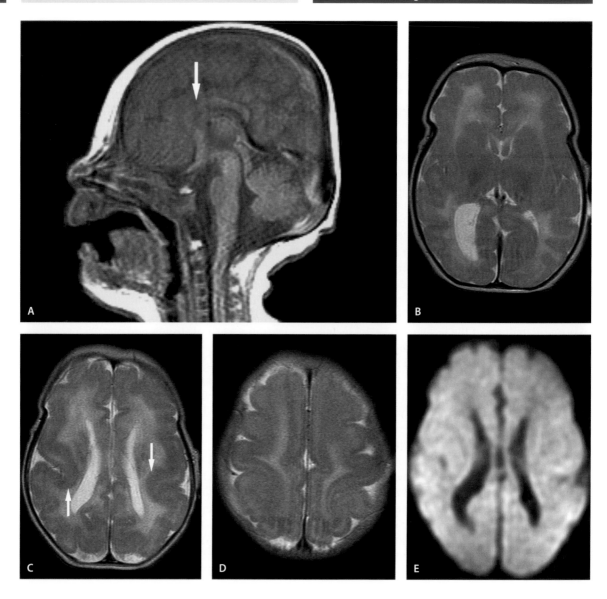

Figure 3.7

Zellweger syndrome

Zellweger Syndrome

Clinical Presentation

A 4-week old female infant presents with hypotonia and seizures. She also has pulmonary hypertension and multiple cysts in the kidneys.

Images (Fig. 3.7)

A. Sagittal T1-weighted image reveals underdevelopment of the rostrum and genu of the corpus callosum (*arrow*)
B. T2-weighted image shows paucity of cortical gyri that appear broad as seen in pachygyria. The cortex is thick, especially in the frontal and temporal regions. No myelination is seen in the corticospinal tracts

C. T2-weighted image. Polymicrogyria are seen in the poorly developed sylvian fissure regions (*arrows*). There are no germinolytic cysts
D. The cortex reveals also broad and shallow gyri on T2-weighted image. Low volume of white matter is seen in the centrum semiovale. There is lack of myelination in the motor cortex that is usually myelinated at birth
E. No signal abnormality is seen on DW image

Discussion

Zellweger (cerebrohepatorenal) syndrome is a rare, congenital disorder characterized by the reduction or absence of peroxisomes that presents in the neonatal period. Patients are characterized by multiple disturbances of lipid metabolism, profound hypotonia and neonatal seizures, and distinct facial dysmorphism and malformations in the brain. Additional features include mental retardation, liver dysfunction and renal cysts. The disorder is always fatal and most patients die within the first year.

MR imaging is the neuroimaging study of choice. MR imaging demonstrates the unusual combination of abnormalities of neuronal migration disorders with heterotopic gray matter, pachygyria, polymicrogyria, with hypomyelination. Abnormal gyration is most commonly seen in the perisylvian and perirolandic regions. Some authors consider the cortical changes as cortical dysplasia rather than true migration anomaly. Nonspecific subependymal germinolytic cysts may be seen as a result of hemorrhage. The presence of hypomyelination helps in differentiating Zellweger syndrome from neonatal adrenoleukodystrophy. Congenital muscular dystrophies can be differentiating from Zellweger syndrome by absence of facial deformities, seizures and lack of hypotonia.

Suggested Reading

Barkovich AJ, Peck WW (1997) MR of Zellweger syndrome. AJNR Am J Neuroradiol 18:1163–1170
Pueschel SM, Oyer CE (1995) Cerebrohepatorenal (Zellweger) syndrome: clinical, neuropathological, and biochemical findings. Childs Nerv Syst 11:639–642

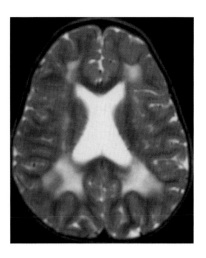

Figure 3.8
Adrenoleukodystrophy

Adrenoleukodystrophy

Clinical Presentation

A 21-month-old male with a history of myopathy.

Image (Fig. 3.8)

A. T2-weighted image shows extensive peritrigonal demyelination with lesser areas of demyelination in the deep white matter anteriorly and around the frontal horns

Discussion

Adrenoleukodystrophy is a rare genetic metabolic disorder characterized by progressive demyelination of nerve cells in the brain, dysfunction of adrenal glands and testes due to impaired peroxisomal function. Adrenoleukodystrophy comprises three subtypes: X-linked recessive disorder, and neonatal and childhood forms. In adrenoleukodystrophy, there is accumulation of high levels of very long-chain fatty acids in various organs due to the absence of peroxisomes. This accumulation is most severe in the brain and adrenal glands resulting in neurological problems and endocrine dysfunction. Neonatal adreno-

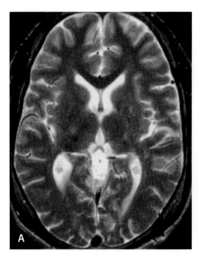 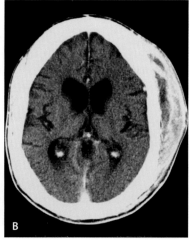

Figure 3.9

Juvenile neuronal ceroid lipofuscinosis with mild radiographic changes

leukodystrophy presents with mental retardation, facial abnormalities, retinal degeneration, weak muscle tone, enlarged liver, and adrenal dysfunction. This form usually progresses rapidly. Neonatal adrenoleukodystrophy is similar to Zellweger syndrome and may actually represent a milder variant of Zellweger syndrome. Neonatal adrenoleukodystrophy has demyelinating with inflammatory cells and foamy microphages whereas Zellweger syndrome patients have hypomyelination.

On T2-weighted MR images, bilateral symmetrical diffuse deep white matter high signal foci are seen in the occipital lobes. A bilateral occipital pattern with involvement of pontomedullary corticospinal tracts is an extremely helpful finding in the diagnosis of adrenoleukodystrophy. Contrast enhancement may be seen and is attributed to the inflammatory process.

Suggested Reading

Barkovich AJ, Ferriero DM, Bass N, Boyer R (1997) Involvement of the pontomedullary corticospinal tracts: a useful finding in the diagnosis of X-linked adrenoleukodystrophy. AJNR Am J Neuroradiol 18:95–100

Chen X, DeLellis RA, Hoda SA (2003) Adrenoleukodystrophy. Arch Pathol Lab Med 127:119–120

Melhem ER, Gotwald TF, Itoh R, Zinreich SJ, Moser HW (2001) T2 relaxation measurements in X-linked adrenoleukodystrophy performed using dual-echo fast fluid-attenuated inversion recovery MR imaging. AJNR Am J Neuroradiol 22:773–776

Neuronal Ceroid Lipofuscinosis (NCL)

Juvenile NCL with Mild Radiographic Changes

Clinical Presentation

A 14-year-old male with juvenile NCL (Spielmeyer-Vogt subtype) with seizures, developmental delay and progressive mental deterioration. He has also von Willebrand's disease.

Images (Fig. 3.9)

A. T2-weighted image at the age of 14 years shows only mild volume loss. The thalami show hypointensity, except the posterior, medial aspect. The putamen also shows hypointensity and is isointense with the globus pallidus' normal low signal

B. CT scan at the age of 19 years shows significant progression of the global atrophy with dilated ventricles and cortical sulci. Note traumatic changes in the subcutaneous tissue on the left

Juvenile NCL with Atrophy

Clinical Presentation

A 15-year-old female with seizures, progressive visual loss and developmental delay. She has juvenile or Spielmeyer-Vogt subtype of NCL.

Images (Fig. 3.10)

A. Sagittal T1-weighted image shows severe cerebellar atrophy
B. T2-weighted image confirms the presence of cerebellar atrophy
C. T2-weighted image through the superior cerebellar peduncles shows significant atrophy
D. T2-weighted image through the basal ganglia shows hypointensity in the putamen with a thin linear hypointensity in both thalami. External capsule shows hyperintensity consistent with demyelination or gliosis
E. Cortical brain atrophy is present on T2-weighted image
F. MRS (TE=35 ms) shows decreased NAA peak with increased myoinositol peak. Cho and Cr peaks are normal

Discussion

NCL represent a group of inherited neurodegenerative disorders with an autosomal recessive inheritance. They are caused by the accumulation of lipopigment within the lysosomes of neurons and other tissues. Several main types have been described: infantile onset (Haltia-Santavuori subtype), late infantile (Jansky-Bielschowsky subtype), and juvenile (Spielmeyer-Vogt or Batten subtype), to adult onset (Kufs subtype) forms, and early juvenile and heterogeneous group atypical forms. The most common types are the infantile and classic juvenile forms. Infantile NCL is progressive and uniformly fatal. The common clinical presentation is seizures, delayed milestones leading to dementia, involuntary movements, ataxia, visual loss and abnormal behavior.

In the infantile type the typical MR imaging findings can be seen even before the clinical signs. In the classic late infantile type, MR imaging is less informative in the early phase. When the disease progresses MR imaging demonstrates global cerebral and cerebellar atrophy, T2-hyperintensity of the lobar white matter and thinning of the cerebral cortex. Hypointensity is seen in the thalami. MR spectroscopy shows reduction of NAA consistent with neuronal damage. An increase of myoinositol and glutamine/glutamate is seen. No lactate is seen, helping in MR imaging differentiation between this disease and the mitochondrial group. The infantile type shows early atrophy and decreased signal in the thalami. A periventricular high-signal rim on T2-weighted MR images is a typical finding. Hypointensity is seen in addition to the thalami also in the corpus striatum. Atrophy, most prominent in the cerebellum, is especially marked in the infantile and late infantile subtypes. Demyelination and gliosis may be seen initially in the external capsules, but later in the cerebral white matter. An autopsy MR imaging correlation study has shown that periventricular changes detected in vivo on MRI are due to severe loss of myelin and gliosis. MR spectroscopy shows reduced levels of NAA.

Suggested Reading

Autti T, Raininko R, Santavuori P, Vanhanen SL, Poutanen VP, Haltia M (1997) MRI of neuronal ceroid lipofuscinosis. II. Postmortem MRI and histopathological study of the brain in 16 cases of neuronal ceroid lipofuscinosis of juvenile or late infantile type. Neuroradiology 5:371–377

D'Incerti L (2000) MRI in neuronal ceroid lipofuscinosis. Neurol Sci 21:71–73

Santavuori P, Vanhanen SL, Autti T (2001) Clinical and neuroradiological diagnostic aspects of neuronal ceroid lipofuscinosis disorders. Eur J Paediatr Neurol [Suppl A]:157–161

Vanhanen SL, Raininko R, Santavuori P (1994) Early differential diagnosis of infantile neuronal ceroid lipofuscinosis, Rett syndrome, and Krabbe disease by CT and MR. AJNR Am J Neuroradiol 15:1443–1453

Vanhanen SL, Raininko R, Autti T, Santavuori P (1995) MRI evaluation of the brain in infantile neuronal ceroid-lipofuscinosis, part 2. MRI findings in 21 patients. J Child Neurol 10:444–450

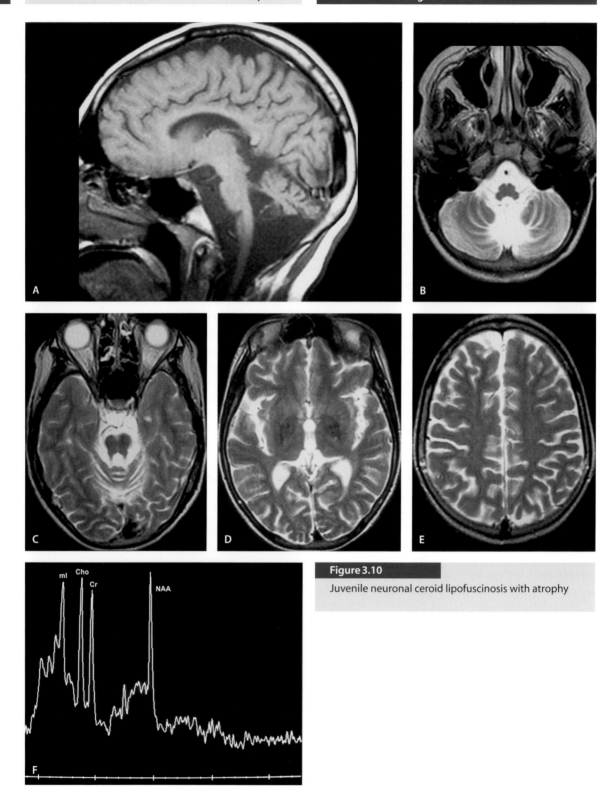

Figure 3.10

Juvenile neuronal ceroid lipofuscinosis with atrophy

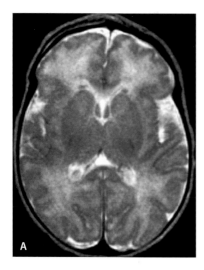
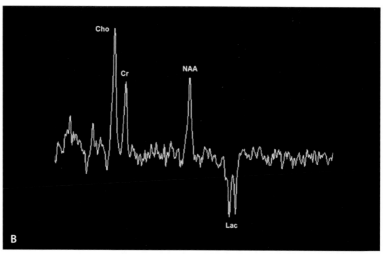

MELAS at 6 days of age

Mitochondrial Disorders

MELAS at Six Days of Age

Clinical Presentation

A 6-day-old female infant with lactic acidosis.

Images (Fig. 3.11)

A. T2-weighted image is unremarkable
B. MRS (TE=135 ms) shows reversed lactate peak at 1.3 ppm. The low NAA and high Cho peaks are normal for a 6-day-old infant

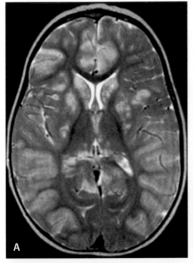

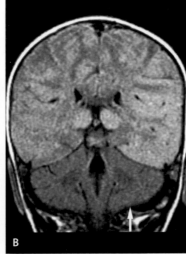

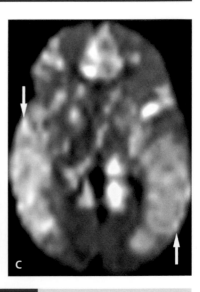

Figure 3.12

MELAS at 20 months of age

MELAS at Twenty Months of Age

Clinical Presentation

A 20-month-old female with lactic acidosis, developmental delay and seizures.

Images (Fig. 3.12)

A. There is increased signal on T2-weighted images diffusely within the cortex of both cerebral hemispheres, within the subcortical white matter bilaterally and also within the basal ganglia, cingular gyrus and thalami bilaterally. Diffuse mass effect upon the sulci is present

B. Coronal FLAIR shows hyperintensity involving both hemispheres and thalami compared to the darker (normal) signal in the cerebellum

C. DW image reveals increased signal in both cerebral hemispheres (*arrows*), cingular gyri and on both thalami

D. MR spectroscopy (TE=135 ms). Single voxel was placed over the subcortical and deep white matter in the right parietal region. There is an inverted lactate peak at 1.3 ppm consistent with increased anaerobic glycolysis. The NAA peak is significantly decreased with normal Cr and Cho peaks

Figure 3.13

Kearns-Sayre syndrome

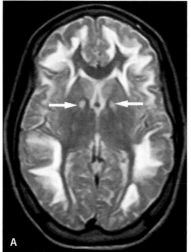
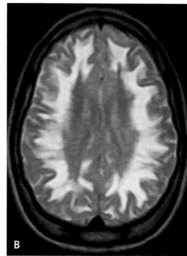

Kearns-Sayre Syndrome

Clinical Presentation

A young adult who has profound deafness since late teens, dementia, ataxia, and ophthalmoplegia.

Images (Fig. 3.13)

A. T2-weighted image through basal ganglia shows subcortical white matter hyperintensity sparing the corpus callosum and optic radiation. The globus pallidi show round hyperintensity bilaterally (*arrows*)
B. T2-weighted image through the centrum semiovale shows the peripheral "new" subcortical white matter involvement sparing the central "older" white matter

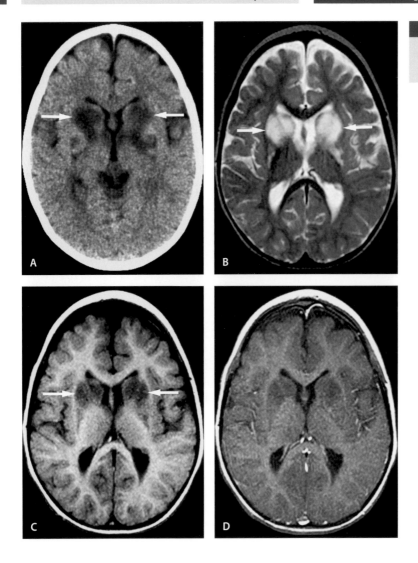

Figure 3.14

Leigh's disease, classic presentation

Leigh's Disease, Classic Presentation

Clinical Presentation

A 2-year-old female with failure to thrive.

Images (Fig. 3.14)

A. Noncontrast CT image shows low densities in the caudate and lentiform nuclei (*arrows*)
B. T2-weighted image demonstrates increased signal within the lentiform nucleus and caudate nuclei bilaterally (*arrows*)
C. T1-weighted image shows low signal in the caudate and lentiform nucleus (*arrows*)
D. Contrast-enhanced T1-weighted image shows no abnormal contrast enhancement

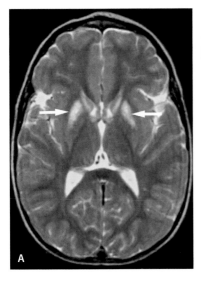
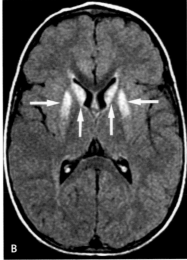
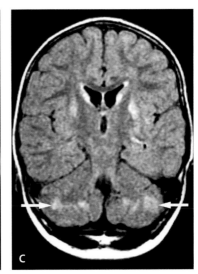

Figure 3.15

Leigh's disease, classic presentation with cerebellar involvement

Leigh's Disease, Classic Presentation with Cerebellar Involvement

Clinical Presentation

A 3-year-old male with arrested development, truncal ataxia and nystagmus since the age of 19 months. He presents with respiratory failure.

Images (Fig. 3.15)

A. T2-weighted image shows increased signal within the caudate nuclei and putamen bilaterally (*arrows*)
B. The hyperintense areas are better seen on axial FLAIR image (*arrows*)
C. Coronal FLAIR image reveals hyperintense lesions symmetrically and diffusely also within the cerebellar hemispheres (*arrows*)

Leigh's Disease, Peripheral Involvement

Clinical Presentation

An 18-year-old female college student with new onset of seizures. She had repeatedly high lactate in the CSF. Brain biopsy was obtained.

Images (Fig. 3.16)

A. T2-weighted image shows hyperintense lesion in the left posterior temporal and parietal region (*arrow*). Another T2 hyperintensity is seen in the periaqueductal gray matter (*arrowhead*)
B. DW image shows hyperintensity in the same lesions
C. ADC map shows increased signal in the left posterior temporoparietal and periaqueductal areas
D. There was no enhancement in the abnormal areas
E. MR spectroscopy (TE=35 ms) from left temporal lesion. Although the image is noisy, it demonstrates the presence of lactate at 1.33 ppm
F. MR spectroscopy (TE=144 ms) from the same area as in E demonstrates an inverted lactate doublet at 1.33 ppm

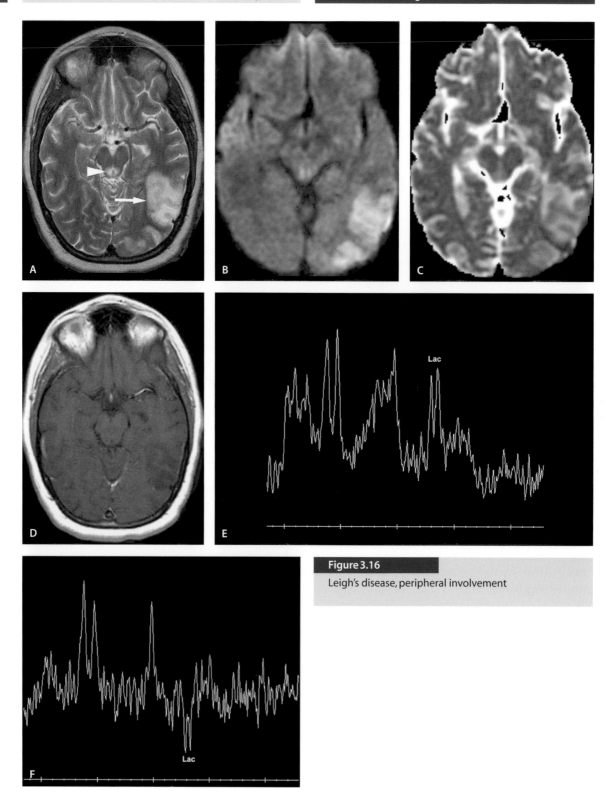

Figure 3.16
Leigh's disease, peripheral involvement

Discussion

Mitochondrial disorders are a clinically heterogeneous group of diseases caused by defects in mitochondrial function and oxidative phosphorylation.

The most common disorder is MELAS (mitochondrial encephalopathy, lactic acidosis, and stroke-like events) which is a multisystem disease associated with specific maternally inherited point mutations of mitochondrial DNA (mtDNA). The most common of these is an A-to-G transition at nucleotide 3243 of the tRNA Leu (UUR) gene. This point mutation is heteroplasmic, i.e. both normal and mutant mtDNA coexist in the tissues of the patient and the clinical symptoms are often related to the proportion of mutant and normal mtDNA in different tissues. The high energy demand of brain and muscle makes them particularly vulnerable to deficient energy production. MELAS is characterized by stroke-like episodes often preceded by treatment-resistant partial seizures. Short stature, diabetes mellitus, and slowly progressive mental impairment leading to dementia are common features. Exercise intolerance is common. Histological examination and muscle biopsy reveals accumulation of abnormal mitochondria and ragged red fibers.

During stroke-like episodes, CT and MR imaging reveal multifocal infarct-like, mainly gray matter lesions, not confined to the vascular territories. MR imaging classically demonstrate signal changes involving both grey and white matter predominantly in the occipital and parietal lobes that strongly mimic stroke lesions. DW imaging shows increased ADC values consistent with predominant extracellular edema in acute lesions in MELAS thereby indicating a nonischemic cause of the strokes seen in MELAS. MR spectroscopy may show lactate peaks suggestive of metabolic damage associated with this disease.

Leigh's syndrome, also known as subacute necrotizing encephalomyelopathy, is included with mitochondrial cytopathies. It is a progressive neurodegenerative disorder associated with several enzyme deficiencies such as pyruvate dehydrogenase complex, pyruvate carboxylase and defects in electron transport chain. Leigh syndromes have a common clinical phenotype, although genetic and biochemical abnormalities are heterogeneous. They are characterized by spongiosis, astrogliosis and capillary proliferation. Three clinical subtypes are identified: infantile type with symptoms occurring in first 2 years of life, juvenile form and adult form. The infantile form presents with hypotonia, vomiting, seizures, and death from respiratory failure. On CT images, non-enhancing hypodense areas are seen in the putamen and caudate nuclei. In the classic form T2-weighted MR images show symmetric hyperintense foci in the globus pallidus, putamen, and caudate nuclei. Putaminal involvement is not a pathognomonic radiological finding. The brain stem tegmentum, particularly the mesencephalon, is characteristically involved on MR imaging in the early and late phases of the illness. Patients who harbor approximately 70–90% mutant mtDNA in their tissues have highly variable manifestations. Patients with over 90% mutations have severe disease, such as Leigh's disease.

Kearns-Sayre syndrome is an autosomal dominant mitochondrial encephalopathy caused by deletion in muscle mtDNA with elevated serum pyruvate. Clinical features include progressive ophthalmoplegia, pigmentary degeneration of the retina, ataxia, myopathy, and cardiac conduction defects. On MR imaging, T2-weighted images show high signal intensity areas in the brain stem, globus pallidus, thalamus, and white matter of the cerebrum and cerebellum. The peripheral ("new") white matter is involved sparing the deep ("old") white matter. The imaging findings may be similar to those seen in Leigh's disease.

Suggested Reading

Abe K, Yoshimura H, Tanaka H, Fujita N, Hikita T, Sakoda S (2004) Comparison of conventional and diffusion-weighted MRI and proton MR spectroscopy in patients with mitochondrial encephalomyopathy, lactic acidosis, and stroke-like events. Neuroradiology 46:113–117

Arii J, Tanabe Y (2000) Leigh syndrome: serial MR imaging and clinical follow-up. AJNR Am J Neuroradiol 21:1502–1509

Heckmann JM, Eastman R, Handler L, Wright M, Owen P (1993) Leigh disease (subacute necrotizing encephalomyelopathy): MR documentation of the evolution of an acute attack. AJNR Am J Neuroradiol 14:1157–1159

Phillips CI, Gosden CM (1991) Leber's hereditary optic neuropathy and Kearns-Sayre syndrome: mitochondrial DNA mutations. Surv Ophthalmol 35:463–472

Schoffner JM (1996) Maternal inheritance and the evaluation of oxidative phosphorylation diseases. Lancet 348:1283–1288

Valanne L, Ketonen L, Majander A, Suomalainen A, Pihko H (1998) Neuroradiological findings in children with mitochondrial disorders. AJNR Am J Neuroradiol 19:369–377

Yonemura K, Hasegawa Y, Kimura K, Minematsu K, Yamaguchi T (2001) Diffusion-weighted MR imaging in a case of mitochondrial myopathy, encephalopathy, lactic acidosis, and stroke like episodes. AJNR Am J Neuroradiol 22:269–272

Zeviani M, Moraes CT, DiMauro S, et al (1988) Deletions of mitochondrial DNA in Kearns-Sayre syndrome. Neurology 38:1339–1346

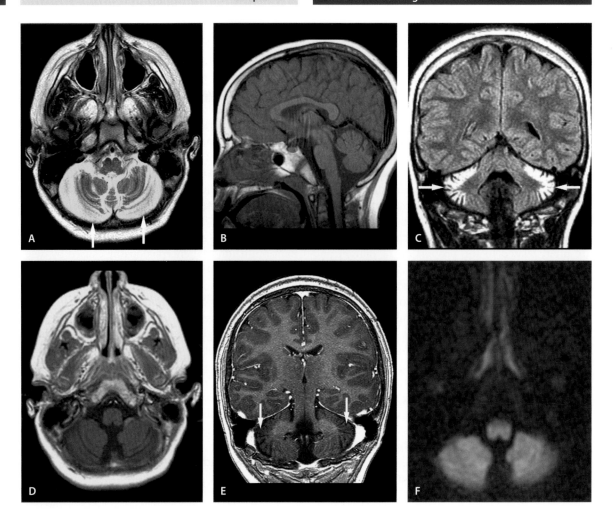

Figure 3.17

Cerebellar degeneration associated with coenzyme Q10 deficiency

Cerebellar Degeneration Associated with Coenzyme Q10 Deficiency

Clinical Presentation

An 8-year-old male with episodic seizures and ataxia.

Images (Fig. 3.17)

A. Axial T2-weighted image through posterior fossa shows marked atrophy of cerebellum with abnormal hyperintensity (*arrows*)

B. Sagittal T1-weighted image also shows cerebellar atrophy

C. Coronal FLAIR shows significant cerebellar cortical hyperintensity with normal-appearing white matter (*arrows*)

D. Axial contrast-enhanced T1-weighted image shows no significant enhancement in the cerebellum

E. Coronal contrast-enhanced gradient echo (SPGR) image reveals cortical low signal intensity in the cerebellum (*arrows*). No abnormal enhancement is present

F. DW image through posterior fossa shows no significant abnormality

Discussion

Coenzyme Q10 is an essential lipophilic component of an electron transport chain that has oxidoreductase functions. It also serves as an antioxidant and membrane stabilizer and has been found to protect cultured cerebellar neurons against both spontaneous and toxin-induced degeneration.

Primary coenzyme Q10 deficiency is a mitochondrial encephalopathy with a heterogeneous clinical presentation. It was first reported as a predominantly myopathic form in two sisters in 1989 characterized by the triad of exercise intolerance, recurrent myoglobinuria, and neurological manifestations. However, the most frequent ataxic form is dominated by ataxia and cerebellar atrophy, and is variously associated with seizures, developmental delay, weakness, pyramidal signs, or peripheral neuropathy. A third less-common form with fatal infantile encephalomyopathy and renal involvement has also been described. Usually the presentation is in childhood, but sometimes it may be delayed in onset until even fifth decade of life.

On imaging, atrophy of the cerebellar hemispheres as well as the vermis is the hallmark of primary CoQ10 deficiency. MR imaging is the modality of choice to demonstrate such atrophy. Primary coenzyme Q10 deficiency is important to diagnose, as its clinical spectrum continues to expand and more importantly such patients may improve with early administration of CoQ10 supplementation.

Suggested Reading

Favit A, Nicoletti F, Scapagnini U, Canonico PL (1992) Ubiquinone protects cultured neurons against spontaneous and excitotoxin-induced degeneration. J Cereb Blood Flow Metab 12:638–645

Gironi M, Lamperti C, Nemmi R, et al (2004) Late-onset cerebellar ataxia with hypogonadism and muscle coenzyme Q10 deficiency. Neurology 62(5):818–820

Lamperti C, Naini A, Hirano M, et al (2003) Cerebellar ataxia and coenzyme Q10 deficiency. Neurology 60:1206–1208

Musumeci O, Naini A, Slonim AE, et al (2001) Familial cerebellar ataxia with muscle coenzyme Q10 deficiency. Neurology 56:849–855

Ogasahara S, Engel AG, Frens D, Mack D (1989) Muscle coenzyme Q deficiency in familial mitochondrial encephalomyopathy. Proc Natl Acad Sci U S A 86:2379–2386

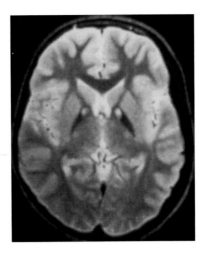

Figure 3.18
Hallervorden-Spatz disease, classical presentation

Hallervorden-Spatz Disease

Clinical Presentation

A 12-year-old girl with visual symptoms and progressive spasticity and choreoathetosis.

Image (Fig. 3.18)

A. T2-weighted image shows dark signal in the globus pallidus with symmetric hyperintense foci in medial globus pallidus. This is "classical eye-of-the-tiger" imaging appearance in this entity

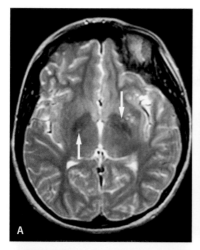

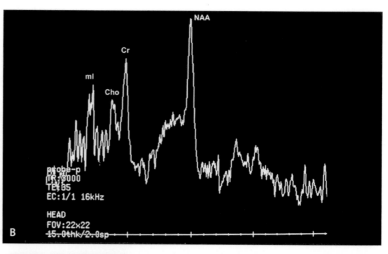

Figure 3.19

Hallervorden-Spatz disease, asymmetric presentation

Asymmetric Presentation

Clinical Presentation

A 15-year-old girl with visual symptoms, dysarthria and seizures.

Images (Fig. 3.19)

A. T2-weighted image shows (more than expected) low signal in the globus pallidi with a central high signal (*arrows*), the so called "eye-of-the-tiger". The high signal areas in the globus pallidi are slightly asymmetric

B. MR spectroscopy (TE=35 ms) reveals decreased NAA with increased myoinositol peaks. Cho is also low

C. T2-weighted image demonstrates the voxel location over the left basal ganglia

Discussion

Hallervorden-Spatz disease (synonym: neurodegeneration with brain iron accumulation, pantothenate kinase-associated neurodegeneration) is a rare neurodegenerative disorder characterized by iron accumulation in the basal ganglia, progressive extrapyramidal dysfunction and dementia. The exact pathogenesis is unknown. Mutations in the pantothenate kinase 2 gene (PANK2) have been shown to lead to pantothenate kinase-associated neurodegeneration by influencing mitochondrial function. This may lead to abnormal iron accumulation in the globus pallidus and reticular substantia nigra and cause late-onset neurodegenerative disorders.

Noncontrast-enhanced CT shows bilateral low densities in the globus pallidus and substantia nigra. T2-weighted MR images demonstrate hypointense signals due to iron accumulation. Areas of gliosis, demyelination, neuronal loss, and axonal swelling are seen as high signal intensity areas on T2-weighted MR images. Initially hyperintense areas are seen in the globus pallidi and substantia nigra. Later as the disease progresses, a hypointense rim is seen around it, due to iron deposition, causing the characteristic "eye-of-the-tiger" sign.

Suggested Reading

Johnson MA, Kuo YM, Westaway SK, Parker SM, Ching KH, Gitschier J, Hayflick SJ (2004) Mitochondrial localization of human PANK2 and hypotheses of secondary iron accumulation in pantothenate kinase-associated neurodegeneration. Ann N Y Acad Sci 1012:282–298

Nuri Sener R (2003) Pantothenate kinase-associated neurodegeneration: MR imaging, proton MR spectroscopy, and diffusion MR imaging findings. AJNR Am J Neuroradiol 24:1690–1693

Sethi N, Sethi PK (2003) Eye-of-the-tiger sign. J Assoc Physicians India 51:486

Swaiman KF (2001) Hallervorden-Spatz syndrome. Pediatr Neurol 25:102–108

Trimble M (2003) Magnetic resonance imaging and Hallervorden-Spatz syndrome. CNS Spectr 8:420

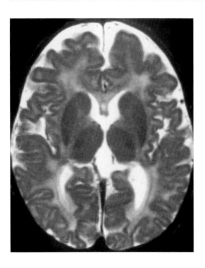

Figure 3.20

Pelizaeus-Merzbacher disease with lack of normal myelination

Defects in Genes Encoding the Myelin Proteins

Pelizaeus-Merzbacher Disease

Pelizaeus-Merzbacher Disease with Lack of Normal Myelination

Clinical Presentation

A 10-month-old male with nystagmus and developmental delay presents for MR imaging evaluation.

Image (Fig. 3.20)

A. T2-weighted image demonstrates diffuse hyperintensity in the white matter including the corpus callosum and internal capsule. This is consistent with near-total lack of normal myelination. Severe white matter atrophy is present with normal-appearing cortical ribbon

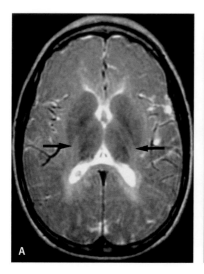 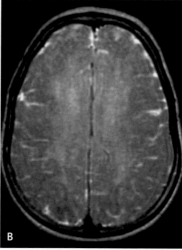

Figure 3.21

Pelizaeus-Merzbacher disease with delayed myelination

Pelizaeus-Merzbacher Disease with Delayed Myelination

Clinical Presentation

An 11-month-old male with developmental delay, ataxia, visual symptoms and spasticity. He has a 3-year-old brother with similar symptoms and hypomyelination on MRI.

Images (Fig. 3.21)

A. T2-weighted image fails to show myelination in posterior limbs of internal capsules (*arrows*) usually present by 2 months of age
B. Brain myelination is inappropriate for an 11-month-old, since no myelination is present on T2-weighted image

Pelizaeus-Merzbacher Disease with Prominent Cerebellar Involvement

Clinical Presentation

A 9-year-old male with developmental delay and hypotonia.

Images (Fig. 3.22)

A. Noncontrast CT scan at the age of 1 year shows significant hypodensity in the white matter tracts
B. The white matter tracts show unusual low density also in the supratentorial area on noncontrast CT image
C. T2-weighted image at the age of 9 years shows abnormal hyperintensity in the cerebellum
D. T2-weighted image fails to show any myelination in the corticospinal fibers as expected. The centrum semiovale is abnormally hyperintense

Discussion

Pelizaeus-Merzbacher disease is an X-linked recessive leukodystrophy caused by a mutation in the proteolipid protein gene on chromosome Xq22. It is characterized by hypotonia, respiratory distress, stridor, nystagmus, and profound myelin loss. It has been divided into a number of subtypes.

Figure 3.22

Pelizaeus-Merzbacher disease with prominent cerebellar involvement

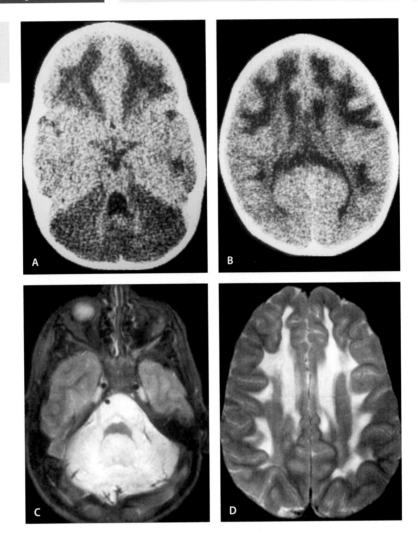

On CT images, mild nonspecific cerebral and cerebellar atrophy is seen. T2-weighted MR images show extensive white matter hypomyelination. Severe cases may show near-total lack of myelination which extends peripherally to involve the arcuate fibers. The white matter has often a "tigroid" appearance. There is no histological evidence of demyelination. The brain stem, diencephalon, cerebellum, and subcortical white matter may show preservation of myelin. MR spectroscopy may show decreased choline peaks in the white matter resulting in markedly high NAA/Cho ratios, and low Cho/Cr ratios representing deficient myelination. Diffusional anisotropy in the corpus callosum, internal capsule and white matter of the frontal lobes has been reported.

p10 p9 Translocation

Clinical Presentation

A 13-month-old female with chromosome disorder: translocation of p10 and p9. She had abnormal prenatal ultrasound and postnatal CT scan. She has cardiac, visceral and skeletal abnormalities, developmental delay and cleft palate.

Images (Fig. 3.23)

A. Sagittal T1-weighted image demonstrates vermian hypoplasia with a prominent retrocerebellar CSF space. This CSF space communicates with the fourth ventricle (*arrow*). The corpus callosum is present but hypoplastic

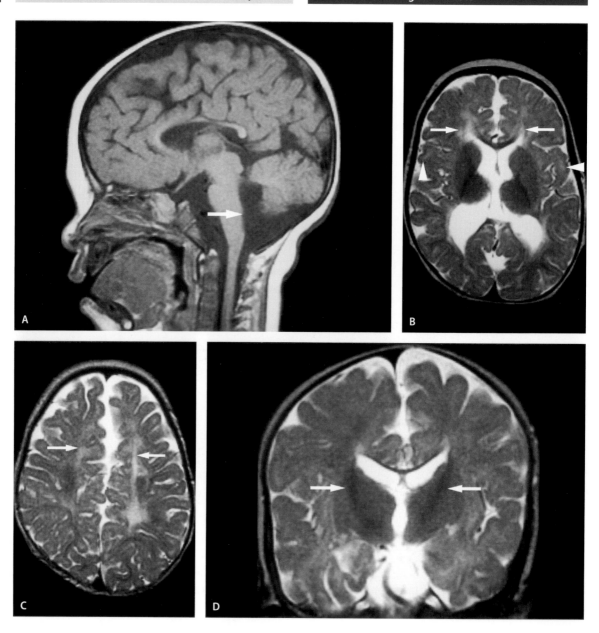

Figure 3.23

p10 p9 translocation

B. Significant areas of the periventricular white matter demonstrate an abnormal high signal on T2-weighted image (*arrows*). Patchy areas of abnormal high signal are seen also in the subcortical white matter (*arrowheads*). The internal capsules show normal myelination and the thin genu of the corpus callosum is myelinated

C. T2-weighted image reveals prominent extra-axial CSF space bilaterally. The falx is absent. The white matter volume is low. The centrum semiovale white matter is still abnormally bright (*arrows*)

D. Coronal T2-weighted image demonstrates normal myelination in the anterior limb on the internal capsules (*arrows*). The sylvian fissures are open

Figure 3.24

18q syndrome

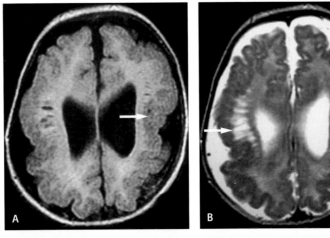

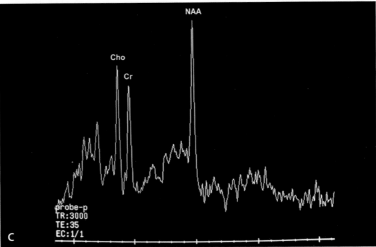

and the extra-axial CSF spaces are prominent. There is lack of maturity of subcortical white matter. The white matter volume is also decreased. No falx is visualized

18q Syndrome

Clinical Presentation

A 15-month-old male who presents with microcephaly, developmental delay and hypotonia.

Images (Fig. 3.24)

A. T1-weighted image shows microcephaly, low white matter volume, abnormal gyration and lack of normal operculum formation (*arrow*)

B. T2-weighted image confirms the findings in A. Additionally prominent perivascular spaces (*arrows*) are better appreciated

C. MR spectroscopy (TE=35 ms) placing voxel over right centrum semiovale reveals no abnormal metabolites. Relatively low NAA reflects patient's age rather than abnormality

Discussion

Leukodystrophies are a heterogeneous group of disorders that affect the central and sometimes the peripheral nervous systems and predominantly involve the white matter. A typical feature is abnormal myelin formation and/or maintenance of normal formed myelin. Although destruction is seen typically in demyelinating diseases, this may also be seen in the leukodystrophies.

Very little has been described in the literature regarding the CNS imaging findings in patients with 10p, 9p syndrome. A case of an 18-week fetus with trisomy 9p and 10p has been reported. Ultrasound of the brain and fetus at that time showed cleft lip/palate, club feet, structural anomalies of the cerebellum and cystic kidneys. No brain MR imaging findings were reported.

White matter alterations in chromosomal disorders have been reported mainly in 18q syndrome. This syndrome is a prototype of hypomyelination. Chromosome analysis reveals partial deletion of the long arm of chromosome 18 including myelin basic protein genes. Typical imaging findings show small brain volume and poor delineation of gray/white matter. In a case report of 18q syndrome three serial magnetic resonance images demonstrated that myelination in the central nervous system was delayed except for the corpus callosum and brainstem. MR spectroscopy has been reported to be normal.

A small series of patients with sex chromosomal and autosomal chromosomal disorders has been reported to have white matter changes in the periventricular and subcortical region seen in T2-weighted and FLAIR images. These lesions were isolated or confluent hyperintensities. Normal myelination progresses in an orderly fashion and usually by 2 years of age the pattern of myelination is similar to that of an adult. Alterations of the cerebral white matter due to specific genes directly involved in the central nervous system myelination process have recently been published. The prevalence of white matter changes in different chromosomal abnormalities appears to be high, even though they have not been well reported in the literature. Some authors hypothesize that unknown factors related to the myelination processes may be localized in different chromosomes.

Suggested Reading

Garcia-Cazorla A, Sans A, Baquero M, et al (2004) White matter alterations associated with chromosomal disorders. Dev Med Child Neurol 3:148–153

Hengstschlager M, Bettelheim D, Repa C, Lang S, Deutinger J, Bernaschek G (2002) A fetus with trisomy 9p and trisomy 10p originating from unbalanced segregation of a maternal complex chromosome rearrangement t(4;10;9). Fetal Diagn Ther 4:243–246

Koeppen AH, Robitaille Y (2002) Pelizaeus-Merzbacher disease. Neuropathol Exp Neurol 61:747–759

Loevner LA, Shapiro RM, Grossman RI, Overhauser J, Kamholz J. (1996) White matter changes associated with deletions of the long arm of chromosome 18 (18q-syndrome): a dysmyelinating disorder? AJNR Am J Neuroradiol 10:1843–1848

Ono J, Harada K, Hasegawa T, et al (1994) Central nervous system abnormalities in chromosome deletion at 11q23. Clin Genet 6:325–329

Ono J, Harada K, Yamamoto T, Onoe S, Okada S (1994) Delayed myelination in a patient with 18q-syndrome. Pediatr Neurol 1:64–67

Plecko B, Stockler-Ipsiroglu S, Gruber S, et al (2003) Degree of hypomyelination and magnetic resonance spectroscopy findings in patients with Pelizaeus Merzbacher phenotype. Neuropediatrics 34:127–136

Sener RN (2004) Pelizaeus-Merzbacher disease: diffusion MR imaging and proton MR spectroscopy findings. J Neuroradiol 31:138–141

Disorders in Amino Acid and Organic Acid Metabolism

Phenylketonuria (PKU)

Clinical Presentation

A 22-year-old male presented with mental retardation. Serum phenylalanine was 11 mg/dl.

Images (Fig. 3.25)

A. T2-weighted image shows hyperintense lesion in bilateral periventricular white matter. The white matter abnormalities involve the regions around the frontal horns, bodies and atria and occipital horns of the lateral ventricles

B. Contrast-enhanced T1-weighted image shows no significant enhancement

C. DW image shows marked hyperintense periventricular lesions

D. ADC map shows hypointensity indicating cytotoxic edema and restricted diffusion as seen in intramyelinic edema

Discussion

PKU is the most common congenital disorder of amino acid metabolism due to deficiency of the enzyme phenylalanine hydroxylase. Untreated patients typically develop a characteristic clinical picture that may include mental retardation, seizures, growth retardation, hyperreflexia, eczematous dermatitis, and hypopigmentation. Treatment consists of dietary control with restricted intake of phenylalanine.

Figure 3.25

Phenylketonuria

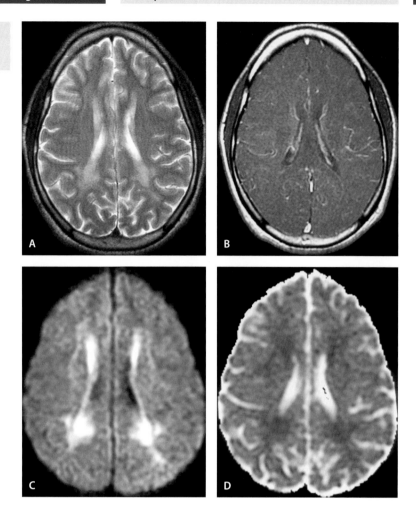

With elevated phenylalanine levels (>600 µmol/l), patients with PKU generally demonstrate symmetric patchy and/or band-like areas of enhanced signal intensity on T2-weighted MR images. The changes predominantly affect the posterior/periventricular white matter. In more severely affected patients, the lesions extend to the frontal and subcortical white matter, including corpus callosum and the area of the association fibers. The etiology of T2 hyperintensity is thought to be due to increased water content due to edema associated with myelination or gliosis. On DW images, these increased signal intensity areas show restricted diffusion indicating cytotoxic edema, such as that seen in intramyelinic edema.

Suggested Reading

Brismar J, Aqeel A, Gascon G, Ozand P (1990) Malignant hyperphenylalaninemia: CT and MR of the brain. AJNR Am J Neuroradiol 11:135–138

Moller HE, Weglage J, Bick U, Wiedermann D, Feldmann R, Ullrich K (2003) Brain imaging and proton magnetic resonance spectroscopy in patients with phenylketonuria. Pediatrics 112:1580–1583

Pearsen KD, Gean-Marton AD, Levy HL, Davis KR (1990) Phenylketonuria: MR imaging of the brain with clinical correlation. Radiology 177:437–440

Phillips MD, McGraw P, Lowe MJ, Mathews VP, Hainline BE (2001) Diffusion-weighted imaging of white matter abnormalities in patients with phenylketonuria. AJNR Am J Neuroradiol 22:1583–1586

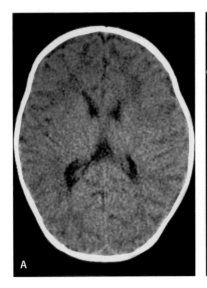

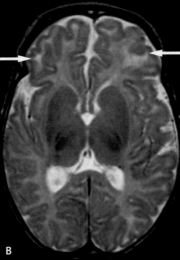

Figure 3.26

Propionic acidemia

Propionic Acidemia

Clinical Presentation

A 9-week-old with propionic acidemia now with recurrent seizures.

Images (Fig. 3.26)

A. CT at the age of 8 weeks following a seizure. There are patchy hypodensities of the peripheral white matter in the frontal regions
B. T2-weighted image shows patchy and confluent white matter hyperintense signal changes in the subcortical white matter of the frontal lobes (*arrows*) and to the lesser degree in the parietal and occipital lobes

Discussion

Propionic acidemia is an autosomal recessive disorder of organic acid metabolism caused by a genetic deficiency of mitochondrial propionyl-CoA carboxylase. Patients with propionic acidemia usually present in the neonatal period with life-threatening ketoacidosis, failure to thrive, and developmental delay.

CT and MR imaging show white matter changes in the form of low attenuation areas (CT) and T2 hyperintensity with predominant symmetric involvement of the basal ganglia region and subcortical white matter. With progression of the disease, widening of sulci and fissures may be seen. Rarely, fatal rapid necrosis of the caudate, globus pallidus and putamen may also be seen.

Suggested Reading

Brismar J, Ozand PT (1994) CT and MR of the brain in disorders of the propionate and methylmalonate metabolism. AJNR Am J Neuroradiol 15:1459–1473

Gebarski SS, Gabrielsen TO, Knake JE, Latack JT (1983) Cerebral CT findings in methylmalonic acid propionic acidemias. AJNR Am J Neuroradiol 4:955–957

Haas RH, Marsden DL, Capistrano-Estrada S, et al (1995) Acute basal ganglia infarction in propionic acidemia. J Child Neurol 10:18–22

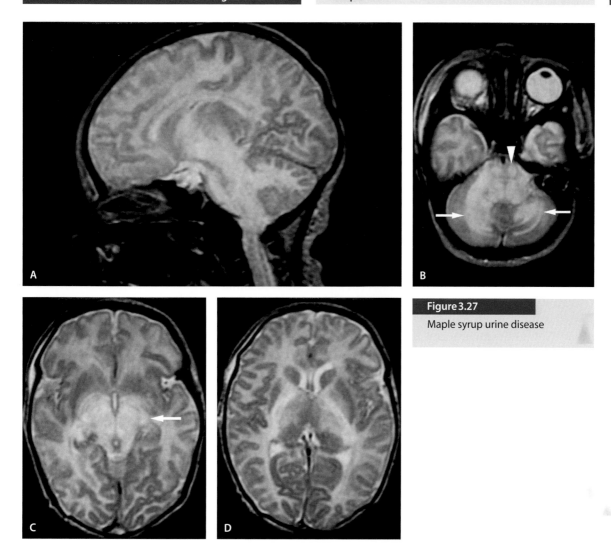

Figure 3.27

Maple syrup urine disease

Maple Syrup Urine Disease (MSUD)

Clinical Presentation

A 12-day-old girl with clinical suspicion of infection presents for MR imaging with fever, poor feeding, and lethargy.

Images (Fig. 3.27)

A. Sagittal T2-weighted image demonstrates "full posterior fossa" with poorly visualized fourth ventricle and prepontine cistern

B. Axial T2-weighted image demonstrates diffuse cerebellar white matter (*arrows*) and brainstem edema. Atypically this case shows both ventral and dorsal pons edema (*arrowhead*)

C. Midbrain edema is seen on the T2-weighted image (*arrow*)

D. Edema extends to the posterior limb of internal capsules and thalami, but spares the pulvinar area

Discussion

MSUD is a heterogeneous disorder with four different phenotypes. All forms have an autosomal recessive mode of inheritance. It is caused by a defect in the oxidative decarboxylation of the branched-chain ketoacids. As a result of the enzymatic defect, branched-chain amino acids, leucine, isoleucine and valine, accumulate in serum, CSF, and urine. The characteristic odor of the urine of the affected child resembles maple syrup, thus the name maple syrup urine disease. In the classic form children born with this disease appear normal at birth but start manifesting the symptoms by the end of the first week of life. The symptoms include lethargy, poor feeding, sometimes vomiting, and coma. Early treatment may halt or reverse neurological abnormalities, but mental and neurological residua are common even in treated patients. In the intermittent form symptoms are seen between 2 months and 40 years of age, and are triggered by stress, such as vaccination, infection, operation and the like.

In the classic form CT and MR imaging show signs of diffuse edema seen as areas of hypodensity on CT and hyperintensity on T2-weighted images. The characteristic intense local edema (called MSUD edema) involves the deep cerebellar white matter, posterior brain stem, cerebral peduncles, thalami, posterior limb of internal capsules and posterior centrum semiovale. All these areas are myelinated at this age, and show hyperintensity. Edema may be difficult to recognize in the T2 weighted image as immature, nonmyelinated brain is also bright. DWI shows these abnormalities more extensively with a markedly reduced ADC value thereby suggesting cytotoxic edema. Fractional anisotropy maps may reveal decreased values in the affected areas, indicating fiber destruction and/or demyelination.

Suggested Reading

Brismar J, Aqeel A, Brismar G, Coates R, Gascon G, Ozand P (1990) Maple syrup urine disease: findings on CT and MR scans of the brain in 10 infants. ANJR Am J Neuroradiol 11:1219–1228

Cavalleri F, Berardi A, Burlina AB, Ferrari F, Mavilla L (2002) Diffusion-weighted MRI of maple syrup urine disease encephalopathy. Neuroradiology 44:499–502

Jan W, Zimmerman RA, Wang ZJ, Berry GT, Kaplan PB, Kaye EM (2003) MR diffusion imaging and MR spectroscopy of maple syrup urine disease during acute metabolic decompensation. Neuroradiology 45:393–399

Parmar H, Sitoh YY, Ho L (2004) Maple syrup urine disease: diffusion-weighted and diffusion-tensor magnetic resonance imaging findings. J Comput Assist Tomogr 28:93–97

Galactosemia

Clinical Presentation

A 6-month-old female with refusal to feed, vomiting and hypotonia.

Images (Fig. 3.28)

A. Hyperintense white matter lesions are difficult to appreciate at this age, since normal myelin is still immature and high signal; however, foci of more hyperintense white matter lesions in the bilateral frontal and temporal lobes are seen (*arrows*) on this T2-weighted image. Mild prominence of the cortical CSF spaces is present

B. Coronal T2-weighted image shows bilateral hyperintense foci in the bilateral periventricular white matter and temporal lobes

Figure 3.28

Galactosemia

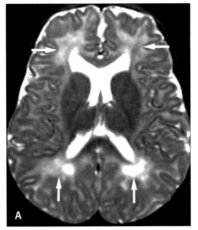
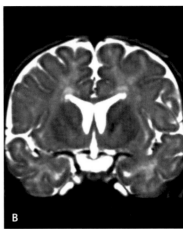

Discussion

Three major types of galactosemia can be seen, based on three different enzyme deficiencies. Classical galactosemia is an autosomal recessive disorder of galactose metabolism caused by deficiency of galactose-1-phosphate uridyltransferase. The gene encoding this enzyme deficiency has been mapped to chromosome 9. Affected infants are normal at birth. Signs of toxicity usually occur after the initiation of milk feedings; presenting symptoms, however, may vary with age and in severity. In the neonatal age, clinical manifestations include lethargy, jaundice, vomiting, failure to thrive, and frequently *E. coli* sepsis. In later infancy or early childhood, cataracts, cirrhosis of the liver, and mental deficiency are the classical features. Pathologically, as the concentration of galactitol increases, cerebral edema occurs due to osmosis. Raised intracranial pressure may be the presenting symptom in some patients. If milk is not withdrawn, the infant may die. A galactose-free diet causes striking disappearance of symptoms. However, the long-term prognosis is less favorable. Many patients have subnormal intelligence and at the end of first decade develop tremor and ataxia. Many children have speech problems. On neuropathology diffuse white matter gliosis can be seen. The findings are mainly seen in the periventricular area.

CT may show diffuse cerebral edema. On T2-weighted MR images, abnormal hyperintense white matter foci suggestive of deficient myelination are seen in cerebral white matter. This high signal intensity is thought to be due to increase in the amount of water in the cerebral white matter. The signal intensity from the internal capsule and corpus callosum is not affected, since the axon bundles are coherent and tightly packed together. Mild cerebral and cerebellar atrophy may also be seen.

Suggested Reading

Belman AL, Moshe SL, Zimmerman RD (1986) Computed tomographic demonstration of cerebral edema in a child with galactosemia. Pediatrics 78:606–609

Marano GD, Sheils WS Jr, Gabriele OF, Klingberg WG (1987) Cranial CT in galactosemia. AJNR Am J Neuroradiol 8:1150–1151

Nelson MD Jr, Wolff JA, Cross CA, Donnell GN, Kaufman FR (1992) Galactosemia: evaluation with MR imaging. Radiology 184:255–261

Late-Onset Type of Ornithine Transcarbamylase (OTCD) Deficiency with a Recent Occipital Infarct

Clinical Presentation

A now young adult female has suffered for years with episodic symptoms: headache, irritability, bizarre behavior, lethargy and seizures. Now she presents with new visual symptoms for MR imaging.

Images (Fig. 3.29)

A. FLAIR image shows asymmetric abnormal high signal intensity in the cortex with minimal signal abnormality in the periventricular white matter and forceps minor. Multiple cystic lesions that follow the CSF signal are seen in the gray/white junction (*arrows*). These hyperintense cortical areas are consistent with old ischemic events
B. FLAIR image shows abnormal hyperintensity involving both optic tracts (*arrows*)
C. Coronal FLAIR shows multiple small cystic lesions at the gray/white matter junction making the cortex appear lace-like
D. DW image fails to show abnormal diffusion in the cortical FLAIR abnormality
E. DW image. The right occipital lobe shows an area of restricted diffusion without corresponding FLAIR abnormality. This is consistent with acute infarct and is responsible for the patient's current symptoms
F. MR spectroscopy (TE=35 ms) placing the voxel over the right occipital signal abnormality (in E) reveals the lactate peak. There are low choline and myoinositol peaks with a mildly decreased NAA peak

Discussion

OTCD is the most common inborn error of metabolism of the urea cycle. It is an X-linked disorder characterized by signs and episodic symptoms of encephalopathy that is induced by accumulation of precursors of urea, principally ammonia and glutamine. Patients present with episodic headaches, vomiting, irritability, bizarre behavior, tremors and seizures. The most severe clinical form is seen in newborns after an unremarkable 24–48 hours. Milder forms can present any time from infancy to adulthood. The late-onset form appears usually in women who have a mutation at one of their X-chromosomes. The late-onset form of OTCD resembles an ischemic stroke. Laboratory investigations show hyperammonemia. It is possible to establish a diagnosis antenatally from the amniotic fluid. Pathologically symmetric cystic lesions at the gray/white matter junction are seen. The same cystic lesions are seen in the MR image and they follow the CSF signal.

MR spectroscopy is a clinically useful diagnostic tool, since alterations in brain metabolites can be seen. The appearance of the MR spectroscopy varies depending on the patient's clinical presentation and accumulation of various metabolites. NAA and creatine concentrations have been reported to be normal in all patients. The glutamine and glutamate peak has been reported to be increased in proportion to the clinical disease stage. Myoinositol is decreased with decreased choline concentration. It has been found that early brain changes are reversible, thus early treatment could minimize or completely prevent neurological symptoms.

Suggested Reading

Bajaj SK, Kurlemann G, Schuierer G, Peters PE (1996) CT and MRI in a girl with late-onset ornithine transcarbamylase deficiency: case report Neuroradiology 8:796–799

Takanashi J, Kurihara A, Tomita M, Kanazawa M, Yamamoto S, Morita F, Ikehira H, Tanada S, Kohno Y (2002) Distinctly abnormal brain metabolism in late-onset ornithine transcarbamylase deficiency. Neurology 2:210–214

Takanashi J, Barkovich AJ, Cheng SF, Weisiger K, Zlatunich CO, Mudge C, Rosenthal P, Tuchman M, Packman S (2003) Brain MR imaging in neonatal hyperammonemic encephalopathy resulting from proximal urea cycle disorders. AJNR Am J Neuroradiol 6:1184–1187

Takanashi J, Barkovich AJ, Cheng SF, Kostiner D, Baker JC, Packman S (2003) Brain MR imaging in acute hyperammonemic encephalopathy arising from late-onset ornithine transcarbamylase deficiency. AJNR Am J Neuroradiol 3:390–393

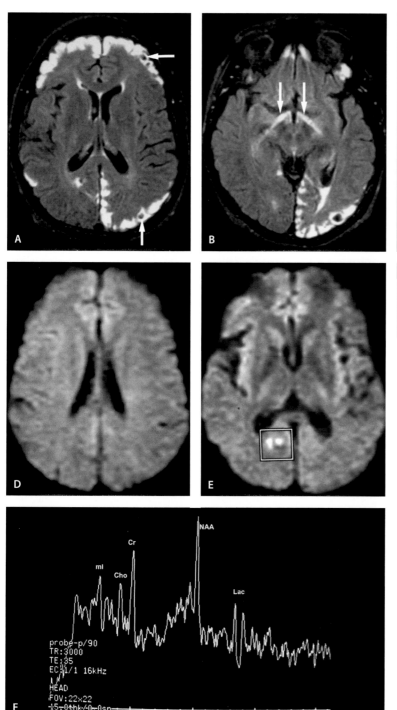

Figure 3.29

Late-onset type of ornithine transcarbamylase deficiency with a recent occipital infarct

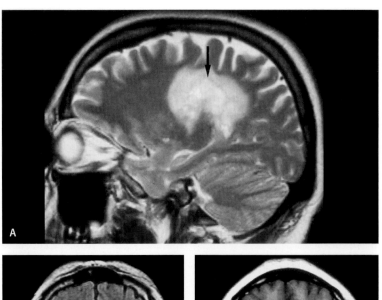

Figure 3.30
Multiple sclerosis

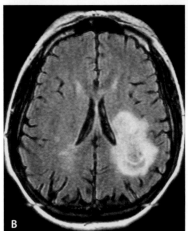

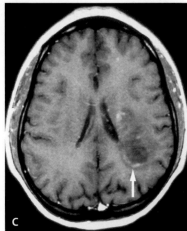

Miscellaneous

Multiple Sclerosis (MS)

Multiple Sclerosis, Possible Schilder's Disease

Clinical Presentation

A 15-year-old female presents with seizures, rapid onset of right-sided weakness and tingling in right extremities.

Images (Fig. 3.30)

A. Sagittal T2-weighted image shows a single round-ed hyperintensity in the occipitoparietal region. There is marked hyperintensity in the central part, surrounded by a lower signal intensity rim (*arrow*) and then a second zone of less-intense hyper-intensity. The subcortical U-fibers are spared

B. FLAIR image demonstrates also the different "lay-ers" of signal intensity in the large left white matter lesion. Vague hyperintensities are also seen in the right occipitoparietal region

C. Contrast-enhanced T1-weighted image demon-strates peripheral enhancement (*arrow*). Note the lack of mass effect for the size of the lesion. An-other tiny enhancing lesion is seen in the frontal lobe

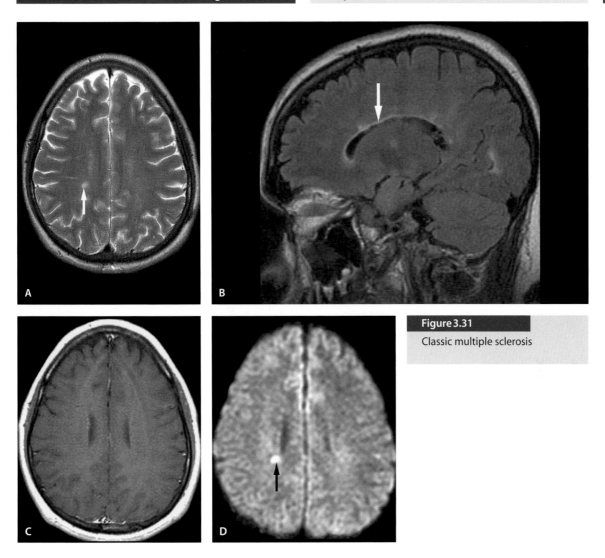

Figure 3.31
Classic multiple sclerosis

Classic Multiple Sclerosis

Clinical Presentation

A young adult with acute onset of optic neuritis. There is a past history of transient extremity numbness.

Images (Fig. 3.31)

A. T2-weighted image shows an oval periventricular hyperintensity (*arrow*)
B. Sagittal FLAIR image demonstrates the typical location of hyperintensity in the callososeptal interface (*arrow*). Multiple ovoid hyperintense lesions are seen in the periventricular white matter. These lesions are typical MS lesions and have a perpendicular orientation toward the ventricular surface ("Dawson's fingers")
C. Contrast-enhanced T1-weighted image fails to demonstrate enhancement. Only acute plaques enhance with contrast
D. The MS plaque seen on A is hyperintense on DW image. This, however, does not have a low ADC value

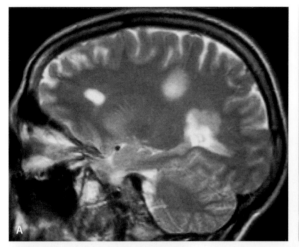

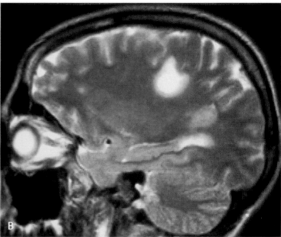

Figure 3.32
Acute multiple sclerosis with ring-enhancing lesion

Acute Multiple Sclerosis with Ring-Enhancing Lesion

Clinical Presentation

A young adult with right extremity weakness and numbness. There is a past history of optic neuritis.

Images (Fig. 3.32)

A. Parasagittal T2-weighted image reveals multiple ovoid areas of T2 hyperintensity in the periventricular and periatrial white matter
B. Hyperintense lesions are also seen in the contralateral side on sagittal T2-weighted image. Note the two signal intensities in the large parietal lesion with a more hyperintense central core
C. Contrast enhanced T1-weighted image demonstrates ring-enhancing lesion. Note the lack of mass effect

Discussion

MS is the most common demyelinating disease of the CNS. It is uncommon in childhood and the peak incidence is at 30 years of age in adults, although 13% of patients present before the age of 20 years. The average onset of MS in children is 11–14 years, but it has been reported as early as at 10 months of age. In adults it is twice as common in females as in males and in children the ratio is even higher. MS has a strong geographical distribution: it is rare in the tropics and increases in frequency at higher latitudes. A number of subtypes can be distinguished: classical MS, neuromyelitis optica (Devic's disease), concentric sclerosis (Baló's disease) and diffuse sclerosis (Schilder's disease).

The diagnosis of MS is usually made on the basis of clinical, laboratory and radiological findings. MS is distinguished from ADEM by a characteristic clinical history of multiple neurological deficits and a chronic, relapsing course, contrary to ADEM that is a monophasic disease. Schilder's myelinoclastic diffuse sclerosis is a rare sporadic demyelinating disease that usually affects children between 5 and 14 years of age. The disease often mimics intracranial neoplasm or abscess. Pathologically MS is a disease of oligodendroglia and results in multifocal areas of demyelination with little or no axonal degeneration.

MR imaging is the most sensitive imaging method. CT imaging provides limited information in MS. Although MR imaging is a sensitive method, it is at the same time nonspecific. Additionally, there is poor correlation between the appearance of a plaque and clinical symptoms. T2 and FLAIR images typically show hyperintensities in the periventricular white matter and/or cervical spine. The disease usually spares the subcortical U-fibers. Because the demyelination is perivenular, the hyperintensity follows the veins and radiates out from the ventricles ("Dawson's fingers"). Schilder's disease shows one or two large demyelinating lesions in parietooccipital region that spare the U-fibers, but are contiguous with the corpus callosum. MS plaques demonstrate increased diffusion and acute plaques have significantly higher ADCs than do chronic plaques. Mean diffusivity and fractional anisotropy histograms have been used to distinguish between plaques in different severity and stage.

MR spectroscopy has been used as a sensitive imaging modality for studying the biochemical behavior of MS plaques in vivo. Relative to normal-appearing brain, the MS plaques show reduction of the NAA peak as an indicator of axonal damage. Additionally Cho and myoinositol have been found to be elevated within MS plaques, suggesting enhanced membrane turnover. Lactate may be seen in the acute phase.

Suggested Reading

Banwell BL (2004) Pediatric multiple sclerosis. Curr Neurol Neurosci Rep 4:245–252

Bitsch A, Bruhn H, Vougioukas V, et al (1999) Inflammatory CNS demyelination: histopathologic correlation with in vivo quantitative proton MR spectroscopy. AJNR Am J Neuroradiol 20:1619–1627

Castriota Scanderbeg A, Tomaiuolo F, Sabatini U, Nocentini U, Grasso M, Caltagirone C (2000) Demyelinating plaques in relapsing-remitting and secondary-progressive multiple sclerosis: assessment with diffusion MR imaging AJNR Am J Neuroradiol 21:862–868

Kurul S, Cakmakci H, Dirik E, Kovanlikaya A (2003) Schilder's disease: case study with serial neuroimaging. J Child Neurol 1:58–61

Schaefer PW, Grant PE, Gonzalez RG (2000) Diffusion-weighted MR imaging of the brain. Radiology 217:331–345

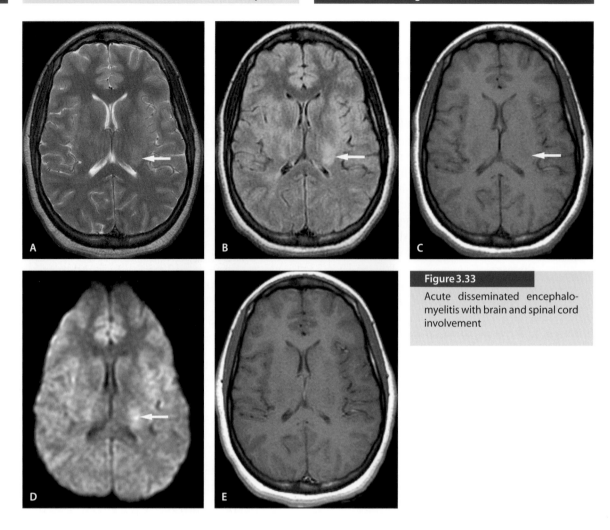

Figure 3.33

Acute disseminated encephalo-myelitis with brain and spinal cord involvement

Acute Disseminated Encephalomyelitis (ADEM)

ADEM with Brain and Spinal Cord Involvement

Clinical Presentation

A 15-year-old female with a 2-day history of extremity weakness and confusion. Patient has also spinal cord involvement (see chapter 10, page 433).

Images (Fig. 3.33)

A. T2-weighted image shows a hyperintense lesion in the left internal capsule (*arrow*)
B. FLAIR image at the same level as A. The left internal capsule lesion is better appreciated (*arrow*)
C. The left internal capsule lesion is hypointense in the T1-weighted image (*arrow*)
D. DW image shows a hyperintense lesion in the left internal capsule which may be due to T2 shine-through effect (*arrow*)
E. Postcontrast T1-weighted image shows no contrast enhancement

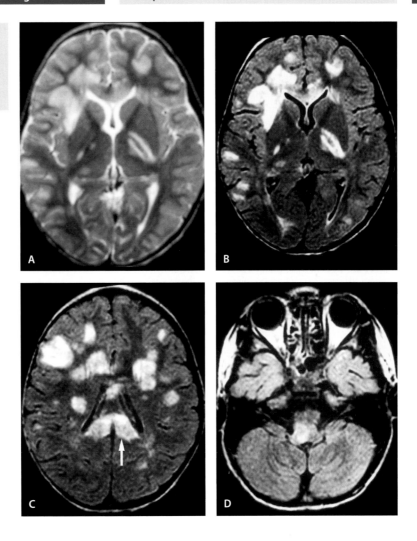

ADEM with Hemispheric White Matter and Basal Ganglia Involvement

Clinical Presentation

A 4-year-old male presents in emergency room with low-grade fever and mental status change. He has a history of viral infection 3 weeks earlier.

Images (Fig. 3.34)

A. T2-weighted image through the basal ganglia demonstrates patchy and asymmetric hyperintensities in the subcortical and periventricular white matter as well as along the internal capsules. The lesions lack mass effect

B. FLAIR image at the same level as A. The hyperintense lesions are better appreciated on FLAIR image

C. FLAIR image through the lateral ventricles demonstrates corpus callosum swelling and hyperintensity (*arrow*). Patchy white matter changes are again seen

D. FLAIR image also shows hyperintense lesion in the right side of the medulla

Discussion

ADEM is the most common post-infectious disorder triggered by an inflammatory response to viral infections or vaccinations. Children are more often affected than adults, but all ages can be affected. The disease process is usually monophasic, contrary to other demyelinating diseases. ADEM is an immunomediated demyelinating condition affecting the central nervous system. It usually has an acute onset 1 to 3 weeks following the viral illness or vaccination. It also may occur in the absence of an identifiable viral infection. On imaging, multifocal lesions of the white matter of the brain, cerebellum and brain stem are seen. Also the spinal cord may be involved (see Chapter 10). Microscopically perivenular lymphocytic and monocytic infiltration and demyelination are seen. MR imaging shows patchy bilateral often-asymmetric areas of T2 hyperintensity in the subcortical and deep white matter of the cerebral hemispheres. Cerebellar and brain stem lesions are also seen. Although it is mainly a white matter disease, deep gray matter nuclei are also seen. Following the contrast injection variable contrast enhancement is seen. The enhancement can be diffuse or nodular; however, peripheral enhancement is often seen.

Although ADEM is a monophasic illness, not all lesions will appear at the same time and also the enhancement pattern can be seen through an extensive period of time. Typically the lesions demonstrate relatively little mass effect compared to the size of the lesion. Resolution of the lesions is often complete. The signal intensity on DW images is variable depending on the severity and phase of the lesions. Decreased NAA has been reported in ADEM.

Suggested Reading

Bernarding J, Braun J, Koennecke HC (2002) Diffusion- and perfusion-weighted MR imaging in a patient with acute demyelinating encephalomyelitis (ADEM). J Magn Reson Imaging 15:96–100

Bizzi A, Ulug AM, Crawford TO, et al (2001) Quantitative proton MR spectroscopic imaging in acute disseminated encephalomyelitis. AJNR Am J Neuroradiol 22:1125–1130

Inglese M, Salvi F, Iannucci G, Mancardi GL, Mascalchi M, Filippi M (2002) Magnetization transfer and diffusion tensor MR imaging of acute disseminated encephalomyelitis. AJNR Am J Neuroradiol 23:267–272

Kesselring J, Miller DH, Robb SA, et al (1990) Acute disseminated encephalomyelitis. MRI findings and the distinction from multiple sclerosis. Brain 113:291–302

Kuker W, Ruff J, Gaertner S, Mehnert F, Mader I, Nagele T (2004) Modern MRI tools for the characterization of acute demyelinating lesions: value of chemical shift and diffusion-weighted imaging. Neuroradiology 46:421–426

Perisylvian Syndrome

Clinical Presentation

A 5-week-old male (ex 34-week premature infant) presents with hypertonicity and stridor.

Images (Fig. 3.35)

A. Sagittal T1-weighted image demonstrates normal midline structures, including corpus callosum
B. T2-weighted image reveals polymicrogyria in the bilateral perisylvian regions (*arrows*). There are multiple small gyri in these regions resulting in an irregular bumpy appearance of the brain surface. The opercula are wide bilaterally
C. T2-weighted image shows cavum septum pellucidum and vergae. The frontal area appears pachygyric with polymicrogyria in the sylvian region
D. T1 FLAIR image shows the irregular cortex, mainly on the left (*arrow*)
E. Coronal FLAIR image shows the wide opercula with irregular cortex, but no parenchymal signal changes
F. DW image shows normal parenchymal signal

Discussion

Wide use of MR imaging has increased our knowledge of cortical development. Recently several syndromes have been described in which patients have fairly specific symptoms associated with radiological findings of polymicrogyria. These include congenital bilateral perisylvian syndrome (CBPS), bilateral posterior parietal polymicrogyria (BPPP) and bilateral frontal polymicrogyria. Bilateral perisylvian syndrome is a homogeneous clinical- radiological entity. It is characterized by bilateral perisylvian polymicrogyria. The clinical spectrum of this syndrome is much wider than previously believed and may vary from minor speech difficulties to severe disablement. Suprabullar paresis, mild tetraparesis, cognitive impairment, and epilepsy are frequently associated. Although evidence in the literature suggests a vascular etiology, a number of familial cases raise the possibility of a genetic cause.

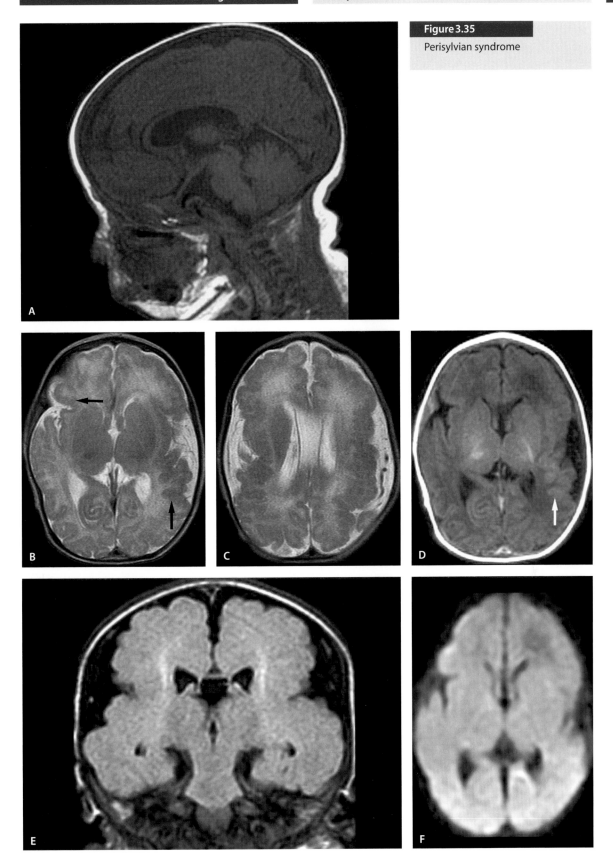

Figure 3.35
Perisylvian syndrome

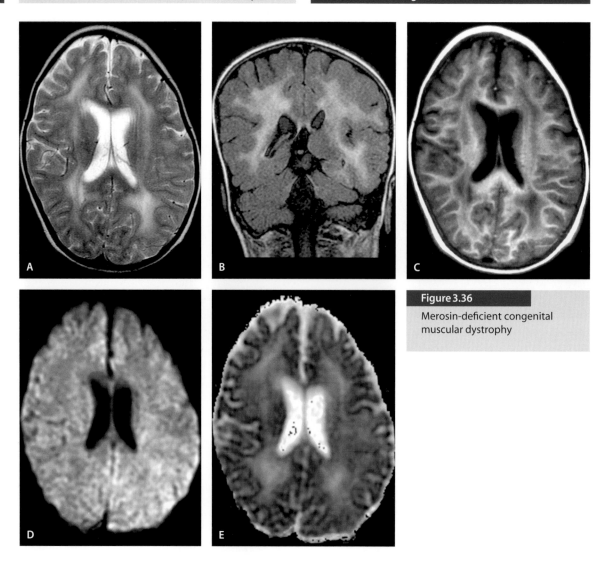

Figure 3.36

Merosin-deficient congenital muscular dystrophy

The diagnosis is best made with MR imaging by analyzing the gyral pattern, cortical thickness and irregularity on the cortical/white matter junction. Functional mapping is useful in analyzing the functional areas in abnormal cortex.

Suggested Reading

Barkovich JA, Hevner R, Guerrini R (1999) Syndromes of bilateral symmetrical polymicrogyria. AJNR Am J Neuroradiol 20:1814–1821

Paetau R, Saraneva J, Salonen O, Valanne L, Ignatius J, Salenius S (2004) Electromagnetic function of polymicrogyric cortex in congenital bilateral perisylvian syndrome. Neurol Neurosurg Psychiatry 5:717–722

Merosin-Deficient Congenital Muscular Dystrophy (CMD)

Clinical Presentation

A 6-year-old female with known merosin-negative CMD presents with new onset of seizures.

Images (Fig. 3.36)

A. T2-weighted image shows bilateral high signal lesions in the white matter. There is frontal predominance. The ventricles are slightly prominent consistent with mild volume loss. The cortex is normal

B. Coronal FLAIR image demonstrates extensive white matter involvement and mild hyperintensity is also seen involving the corpus callosum. The cerebellar white matter is intact

C. T1 FLAIR image reveals the distribution of the white matter changes to be limited to the periventricular and deep white matter sparing the corpus callosum and subcortical U-fibers. The occipital white matter is better preserved

D. DW image is unremarkable

E. ADC map shows high signal lesions in the bilateral white matter. Isointensity on DW image (D) is due to balance between T2 prolongation and increased diffusibility

Discussion

CMDs are a heterogeneous group of congenital myopathies that are hereditary and progressive disorders. CMD with macrocephaly and white matter abnormalities without cortical dysplasia is a well-defined disease. It is characterized by weakness and hypotonia at birth, joint contractures, delayed motor development and features of dystrophy on muscle biopsy. In most children the intelligence is normal. Some children develop generalized seizures. Involvement of the central nervous system occurs in some forms of CMD: Fukuyama type, the muscle and brain eye syndrome (Santavuori type CMD), the merosin-negative type with cerebral white matter abnormalities and cerebromuscular syndromes also called "cobblestone CMD".

Merosin is an isoform of laminin that is expressed in the basement membrane of each muscle fiber and of Schwann cells in the peripheral nervous system. Merosin deficiency has been documented in 40–50% of children with classical CMD. MR imaging demonstrates a diffuse and symmetrical increase in white matter T2 signal of the cerebral hemispheres. The precise nature of the white matter lesions is unknown. Increased T2 prolongation is attributed to increased water content in the white matter owing to an abnormal blood-brain barrier rather than to decreased abnormal myelination.

Suggested Reading

Caro PA, Scavina M, Hoffman E, Pegoraro E, Marks HG (1999) MR findings in children with merosin-deficient congenital muscular dystrophy. AJNR Am J Neuroradiol 20:324–326

Echenne B, Rivier F, Jellali AJ, Azais M, Mornet D, Pons F (1997) Merosin positive congenital muscular dystrophy with mental deficiency, epilepsy and MRI changes in the cerebral white matter. Neuromuscul Disord 7:187–190

Miyagoe-Suzuki Y, Nakagawa M, Takeda S (2000) Merosin and congenital muscular dystrophy. Microsc Res Tech 48:181–191

Tan E, Topaloglu H, Sewry C, et al (1997) Late onset muscular dystrophy with cerebral white matter changes due to partial merosin deficiency. Neuromuscul Disord 7:85–89

Vanishing White Matter (VWM) Disease

Clinical Presentation

An 11-year-old male with decreased mental status; essentially he is comatose. He has a history of progressive white matter degeneration during the previous 4 years and he is status post epilepticus. The MR image of 3 years ago showed abnormality involving the entire white matter of the cerebellar hemispheres as well as a cerebellum and the brainstem. Spectroscopy at that time was normal. That time he had marked ataxia and spasticity with spared vision.

Images (Fig. 3.37)

A. Coronal T2-weighted image shows extensive white matter hyperintensity including the cerebellum

B. The white matter hyperintensity extends to the centrum semiovale and includes subcortical U-fibers

C. Coronal SPGR image shows patchy hypointensities in the white matter

D. There is diffuse low signal with cystic changes in the white matter seen in the coronal FLAIR image (*arrow*)

E. DW image reveals diffuse low signal in the white matter

F. ADC map reveals diffuse increased signal with foci of even higher signal in the white mater, most likely due to cystic changes

G. Proton MR spectroscopy (TE=144 ms) of the centrum semiovale white matter reveals low NAA signifying neuronal damage. There are large inverted lactate peaks

H. Localizer demonstrating the MR spectroscopy voxel placement

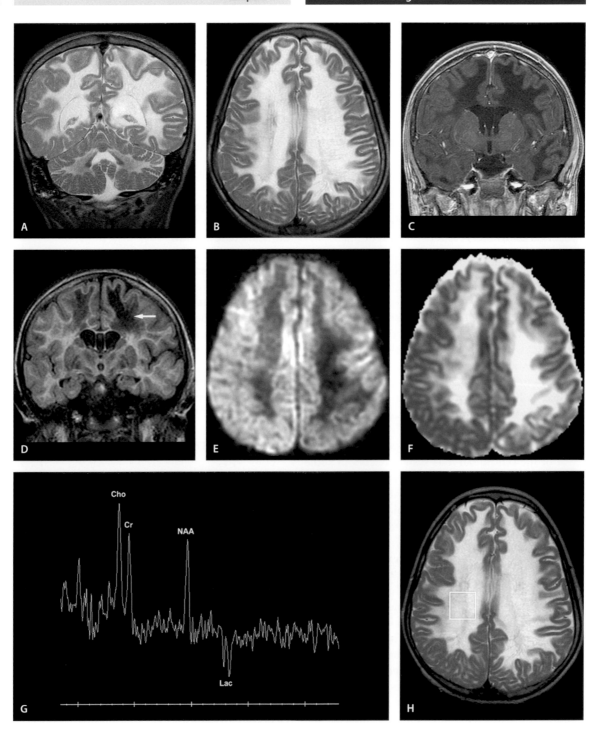

Figure 3.37

Vanishing white matter disease

Discussion

Leukoencephalopathy with VWM is a newly recognized white matter disease. It is an autosomal recessive disorder with normal early development and, usually, childhood-onset neurological deterioration. The clinical symptoms include a slowly progressive cerebellar ataxia, spasticity, variable optic atrophy, and relatively preserved mental capacity. In addition, there are episodes of rapid and major deterioration following infections with fever and minor head trauma. These episodes can end in unexplained coma. Until 1999 the diagnosis of VWM disease was based on clinical examination and the results of repeat MR imaging and MR spectroscopy.

MR imaging shows diffuse cerebral hemispheric leukoencephalopathy with evidence of white matter rarefaction. MR imaging findings suggest that over time, there is a progressive vanishing of the abnormal white matter, which is replaced by cerebrospinal fluid. MR spectroscopy of the abnormal white matter may reveal a profound decrease of all normal signals with the presence of extra signals from lactate and glucose. MR spectroscopy of the white matter in a patient whose disease is at an early stage is much less abnormal.

Suggested Reading

Gallo A, Rocca MA, Falini A, et al (2004) Multiparametric MRI in a patient with adult-onset leukoencephalopathy with vanishing white matter. Neurology 27:323–326

Leegwater PA, Konst AA, Kuyt B, et al (1999) The gene for leukoencephalopathy with vanishing white matter is located on chromosome 3q27. Am J Hum Genet 3:728–734

Leegwater PA, Pronk JC, van der Knaap MS (2003) Leukoencephalopathy with vanishing white matter: from magnetic resonance imaging pattern to five genes. J Child Neurol 18:639–645

Van der Knapp, Kamphorst W, Barth PG, Kraaijeveld CL, Gut E, Valk J (1998) Phenotypic variation in leukoencephalopathy with white matter. Neurology 51:540–547

Megalencephalic Leukoencephalopathy with Subcortical Cysts (MLC) and Normal Development

Clinical Presentation

A 22-month-old infant boy with macrocephaly and normal development. MR imaging at the age of 10 months revealed white matter hyperintensities on T2-weighted images.

Images (Fig. 3.38)

A. T2-weighted image reveals continuous white matter abnormality with abnormal hyperintensity throughout the supratentorial white matter sparing the brainstem and cerebellum. A cystic lesion is seen in the left temporal tip (*arrow*) that was not present in the previous study. This follows CSF signal in all pulse sequences. Basal ganglia signal is normal

B. T2-weighted image slightly higher than A demonstrates widespread white matter abnormality, thin but normal appearing cortical ribbon. A cavum septum pellucidum (*arrow*) is present

C. Coronal contrast-enhanced SPGR image shows bitemporal cystic appearing lesions with CSF signal (*arrows*) not present in the previous scan at the age of 10 months. Cavum septum pellucidum (*arrowhead*) is well seen in the coronal image

D. Gadolinium-enhanced T1-weighted image with magnetization transfer shows anterior temporal tip CSF signal lesions without enhancement

E. DW image confirms the CSF-like signal in the cystic lesions

F. The cystic lesions follow the CSF signal in the ADC map. The white matter demonstrates also hyperintense signal

G. Multivoxel MR spectroscopy (TE=144 ms) over the cortical gray and white matter demonstrates lower NAA peak in the white matter than in the gray matter. No abnormal metabolites are seen

H. Axial image demonstrating the voxel location for the MR spectroscopy seen in G

Figure 3.38 ▼

Megalencephalic leukoencephalopathy with subcortical cysts and normal development

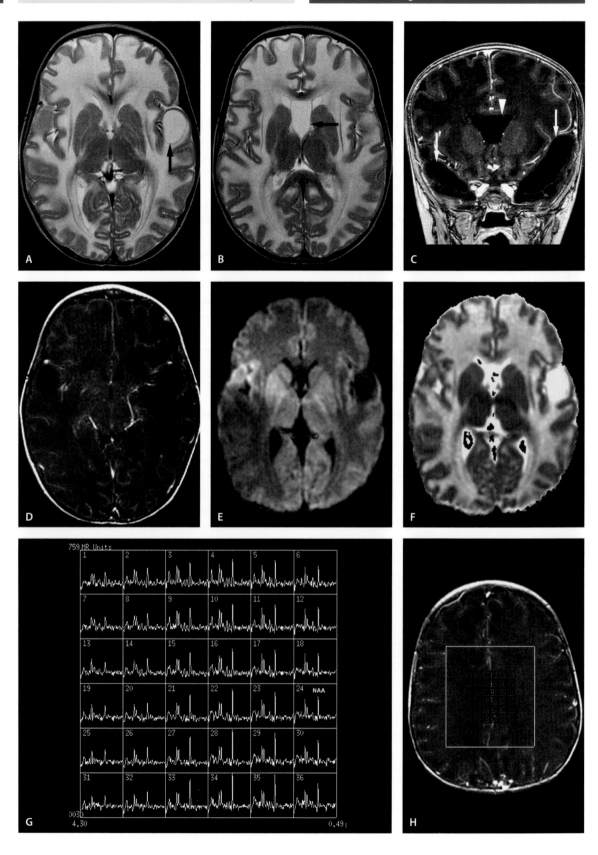

Discussion

MLC is a recently described white matter condition. It demonstrates diffuse hemispheric swelling and typical cysts in the frontoparietal subcortical white matter and the tips of the temporal lobes. It has a very mild disease course. In this condition screening for inborn errors, especially those that cause either megalencephaly or white matter disease have been negative. MR spectra are described to be relatively mildly abnormal. Neurological findings are initially normal or near normal, despite megalencephaly and MR imaging evidence of severe white matter affection. In affected children slowly progressive ataxia and spasticity develop, while intellectual functioning is preserved for years after onset of the disorder. MR imaging characteristics include diffuse abnormality in signal intensity and swelling of the cerebral hemispheral white matter with cyst-like spaces in the frontoparietal and anterior-temporal subcortical areas.

Brain biopsy in one of the patients has been performed. It revealed spongiform leukoencephalopathy without cortical involvement. Most vacuoles were covered by single five-layered membranes. The vacuoles involved the outermost lamellae of myelin sheaths only, whereas the remainder of the myelin sheaths remained undisturbed. The histopathological findings place the disease among the vacuolating myelinopathies, although it is distinct from the well-known forms. MCL has been localized on two different chromosomes demonstrating genetic heterogeneity. Temporal lobe cyst with white matter changes have been described also in another entity: Two patients with leukoencephalopathy and temporal cysts were described, but these patients present with microcephaly. Both patients had a nonprogressive neurological disorder with mental retardation, microcephaly and sensorineural deafness.

Suggested Reading

Gomes AL, Vieira JP, Saldanha J (2001) Non-progressive leukoencephalopathy with bilateral temporal cysts. Eur J Paediatr Neurol 3:121–125

Van der Knaap MS, Barth PG, Stroink H, van Nieuwenhuizen O, Arts WF, Hoogenraad F, Valk J (1995) Leukoencephalopathy with swelling and a discrepantly mild clinical course in eight children. Ann Neurol 3:324–334

Van der Knaap MS, Valk J, Barth PG, Smit LM, van Engelen BG, Tortori Donati P (1995) Leukoencephalopathy with swelling in children and adolescents: MRI patterns and differential diagnosis. Neuroradiology 8:679–686

Van der Knaap MS, Barth PG, Vrensen GF, Valk J (1996) Histopathology of an infantile-onset spongiform leukoencephalopathy with a discrepantly mild clinical course. Acta Neuropathol (Berl) 2:206–212

Delayed Myelination

Clinical Presentation

A 13-month-old male with large head and developmental delay, but progressing all the time.

Images (Fig. 3.39)

A. T2-weighted image at the age of 13 months shows abnormal hyperintensity involving nearly all white matter tracts, but especially in the frontal areas. Normal appearing myelination is seen on the posterior limbs of the internal capsules (*arrows*). Patient had only mild developmental delay compared to significant myelination delay

B. T2-weighted image at the age of 2 years. There is significant progression of myelination. Developmentally patient had also progressed

Discussion

The human brain is not fully developed at birth. Instead, the brains of children undergo an extended period of postnatal maturation. The process of myelination is a predetermined and follows a predictable pattern that starts during the second trimester of gestation. Histologic studies reveal that white matter myelination continues through adolescence into adult life. During the past 15 years, MR imaging has been used to monitor the myelination process in the developing brain. The assessment of whether brain development is at an appropriate level for age has become an integral part of MR imaging reporting in pediatric practice, not only in premature babies, but also in full-term babies and toddlers with developmental delay.

The first descriptions with myelination seen with MR imaging emphasized T1 and T2 shortening monitoring the progression of myelination in the white matter tracts. Genetic abnormalities, perinatal anoxia, inborn errors of metabolism and congenital anomalies are frequently associated with delayed or diminished myelination. No underlying cause is ap-

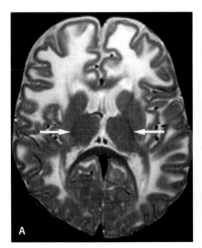 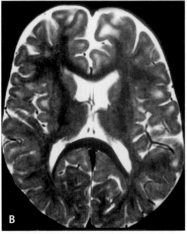

Figure 3.39
Delayed myelination

parent in some children who have delayed myelination. Delayed myelination is rarely the only abnormality in the developing brain; other lesions include low volume of cerebral white matter, thin corpus callosum and cortical atrophy. When delayed myelination is suspected, MR imaging should be performed before the age of 24 months. Eventually the white matter will myelinate and the delayed myelination may not be detected if not imaged early enough. Although myelination can be accurately assessed using the routine T1 and T2 MR imaging sequences, other techniques may prove more accurate. As the white matter myelinates it changes from hypointense to hyperintense to gray matter on T1-weighted images and from hyperintense to hypointense to gray matter on T2-weighted images.

Tables of specific milestones have been generated to help estimate the progression of myelination. As a general rule myelination proceeds from below to cephalad, from posterior to anterior and from central to peripheral. From the early MR imaging studies it is known that there is regional variability in differences in neuronal maturity and myelination, and imaging shows this variability in differences in regional blood flow, glucose uptake, water diffusion and concentration of NAA, choline and creatine. It is important to take these regional differences into consideration when interpreting the imaging studies of young children in order to avoid wrong judgment of maturity. For example, it is well known that normal neonatal ventrolateral thalamus and prerolandic cortex have slightly reduced water diffusion compared with the rest of the brain. MR spectroscopy differences do exist in the developing brain as well. Normal neonatal

frontal white matter has reduced NAA compared with that of the thalamus and may even have some detectable lactate.

Although in general practice it is customary to estimate the degree of myelination by using conventional imaging sequences such as T1, T2 and FLAIR sequences, diffusion and diffusion tensor imaging may provide more sensitive markers of normal brain maturation and deviations of it. Changes in magnitude and anisotropy of water diffusion in myelinated fibers may provide a clinically useful developmental milestone marker for brain maturity. Normal neonatal brain shows much higher ADC values than the adult brain. There is a decrease in ADC during childhood and this may be a combination of several factors: reduction of overall water content of the brain with decrease in extracellular water, cellular maturation, white matter myelination, and proliferation of maturing neurons and glial cells. Also there is physical restriction of water motion by the multiple layers of the myelin membrane. Thus, the motion of water molecules becomes increasingly anisotropic. The difference in maturation between infant and adult brain is visible with ADC, with each age group demonstrating values that would be pathological in another group. Recognizing the baseline difference is important when interpreting DW images particularly in the case of global ischemia, when normal brain may not be available for comparison.

Suggested Reading

Barkovich AJ (2000) Concepts of myelin and myelination in neuroradiology. AJNR Am J Neuroradiol 21:1099–1109

Barkovich AJ, Kjos BO (1988) Normal postnatal development of the corpus callosum as demonstrated by MR imaging. AJNR Am J Neuroradiol 9:487–491

Childs AM, Ramenghi LA, Evans DJ, et al (1998) MR features of developing periventricular white matter in preterm infants: evidence of glial cell migration. AJNR Am J Neuroradiol 19:971–976

Holland BA, Haas DK, Norman D, Brant-Zawadzki M, Newton TH (1986) MRI of normal brain maturation. AJNR Am J Neuroradiol 7:201–208

McGraw P, Liang L, Provenzale JM (2002) Evaluation of normal age-related changes in anisotropy during infancy and childhood as shown by diffusion tensor imaging. AJR Am J Roentgenol 179:1515–1522

Mukherjee P, Miller JH, Shimony JS, et al (2001) Normal brain maturation during childhood: developmental trends characterized with diffusion-tensor MR imaging. Radiology 221:349–358

Sie LT, van der Knaap MS, van Wezel-Meijler G, Valk J (1997) MRI assessment of myelination of motor and sensory pathways in the brain of preterm and term-born infants. Neuropediatrics 28:97–105

Autoimmune Polyglandular Syndrome (APS)

Clinical Presentation

A 19-year-old female presents with acute mental status change. She is known to have APS type I.

Images (Fig. 3.40)

A. Noncontrast CT image reveals bilateral symmetric lentiform nucleus and thalamic calcifications. Additionally scattered gray/white matter junction calcifications are seen (*arrows*)

B. Basal ganglia calcification seen on CT image is difficult to appreciate on T2-weighted image since normal globus pallidus iron presents as low signal intensity

C. FLAIR image reveals mild hyperintensity on the putamen and hypointensity on the globus pallidus (*arrows*), consistent with calcification seen on CT image

D. T1-weighted image shows bilateral hyperintense symmetric lentiform nucleus calcifications (*arrows*). Vague calcifications are also seen in the thalami (*arrowhead*), but not in the gray/white matter junction. These parenchymal calcifications are considered to be a manifestation of hypoparathyroidism with metabolic calcinosis

E. The heaviest calcification on the CT image is seen as dark signal (*arrows*) on DW image

F. Contrast-enhanced T1-weighted image shows no abnormal enhancement

Discussion

APS is caused by an autoimmune process in multiple endocrine glands. Affected individuals develop problems with numerous glands including the thyroid and parathyroid glands, adrenal glands, gonads, and pancreas. This usually results in endocrine gland hypofunction, except for the thyroid gland, in which both hyper- and hypofunction may occur. The syndrome can be classified into two types, type I and type II. Type I PGA syndrome is characterized by hypoparathyroidism, primary adrenal insufficiency and primary ovarian failure. Type II PGA is associated with primary adrenal insufficiency, Hashimoto's thyroiditis and primary ovarian failure.

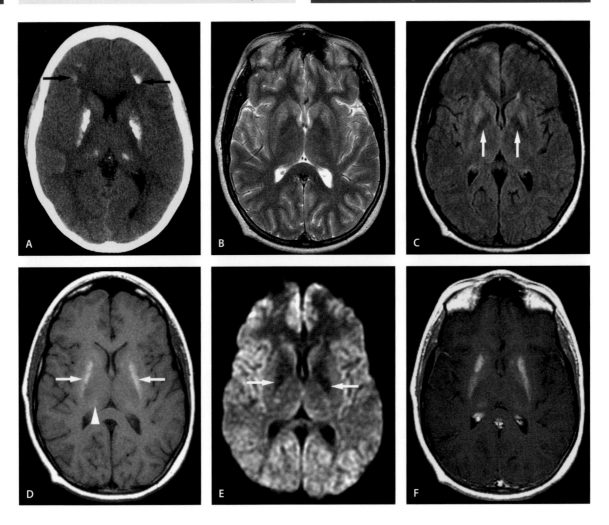

Figure 3.40

Autoimmune polyglandular syndrome

Long-standing type I PGA with endocrine manifestations of hypoparathyroidism leads to extensive calcification of the basal ganglia which may result in extrapyramidal symptoms. The common differential diagnosis of dense basal ganglia calcification includes idiopathic variety, metabolic causes, polyglandular autoimmune syndrome, and Fahr's syndrome. Calcification may be seen in tuberculosis, acquired immunodeficiency syndromes, congenital toxoplasmosis, rubella and cytomegalovirus virus infections, but they are usually more scattered hemispheric calcifications rather than basal ganglia and dentate nucleus calcifications seen in APS type I.

Suggested Reading

Baumert T, Kleber G, Schwarz J, Stabler A, Lamerz R, Mann K (1993) Reversible hyperkinesia in a patient with autoimmune polyglandular syndrome type I. Clin Invest 71: 924–927

Cinaz P, Bideci A, Hazendaroglu A, Ezgu FS, Agaoglu O, Kursaklioglu S (1997) Autoimmune polyglandular syndrome type I. A case report. Turk J Pediatr 39:271–275

Figure 3.41

Osmotic myelinolysis
(extrapontine myelinolysis)

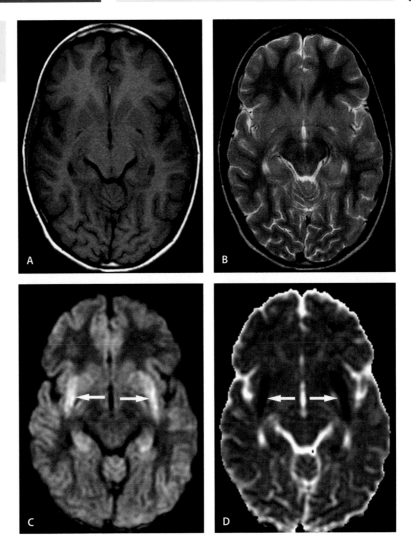

Osmotic Myelinolysis
(Extrapontine Myelinolysis)

Clinical Presentation

A 10-year-old male with hypernatremia that was corrected rapidly presented with ataxia and confusion.

Images (Fig. 3.41)

A and B.   T1- (A) and T2-weighted (B) images show no significant abnormality

C.   DW image shows hyperintense lesions in the bilateral external capsules (*arrows*)

D.   ADC map shows hypointensity in the lesions representing restricted diffusion (*arrows*)

Discussion

Osmotic myelinolysis is a disorder of unknown etiology often related to rapid correction of hyponatremia and liver disease. The most common lesion is in the central pons, but other locations such as thalamus, basal ganglia, external capsules, and cerebellar vermis, have been also reported. Central pontine myelinolysis and extrapontine myelinolysis usually occur together.

Typically, CT scan shows hypodensity in the lesion. MR is superior to CT imaging in detection of the lesions: it shows hypointensity on T1-weighted and hyperintensity on T2-weighted and FLAIR images. On DW imaging, the acute lesions tend to show hyperintensity with decreased ADC representing decreased diffusibility.

Suggested Reading

Brown WD, Caruso JM (1999) Extrapontine myelinolysis with involvement of the hippocampus in three children with severe hypernatremia. J Child Neurol 14:428–433

Cramer SC, Stegbauer KC, Schneider A, Mukai J, Maravilla KR (2001) Decreased diffusion in central pontine myelinolysis. AJNR Am J Neuroradiol 22:1476–1479

Sztencel J, Baleriaux D, Borenstein S, Brunko E, Zegers de Beyl D (1983) Central pontine myelinolysis: correlation between CT and electrophysiologic data. AJNR Am J Neuroradiol 4:529–530

Infection

Introduction

Central nervous system (CNS) infections in pediatric patients continue to be a significant cause of morbidity and mortality. The patient presentation and imaging findings vary depending on the age of the patient and the state of their immune system, the infective agent and the source of infection. Congenital (in utero) infections as well as infections in a very young neonate may have devastating effects on the rapidly developing brain, leading to imaging changes that are distinctly different from inflammatory disease in adults. Infection in the first trimester may result in severe congenital malformations, while later infection in utero may result in destructive changes. As the brain matures, the alterations and the response to the infectious agent become more predictable and similar in appearance to those seen in older children and adults. Understanding the pathology behind infection often allows us to understand the imaging findings and predict some of the inflammatory changes. Certain organisms can cause characteristic inflammatory reactions; however, most lesions are nonspecific and imaging findings cannot be the bases for a specific diagnosis. Thus most diagnoses are based on the clinical presentation and documentation of a microbial pathogen in a child. The role of imaging is often limited to the detection of complications related to the primary inflammatory process.

Head Ultrasound Head ultrasound is often the primary imaging modality in evaluation of a newborn suspected of having an intracranial process. Ventricle size assessment, paraventricular and parenchymal calcifications, areas of infarction, cerebritis and abscess are often easily visualized on real-time ultrasound. These findings, however, are usually nonspecific.

CT Scanning CT scanning is the imaging modality of choice for detection of intracranial calcifications often found in congenital infections. Parenchymal abnormalities during the neonatal time are often better appreciated on CT images than on MR images where white matter is still nonmyelinated and thus appears as a high signal intensity on T2-weighted images.

Congenital infections are transmitted to the fetus through the transplacental route or during birth. Neonatal infections are acquired during the first four weeks of life. During that time, the CNS and immune system are not fully developed and this alters the presenting symptoms and imaging findings. The acronym *TORCH* is often applied to these congenital infections; it stands for "toxoplasmosis", "other" (syphilis, HIV), "rubella", "cytomegalovirus" (CMV), "herpes simplex virus (HSV) type 2". Early insults, during the first or second trimester, result in CNS malformations such as microcephaly, lissencephaly or polymicrogyria. Later during the pregnancy, infections may result in aqueductal stenosis and hydrocephalus, delayed myelination, hydranencephaly, multicystic encephalomalacia, calcifications, hemorrhage and atrophy.

Clinical manifestations of congenital infections not only include CNS malformations but also spontaneous abortion, fetal death, intrauterine growth retardation, developmental delay, hypotonia, other congenital anomalies including microcephaly and ocular abnormalities. The calcifications often present in TORCH infections are better seen in CT images. Progression of myelination is better seen with MR images. Congenital CNS infections can also manifest later in life with developmental delay, seizures, mental retardation, motor symptoms, and microcephaly.

Clinical presentation of CNS infection depends on the compartment involved with the infection. Each compartment can be infected including the calvarium (osteomyelitis), meninges (subdural empyema, epidural abscess), CSF and ependyma (meningitis, ventriculitis), brain parenchyma (encephalitis, parenchymal abscess, ependymitis) and vasculature (vasculitis, mycotic aneurysm, septic thrombophlebitis). The same layers that can be infected also protect the human CNS. The protective mechanism includes the mechanical barriers such as the skin, muscle, bone and fibrous tissue. The blood-brain barrier and blood-CSF barriers limit the penetration of many microorganisms into the CNS. The same protective barriers also may prevent passage of antibiotics, immunoglobulins and other therapeutic molecules entering into the intracranial compartment delaying the healing process.

Knowing the entry route to the CNS, one can predict the causative agent and improve that therapeutic approach. Infectious agents most often gain access to the CNS via the hematogenous route. Direct extension from the adjacent paranasal sinuses or middle ear cavity is a commonly seen entry route. Some more rare entry routes are related to rabies where the pathogen may travel along peripheral nerves from the site of infection to the CNS. In infection with HSV, the entry occurs through the olfactory bulbs.

MR imaging MR imaging is more sensitive than CT scanning in the diagnostic work-up of acute inflammatory disease, especially in older children with mature myelin. However, CT scanning demonstrates more reliably chronic calcifications often seen as a sequela of certain brain infections. Differentiating brain abscesses from cystic or necrotic tumors by CT scanning and MR imaging can be difficult.

MR spectroscopy MR spectroscopy is easy to perform at the same time as the MR imaging study. It is helpful in separating a ring-enhancing abscess from other ring lesions. The pyogenic abscess typically demonstrates resonances from end-products of bacterial breakdown, such as cytosolic amino acids (0.9 ppm,) lactate (1.3 ppm), alanine (1.5 ppm) and acetate (1.92 ppm). Additionally, resonance peaks from valine, leucine and succinate have been reported in abscesses, separating them from necrotic tumors that only demonstrate lipid peaks. Cysticercosis abscess shows also lactate, acetate, succinate and unidentified amino acid peaks. MR spectroscopy can be used to evaluate changes after treatment as the abscess following treatment shows only a lactate peak.

DW imaging DW imaging is a way to evaluate the diffusion properties of water molecules in tissue and has been used in the diagnosis of ischemia, tumors, epilepsy and white matter disorders, including HIV infection (see also Introduction to chapter 6). DW imaging has proved to be a valuable tool in the differential diagnosis of abscess and cystic/necrotic tumors. Abscesses show often characteristic restricted diffusion. However, it is not a specific finding, as low apparent diffusion coefficient (ADC) values can also be seen in metastases. Clinical correlation is usually able to solve this difference. DW imaging takes less time and is more accurate than MR spectroscopy for abscess diagnosis.

Suggested Reading

Barkovich AJ, Girard N (2003) Fetal brain infections. Childs Nerv Syst 7/8:501–507

Burtscher IB, Holtås S (1999) In vivo proton MR spectroscopy of untreated and treated brain abscesses. AJNR Am J Neuroradiol 20:1049–1053

Kauffman WM, Sivit CJ, Fitz CR, Rakusan TA, Herzog K, Chandra RS (1992) CT and MR evaluation of intracranial involvement in pediatric HIV infection: a clinical–imaging correlation. AJNR Am J Neuroradiol 13:949–957

Khong PL, Lam BC, Tung HK, Wong V, Chan FL, Ooi GC (2003) MRI of neonatal encephalopathy. Clin Radiol 11833–11844

Lai PH, Ho JT, Chen WL, et al (2002) Brain abscess and necrotic brain tumor: discrimination with proton MR spectroscopy and diffusion-weighted imaging. AJNR Am J Neuroradiol 23:1369–1377

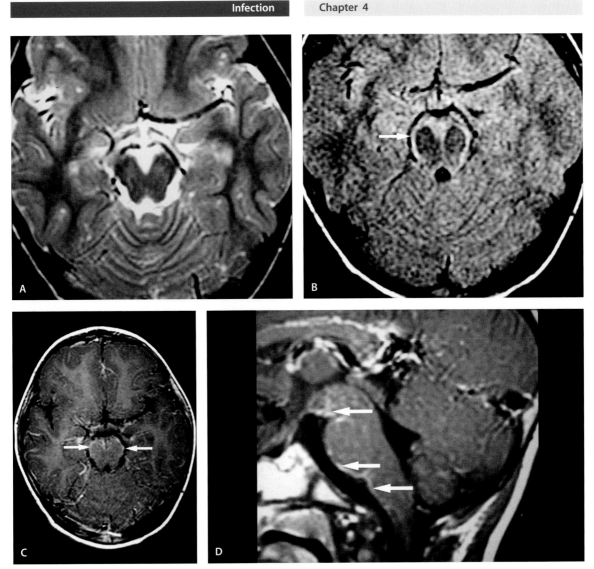

Figure 4.1

Acute pyogenic meningitis

Meningitis and Complications of Meningitis

Acute Pyogenic Meningitis

Clinical Presentation

A 3-year-old male with fever, headache, nausea and vomiting.

Images (Fig. 4.1)

A. T2-weighted image is normal
B. FLAIR image reveals abnormal CSF hyperintensity in the basal cisterns (*arrow*)
C. Contrast-enhanced T1-weighted image demonstrates abnormal leptomeningeal enhancement in the basal cisterns (*arrows*)
D. Sagittal contrast-enhanced T1-weighted image confirms the leptomeningeal enhancement in the ventral surface of the midbrain, pons, and medulla (*arrows*)

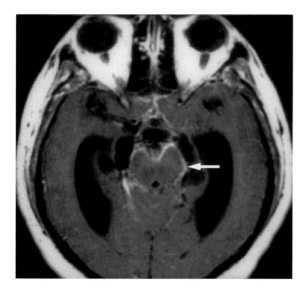

Figure 4.2

Subacute pyogenic meningitis with hydrocephalus

Subacute Pyogenic Meningitis with Hydrocephalus

Clinical Presentation

An 8-year-old male with a 10-day history of fever and headaches.

Images (Fig. 4.2)

A. Contrast-enhanced T1-weighted image shows meningeal enhancement around the basal cisterns (*arrow*). Hydrocephalus is present with significantly dilated temporal horns

Suppurative Meningitis with Subdural Effusions and Cortical Ischemia

Clinical Presentation

A 2-week-old male with group B streptococcal meningitis.

Images (Fig. 4.3)

A. Noncontrast CT scan demonstrates bilateral frontal extra-axial fluid collections. The collections have two different densities, the posterior one showing a slightly higher density than CSF
B. T2-weighted image reveals bifrontal subdural effusions. The frontal cortex is hyperintense bilaterally (*arrowheads*). Additionally there is abnormal hyperintensity in the splenium of the corpus callosum (*arrow*)
C. T1-weighted image demonstrates the subdural effusion to be isointense to CSF
D. Significant leptomeningeal enhancement is seen in the contrast-enhanced T1-weighted magnetization transfer image
E. DW image shows the cortical hyperintensities and corpus callosum lesion to be hyperintense
F. ADC map shows these lesions to be low signal consistent with acute infarcts of the subpial cortex and corpus callosum. In the follow-up MR image 4 years later (not shown) the frontal areas demonstrated volume loss and the patient was severely developmentally delayed

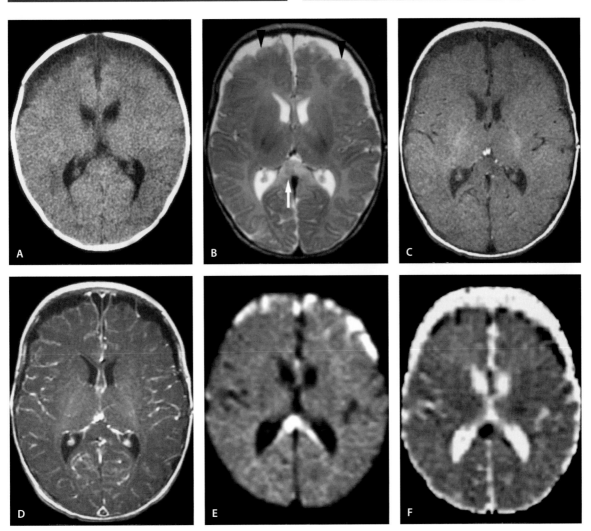

Figure 4.3

Suppurative meningitis with subdural effusions and cortical ischemia

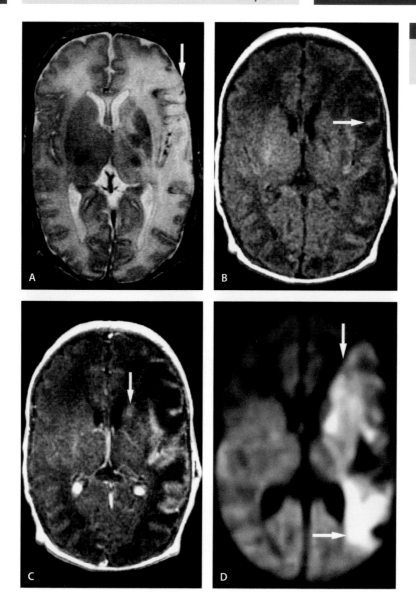

Figure 4.4

Suppurative meningitis and brain infarct

Suppurative Meningitis and Brain Infarct

Clinical Presentation

A 2-month-old male with *Staphylococcus aureus* meningitis presents with hemiparesis.

Images (Fig. 4.4)

A. T2-weighted image shows a swollen cortex with loss of cortical ribbon on left (*arrow*) with increased signal in the underlying white matter

B. T1-weighted image confirms the cortical swelling and shows serpiginous increased signal intensity in the cortex consistent with cortical laminar necrosis (*arrow*)

C. Contrast-enhanced T1-weighted image reveals extensive lepto- and pachymeningeal enhancement with some cortical enhancement. The left caudate head exhibits also enhancement (*arrow*)

D. DW image shows hyperintensity in the left hemisphere in the MCA territory (*arrows*). This is consistent with cytotoxic edema seen in infarcts

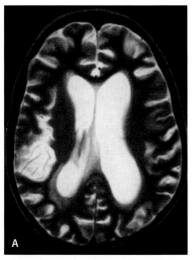
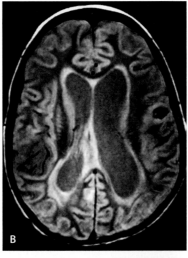

Figure 4.5
Meningitis with multiple infarcts

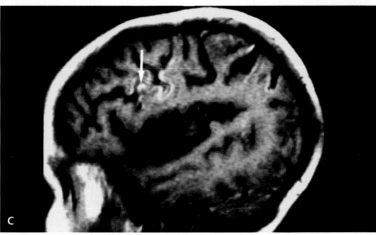
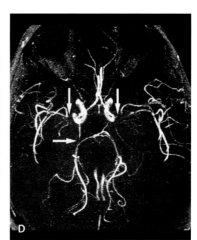

Meningitis with Multiple Infarcts

Clinical Presentation

An 8-year-old girl with acute lymphatic leukemia presents with alpha-hemolytic streptococcal meningitis and gram-negative bacteremia. She is unable to use her left arm.

Images (Fig. 4.5)

A. T2-weighted image shows hyperintensity in the right MCA territory
B. Proton density image demonstrates a signal abnormality in the same location as A. It is isointense to white matter with some linear vascular flow voids through the area
C. Sagittal T1-weighted image reveals the hypointense lesion in the same area. Cortical hyperintensity representing cortical necrosis is also seen (*arrow*)
D. Collapsed image of MR arteriogram (3D TOF) shows limited flow-related enhancement in the vessels at the circle of Willis (*arrows*). This is compatible with vasospasm in the vessels

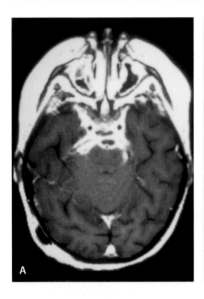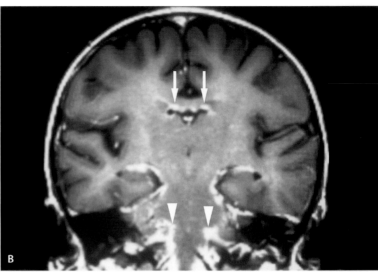

Figure 4.6

Candida meningitis

Candida Meningitis

Clinical Presentation

A 3-year-old girl with acute lymphatic leukemia and *Candida* meningitis.

Images (Fig. 4.6)

A. Axial contrast-enhanced T1-weighted image shows thick nodular enhancement around the basal cisterns and surface of the pons
B. Coronal contrast-enhanced T1-weighted image shows nodular enhancement around the basal cisterns, on the roof of the lateral ventricles (*arrows*) and on the surface of the pons, medulla and spinal cord (*arrowheads*)

Discussion

Acute pyogenic meningitis begins in several ways such as hematogenous spread, local spread from contiguous extracerebral infection from otitis media, mastoiditis, or sinusitis. The types of organisms involved in pyogenic meningitis depend upon the age of the patient. In neonates, group B streptococcus and *Escherichia coli* are the most common organisms. *Haemophilus influenzae* and *Neisseria meningitidis* are common organisms in children.

MR imaging is superior to CT in the evaluation of meningitis. Contrast MR as well as FLAIR sequences are sensitive in the detection of meningitis. Non-contrast T1-weighted images may show obliterated cisterns. Post-gadolinium scans show strong enhancement of the cisterns. Complications can be seen in 50 % of cases. Complications are seen in the form of hydrocephalus, ventriculitis, subdural effusions/empyema, and parenchymal lesions such as cerebritis, abscess, edema and cerebral infarction. The role of imaging is to identify potential complications.

Suggested Reading

Fukui MB, Williams RL, Mudigonda S (2001) CT and MR imaging features of pyogenic ventriculitis. AJNR Am J Neuroradiol 22:1510–1516

Kanamalla US, Ibarra RA, Jinkins JR (2000) Imaging of cranial meningitis and ventriculitis. Neuroimaging Clin North Am 10:309–331

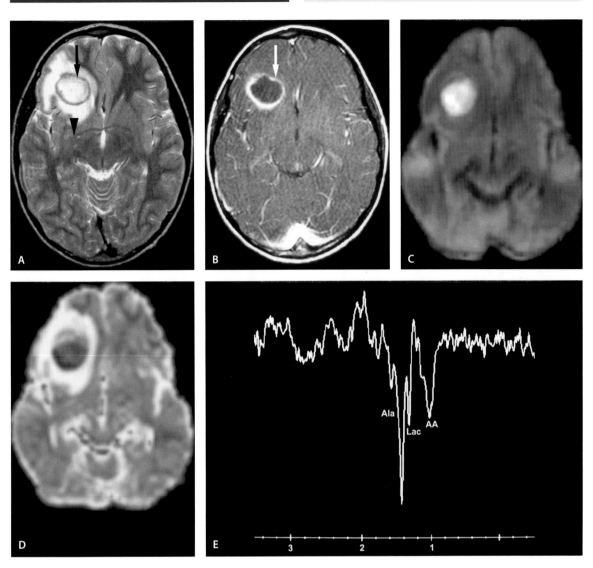

Figure 4.7

Brain abscess

Brain Abscess

Clinical Presentation

A 7-year-old male with chronic streptococcal infection presents with severe headaches.

Images (Fig. 4.7)

A. T2-weighted image shows a well-circumscribed ring lesion centered in the right frontal white matter (*arrow*). The lesion is surrounded by extensive edema. The center of the lesion is isointense to CSF while the periphery shows an inner rim that is slightly hyperintense to gray matter. Note the mass effect upon the anterior commissure (*arrowhead*)

B. Contrast-enhanced T1-weighted magnetization transfer image shows a ring-enhancing lesion. Note that the medial wall is thinner (*arrow*) than the lateral wall

C. DW image shows hyperintense signal in the center of the abscess

D. The central part shows decreased signal on the ADC map

E. Single voxel MR spectroscopy (TE 144ms) centered over the central part of the lesion shows resonance peaks representing alanine, lactate and amino acids. At a TE 144 the phase reversal resonances are well seen at 1.5, 1.3 and 0.9 ppm, which confirm the assignment to alanine, lactate and amino acids, respectively

Discussion

Brain abscess is defined as a focal suppurative process within the brain parenchyma. Brain abscess can originate from contiguous site infections (e.g., chronic otitis media, mastoiditis, sinusitis, meningitis), from distant pathologic states (e.g., cyanotic congenital heart disease, chronic lung infections), after head trauma or neurological procedures, or from a cryptogenic source. Rarely, brain abscess may be seen as a complication of shunt infection.

CT and MR imaging are the essential imaging tools for detection of brain abscess. The imaging findings vary depending upon the stage of the disease. In the cerebritis stage both CT and MR imaging show ill-defined edema and patchy or peripheral enhancement. Cerebral abscesses are characterized by three distinct zones of signal abnormality. The abscess cavity often demonstrate long TI and T2 values whereas the capsule often displays shortening of both T1 and T2 values. Peripherally, a zone of edema is usually present surrounding the lesion. Typically the abscess is surrounded by extensive edema. The abscess wall usually shows a ring enhancement following contrast enhancement. The abscess wall is usually thinner medially. Capsule formation may be altered in immunocompromised patients and neonates and young infants who all demonstrate poor capsule formation and the enhancement may be absent or minimal. Steroids also modify the amount of edema and capsule formation.

A ring-enhancing abscess lesion needs to be differentiated from necrotic/cystic tumors, metastases, resolving hematoma, and granuloma. DW imaging is helpful in differentiating between abscesses and necrotic/cystic brain tumors. Brain abscesses usually show high signal intensity on DW image along with a reduced ADC value. However, in cystic/necrotic tumors, and metastases, DW image shows a low signal with a high ADC value. These features are suggestive, but not specific for the disease pattern. MR spectroscopy may be used in conjunction with DW imaging to establish the correct diagnosis. The presence of amino acids (succinate, acetate, and valine or leucine) and lactate favors abscess rather than tumor/necrotic cavity. It has been reported that following treatment only lactate is present; thus MR spectroscopy is a potential tool for noninvasive establishment of successful brain abscess treatment.

Suggested Reading

Burtscher IM, Holtås S (1999) In vivo proton MR spectroscopy of untreated and treated brain abscesses. AJNR Am J Neuroradiol 20:1049–1053

Nadal Desbarats L, Herlidou S, de Marco G, et al (2003) Differential MRI diagnosis between brain abscesses and necrotic or cystic brain tumors using the apparent diffusion coefficient and normalized diffusion-weighted images. Magn Reson Imaging 21:645–650

Pandey P, Suri A, Singh A, Mahapatra AK (2003) Brain abscess – an unusual complication of ventriculo-peritoneal shunt. Indian J Pediatr 70:833–834

Tsui EY, Chan JH, Cheung YK, Lai KF, Fong D, Ng SH (2002) Evaluation of cerebral abscesses by diffusion-weighted MR imaging and MR spectroscopy. Comput Med Imaging Graph 26:347–351

Figure 4.8
Empyema

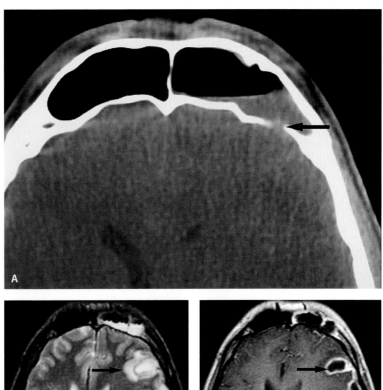

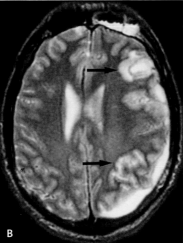

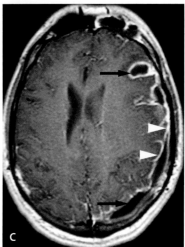

Empyema

Subdural Empyema with Cortical and Meningeal Involvement

Clinical Presentation

A 20-year-old male with a history of sinusitis presents with severe headache, vomiting and fever.

Images (Fig. 4.8)

A. CT scan shows air/fluid level in the frontal sinus with interruption of the posterior wall of the sinus (*arrow*). There appears to be slightly increased density in the epidural space at this location
B. T2-weighted image also demonstrates the air/fluid level in the frontal sinus with extra-axial high intensity over the left hemisphere. There is a mass effect upon the midline structures. The cortex on the left is swollen with an abnormal high signal (*arrows*)

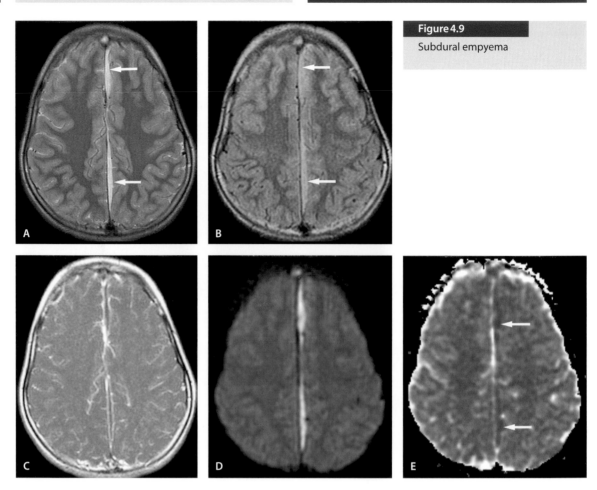

Figure 4.9

Subdural empyema

C. Contrast-enhanced T1-weighted image demonstrates multiple extra-axial fluid collections over the left frontal and parietal lobes (*arrows*) which are slightly hyperintense compared to CSF. There is peripheral enhancement around the margins of these collections. Additionally, dural and leptomeningeal enhancement is seen (*arrowheads*)

Subdural Empyema

Clinical Presentation

A 9-year-old female presents with fever and headaches. She has also edema in the eyelid.

Images (Fig. 4.9)

A. T2-weighted image shows two subtle extra-axial collections along the falx (*arrows*)
B. On FLAIR image these collections are hyperintense (*arrows*)
C. Contrast-enhanced T1-weighted image with magnetization transfer demonstrates peripheral enhancement around the margins of these collections
D. DW image reveals these collections to be hyperintense (restricted diffusion), representing subdural abscesses
E. ADC map shows these lesions as hypointense (*arrows*) compared to CSF

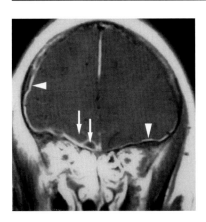

Figure 4.10

Epidural empyema

Epidural Empyema

Clinical Presentation

An 18-year-old male with history of sinusitis, headache and vomiting.

Images (Fig. 4.10)

A. Coronal contrast-enhanced T1-weighted image shows multiple extra-axial fluid collections over the anterior skull base (*arrows*). There is peripheral enhancement around the margins of these collections. Additionally, dural and leptomeningeal enhancement is seen (*arrowheads*)

Discussion

An empyema is a loculated collection of pus within a membrane-bound space. The empyema can occur either in the subdural or epidural space or may involve both spaces simultaneously. Subdural empyema is more common than epidural empyema. Both entities are most commonly seen as a complication of paranasal sinus infection. Other etiologies include mastoiditis, osteomyelitis and intracranial surgery. In infants, meningitis can lead to subdural collection. Complications from this infectious process include cortical vein thrombosis or dural sinus thrombosis with secondary venous infarctions and parenchymal abscess formation. Since the dura is relatively resistant to the penetration of antibiotics, aspiration or drainage of empyema is often mandatory. These procedures are surgical emergencies. On CT scan, these extra-axial fluid collections have either CSF density or are slightly higher density. MR imaging is a more sensitive method to outline the extent of the lesions. The extra-axial fluid is usually isointense or just slightly higher intensity on T1-weighted image compared to CSF. On the T2-weighted image the intensity is often close to that of CSF. On the post-contrast images there is abnormal enhancement in the margins of the collections. The complications in the underlying brain include cerebritis and abscess formation in addition to cortical vein thrombosis and venous infarcts. DW images show the pus in the pyogenic abscess as a hyperintense lesion with relatively low ADC values. Toxoplasmosis abscess may show a variety of signal intensities that may be a reflection of different pathological/morphological subtypes.

Suggested Reading

Desprechins B, Stadnik T, Koerts G, Shabana W, Breucq C, Osteaux M (1999) Use of diffusion-weighted MR imaging in differential diagnosis between intracerebral necrotic tumors and cerebral abscesses. AJNR Am J Neuroradiol 20:1252–1257

Weingarten K, Zimmerman RD, Becker RD, et al (1989) Subdural and epidural empyemas: MR imaging. AJR Am J Roentgenol 152:615–621

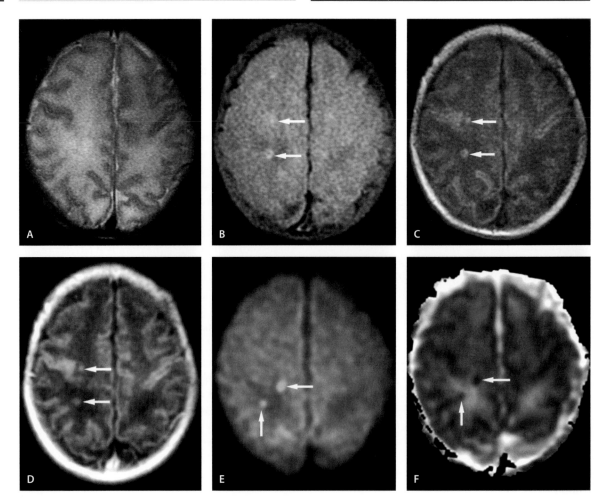

Figure 4.11

Septic emboli

Septic Emboli

Clinical Presentation

A 15-day-old male presents with fever and irritability. He is a former 34-week gestational age premature baby with repeated attacks of apnea. CSF reveals increased a white blood cell count and increased protein. The patient has fungal sepsis of unknown etiology and unknown source. The CSF revealed later *Candida* infection in the CNS.

Images (Fig. 4.11)

A. T2-weighted image is unremarkable

B. FLAIR image shows multiple hyperintense areas (*arrows*) in the right centrum semiovale

C. The same lesions are also hyperintense on T1-weighted image (*arrows*)

D. On T1 FLAIR image the lesions are isointense to the gray matter (*arrows*)

E. DW image shows two hyperintense lesions in the right centrum semiovale (*arrows*)

F. The same lesions are hypointense on the ADC map (*arrows*)

Discussion

The main risk factors for septic emboli are bacterial endocarditis and intrathoracic infections. Cortical branch infarction has been reported to be the most common lesion, which usually involves the distal middle cerebral artery tree. The second most common findings are numerous small embolic lesions in the corticomedullary matter junction some of which are clinically silent and many of which enhance with contrast. Since it can take a few weeks up to several months for septic emboli to develop into an abscess, serial MR imaging with a DW imaging sequence are useful for follow-up of this disease process. Typically the infarction is bright on DW image with decreased ADC. Some patients may develop brain hemorrhage, most commonly subarachnoid hemorrhage. The septic embolus can be large enough to produce a septic infarction with subsequent abscess formation.

Suggested Reading

Bakshi R, Wright PD, Kinkel PR, et al (1999) Cranial magnetic resonance imaging findings in bacterial endocarditis: the neuroimaging spectrum of septic brain embolization demonstrated in twelve patients. J Neuroimaging 2:78–84

Nocardiosis

Clinical Presentation

A 7-year-old male with leukemia presents with fever and confusion.

Images (Fig. 4.12)

A. Proton density-weighted image shows multiple areas of increased signal with minimal mass effect
B. T2-weighted image obtained at the same time as A better shows the hyperintensities in the thalami, white matter and cortex
C. Multiple round enhancing nodules are seen on contrast-enhanced T1-weighted image. No ring lesions are present
D. Noncontrast CT scan at the same time as A, B and C demonstrates multiple scattered hyperdense lesions in addition to white matter edema
E. Contrast enhanced CT scan shows some enhancement in dense lesions

F. Five months later contrast-enhanced T1-weighted image shows significant decrease in previously seen (C) enhancing lesions
G. Nine months later T2-weighted image continues to show minor signal abnormality in both thalami (*arrows*), the previously seen multiple hyperintense lesions and white matter edema are no longer present

Discussion

Nocardia is an uncommon bacterial cause of intracranial abscess, comprising 1 to 2% of cerebral abscesses. Approximately 80% of *Nocardia* infections are due to *N. asteroides* complex. *Nocardia* was previously considered a fungal infection, but it is a filamentous bacteria. It was formerly rare but it is becoming more common and is usually seen in immunocompromised hosts. Most infections begin in the lung following inhalation of *Nocardia* organisms or in the skin after local traumatic inoculation. Infections may be self-limited or progressive. Hematogenous dissemination, usually from a primary pulmonary focus, most commonly involves the CNS and skin, although any organ may be affected. CNS is the most common secondary site of infection. Approximately one-third of patients with *Nocardia* infection will have CNS involvement. The mortality is approximately 40% in patients with CNS involvement. A known predisposing factor is present in half of the cases: steroid therapy, leukemia, lymphoma, cytotoxins, immunosuppression, diabetes, collagen diseases, sarcoid and chronic granulomatous diseases of childhood. Another 30% have defects in cellular immunity and in 20% of patients no known predisposing factors are seen. Mortality is higher in *Nocardia* abscesses than in pyogenic abscesses.

Imaging findings depend upon the stage of the abscess. Noncontrast CT scan usually shows ill-defined hypodense areas which may mimic ischemic or demyelinating lesions. On contrast-enhanced CT and MR images, nocardial abscesses typically appear as nonspecific ring-enhancing lesions surrounded by edema. Budding appearance of ring-enhancing lesions may also be seen. There is little fibrosis and these abscesses are poorly encapsulated. Multiple abscesses may be seen in 40% to 50% of patients. Rarely, nocardial infection of the brain can occur with symptoms of stroke. The differential diagnosis for ring-enhancing lesions includes metastatic deposits, primary necrotic neoplasm such as glioblastoma multiforme, and resolving hematoma.

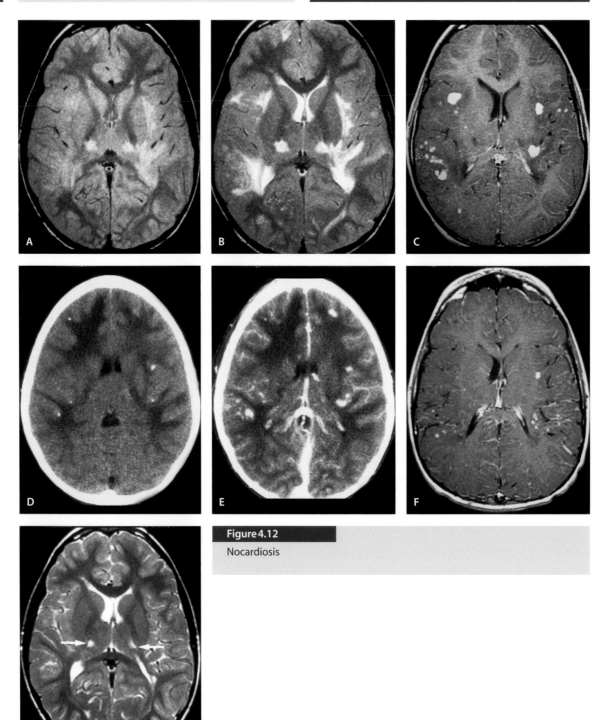

Figure 4.12

Nocardiosis

Suggested Reading

Boerm W (2004) Nocardia brain abscess misinterpreted as cerebral infarction. J Clin Neurosci 11:348

Shin JH, Lee HK (2003) Nocardial brain abscess in a renal transplant recipient. J Clin Imaging 27:321–324

Figure 4.13

Citrobacter meningitis
and cerebritis

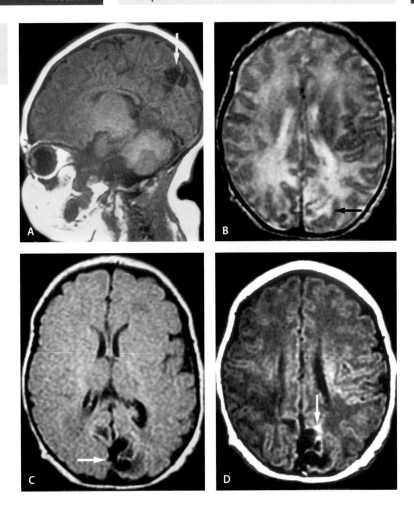

Images (Fig. 4.13)

A. Sagittal T1-weighted image shows hypointense lesion in the left parieto-occipital area (*arrow*)
B. T2-weighted image shows hyperintensity in the
   left occipital area (*arrow*) involving both gray and
   white matter
C. FLAIR reveals areas of low signal in the left occipital area (*arrow*) consistent with cavitary lesions
D. Contrast-enhanced T1-weighted image shows enhancement in the wall of the cavitary lesions (*arrow*). This is consistent with "square" abscess and
   necrotic cavity typically seen in *Citrobacter*
   meningitis and encephalitis

Citrobacter Infections

Citrobacter Meningitis and Cerebritis

Clinical Presentation

A 24-day-old female with *Citrobacter* sepsis and
cerebritis.

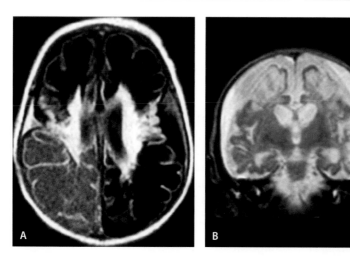
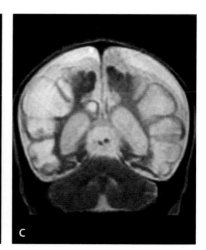

Figure 4.14

Chronic *Citrobacter* cerebritis

Chronic *Citrobacter* Cerebritis

Clinical Presentation

A 6-week-old female with history of newborn *Citrobacter* cerebritis. The patient developed cystic encephalomalacia as an end-stage of the disease.

Images (Fig. 4.14)

A. FLAIR image through the ventricles shows bilateral large cystic spaces replacing the brain parenchyma
B. Coronal T2-weighted image through the basal ganglia shows relative sparing of the basal ganglia. The ventricles are enlarged
C. The end-stage cystic changes are well seen in the T2-weighted image posterior to B

Discussion

Citrobacter diversus is a gram-negative enteric bacillus, a pathogen from the gastrointestinal tract. It has been associated with nosocomial infections, usually of the urinary and respiratory tracts, in very young patients and debilitated patients, in addition to endocarditis and hospital-acquired bacteremia. *Citrobacter* CNS infection in the newborn is rare after 1 month of age. In neonates, *Citrobacter* strains are an important cause of meningitis. Neonatal meningitis or cerebritis caused by *C. diversus* is complicated by abscess formation in 40–80% of patients. Multiple abscesses are seen. Neonatal white matter offers little resistance to infection and multicystic encephalomalacia may develop secondary to *Citrobacter* neonatal brain infection. Findings include parenchymal loss, ventricular enlargement, and cystic areas. About 50% of meningitis and abscess survivors have significant brain damage. About 30% of neonates with *Citrobacter* meningitis die.

Contrast-enhanced CT scan may show enhancing meninges. Abscess is seen as rim-enhancing lesions surrounded by edema on both CT scan and MR image. The abscesses are typically "square" in appearance. Not all enhancing lesions in these patients are abscesses; some are white matter necrosis and liquefaction. The abscesses typically replace (not displace) the white matter. MR imaging is more sensitive in detection of early changes of cerebritis.

Suggested Reading

Feferbaum R, Diniz EM, Valente M, et al (2000) Brain abscess by *Citrobacter diversus* in infancy: case report. Arq Neuropsiquiatr 58:736–740

Leggiadro RJ (1996) Favorable outcome possible in *Citrobacter* brain abscess. Pediatr Infect Dis J 15:557

Levine RS, Rosenberg HK, Zimmerman RA, Stanford (1983) Complications of citrobacter neonatal meningitis: assessment by real-time cranial sonography correlated with CT. AJNR Am J Neuroradiol 4:668–671

Herpes Simplex Virus Encephalitis

Neonatal Herpes Simplex Virus Encephalitis Type 2

Clinical Presentation

A 57-day-old infant, who was an ex-27-week gestational age premature infant, immediately after birth suffered HSV encephalitis and received two courses of acyclovir treatment.

Images (Fig. 4.15)

A. Noncontrast CT shows enlarged ventricles, calcifications in the bilateral basal ganglia (*arrows*) and dystrophic calcification along the right lateral ventricle (*arrowhead*). The gyration is immature with widely open sylvian fissures

B. T1-weighted image. Much of the brain parenchyma has been lost with some the inferior frontal, occipital and temporal lobe persisting. The rest of the cranium is filled with CSF (see D)

C. T2-weighted image at the same level as B shows low-signal basal ganglia calcifications. No myelination is seen in the white matter at this age

D. Sagittal midline T1-weighted image reveals lack of brain parenchyma above the low temporal, occipital and frontal lobes. Note the hypoplastic midbrain, pons and medulla. The cerebellar hemispheres are also hypoplastic

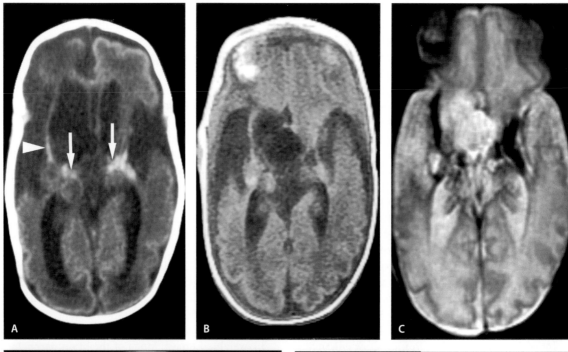

Figure 4.15

Neonatal herpes simplex virus encephalitis type 2

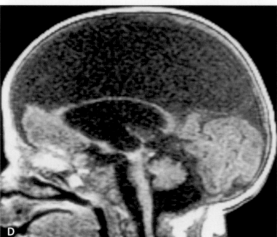

Neonatal Herpes Simplex Virus Encephalitis Type 2

Clinical Presentation

A 2-week-old male with new onset of seizures, fever and irritability. He received acyclovir treatment. However, he has increased tone and continues to have seizures. The follow-up MR image is obtained at the age of 7 weeks. At the age of 22 months the child is severely developmentally delayed.

Images (Fig. 4.16)

A. T2-weighted image at the age of 2 weeks shows swollen cortex, especially in the left hemisphere with poorly defined cortical ribbon (*arrows*). Only the occipital lobes are uninvolved. Abnormal high signal is also seen in the thalami and right basal ganglia

B. T1-weighted image confirms the presence of diffuse cortical and subcortical edema

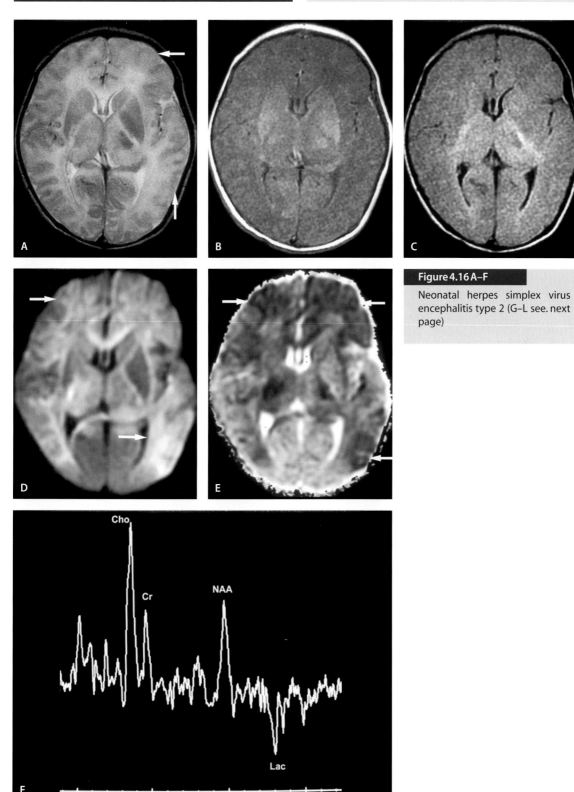

Figure 4.16 A–F

Neonatal herpes simplex virus encephalitis type 2 (G–L see. next page)

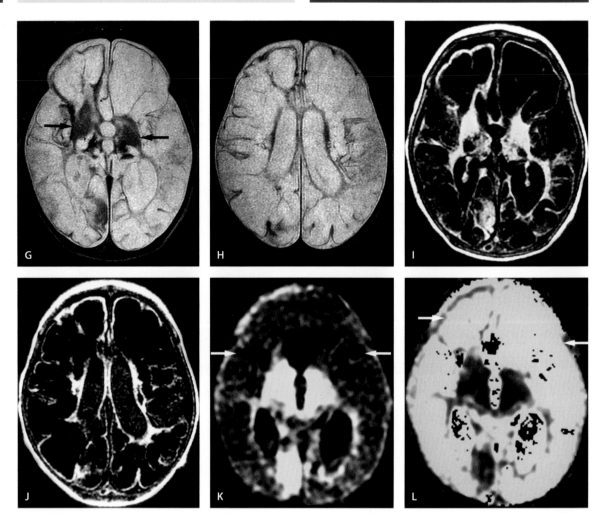

Figure 4.16 G–L

Neonatal herpes simplex virus encephalitis type 2

C. Diffuse brain swelling is also seen on FLAIR image, although brain edema is difficult to detect in the unmyelinated brain

D. DW image reveals diffuse abnormal high signal in the bilateral white and cortical gray matter (*arrows*). Only the occipital lobes display normal signal

E. The abnormal signal seen on the DW image (D) is hypointense on the ADC map consistent with restricted diffusion from cytotoxic edema (*arrows*)

F. Single voxel proton MR spectroscopy (TE 144 ms) placed over the right thalamus reveals a prominent lactate peak. The low NAA and high Cho peaks are normal in this age group

G. T2-weighted image at the age of 7 weeks shows extensive encephalomalacia involving both hemispheres, but sparing some basal ganglia structures (*arrows*). The follow-up MR image (not shown) at the age of 22 months was unchanged

H. T2-weighted image through the ventricles shows multicystic encephalomalacia. The signal in the cysts is isointense to CSF

I. T1-weighted image through the basal ganglia confirms the extensive encephalomalacia with minimal gliotic basal ganglia

J. T1-weighted image through the ventricles confirms the extensive parenchymal loss

K. DW image shows diffuse hypointensity in the areas of multicystic encephalomalacia (*arrows*)

L. ADC map reveals normal signal in the small area of residual brain tissue in the right occipital region and basal ganglia. Areas of encephalomalacia show hyperintensity similar to CSF representing increased diffusibility (*arrows*)

Herpes Simplex Virus Encephalitis Type 1

Clinical Presentation

A 4-year-old female with fever, headache and altered mental status. HSV encephalitis was diagnosed with a PCR test and CT scans. MR imaging was done 6 days after the onset of symptoms.

Images (Fig. 4.17)

A. Noncontrast CT scan 3 days after the onset of symptoms reveals bitemporal edema, left side greater than right. The initial CT scan was normal

B. T2-weighted image shows bitemporal hyperintense edema (*arrows*). The edema involves mainly the medial and anterior temporal lobes. There is another area of less hyperintensity in the left posterior temporal lobe white matter (*arrowhead*). This area shows restricted diffusion on DW image (D)

C. Coronal FLAIR image better outlines the extent of the edema: both temporal lobes and insular cortex bilaterally (*arrows*) are involved. The left side is significantly more involved

D. DW image reveals hyperintensity in the posterior aspect of the left temporal lobe. The anterior temporal lobe is minimally hyperintense

E. ADC map shows hypointensity in the areas of hyperintensity on DW image (D) consistent with restricted diffusion

F. Contrast-enhanced T1-weighted magnetization transfer image shows mild bilateral leptomeningeal enhancement without significant parenchymal enhancement

G. Follow-up noncontrast CT scan at 5 months shows development of significant atrophy

Discussion

Herpes viruses represent a large group of viruses, including herpes simplex virus type 1, HSV type 2, CMV, Epstein-Barr virus, varicella zoster virus, B virus, herpesvirus 6 and herpesvirus 7. Herpes virus encephalitis is the most common type of acute viral infection, with an incidence of 1/250,000. Herpes encephalitis in infants is caused by HSV type 2 whereas herpes encephalitis seen in children and adults is caused by HSV type 1. HSV type 1 has particular predilection for the limbic system with localization of infection to the temporal lobes, insular cortex, subfrontal area, and cingulated gyri. Although the infection usually spares the basal ganglia, it may be present. Patients usually present with mental deterioration, hallucinations, fever, headaches, and seizures.

HSV type 2 infection is a sexually transmitted disease and is associated with genital lesions. The congenital infection is usually transmitted at birth from contact with infected secretions. CNS involvement is seen in 30 % of these children and 80 % do not survive the infection. True congenital infection acquired in utero is rare. Infants infected in utero may have skin lesions at birth, chorioretinitis, microphthalmos, severe CNS damage manifested by microphthalmos and hydranencephaly.

Neonatal HSV encephalitis is practically always symptomatic. HSV type 2 infection is a diffuse and nonfocal disease, in contrast to HSV encephalitis type 1 disease. It results in widespread brain destruction. Severe neurological sequelae include seizures, microcephaly, microphthalmos, ventriculomegaly and multicystic encephalomalacia. CT and MR imaging findings are nonspecific and early on may even be negative. Early findings include loss of gray/white matter contrast. In the early phase there may be increased cortical blood flow but with progression of disease there is focal hemorrhagic necrosis and parenchymal calcification,

CT scanning in HSV encephalitis type 1 infection shows the earliest findings at 3 days after the onset of symptoms. After 3 days the noncontrast CT scan may show ill-defined low-density areas with patchy or gyral enhancement on contrast enhancement. MR imaging is more sensitive than CT scanning in detecting early changes. Typical early findings include gyral edema, seen as a low-intensity signal on T1-weighted and high-signal intensity in the temporal lobes, and cingulated gyrus on T2-weighted MR images. The signal abnormality often extends into the insular cortex and spares the putamen. Areas of petechial hem-

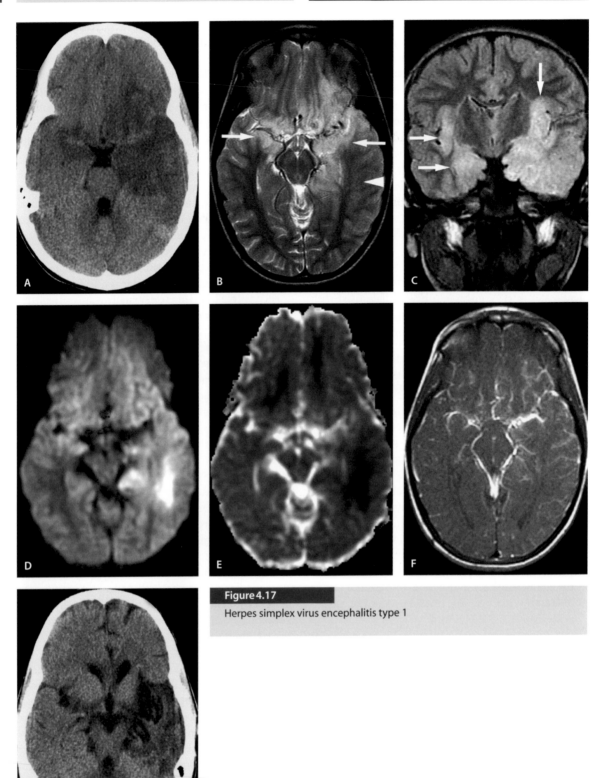

Figure 4.17

Herpes simplex virus encephalitis type 1

orrhage may be seen. Post-contrast studies may show mild enhancement. Involvement may be unilateral in the early stage; however, sequential development of contralateral changes is highly suggestive of the disease. DW imaging is far superior to conventional MR imaging for detection of early subtle findings of herpes encephalitis. Detection of parenchymal and gyral enhancement may be improved with magnetization transfer saturation imaging. As with other chronic processes in the brain, a late sequela of herpes infection is atrophy. Neurosyphilis and primary central system lymphoma are rare mimickers of the disease.

Suggested Reading

Bash S, Hathout GM, Cohen S (2001) Mesiotemporal T2-weighted hyperintensity: neurosyphilis mimicking herpes encephalitis. AJNR Am J Neuroradiol 22:314–316

Burke JW, Mathews VP, Elster AD, Ulmer JL, McLean FM, Davis SB (1996) Contrast-enhanced magnetization transfer saturation imaging improves MR detection of herpes simplex encephalitis. AJNR Am J Neuroradiol 17:773–776

Sener RN (2001) Herpes simplex encephalitis: diffusion MR imaging findings. Comput Med Imaging Graph 25:391–397

Shaw DW, Cohen WA (1993) Viral infections of the CNS in children: imaging features. AJR Am J Roentgenol 160:125–133

Congenital Cytomegalovirus Infection

Clinical Presentation

A 1-day-old male with congenital hydrocephalus.

Images (Fig. 4.18)

A. T2-weighted image shows hydrocephalus. Especially the occipital horns are asymmetric and significantly dilated with no visualized brain parenchyma posteriorly. The gyration is poorly developed and the sylvian fissures are open (*arrows*)
B. T1-weighted image confirms the presence of hydrocephalus. Subependymal calcifications are seen (*arrows*). Note the deviation of the straight sinus (*arrowheads*)
C. FLAIR image confirms the hydrocephalus, poor gyration and widely open sylvian fissures
D. DW image reveals presence of periventricular calcifications (*arrows*)

Discussion

Congenital CMV is the most common cause of congenital virus infection. Among infected neonates, 90–95 % are asymptomatic at birth, but almost 30 % develop late complications in the 1st year of life. The periventricular subependymal germinal matrix cells are most frequently affected.

A variety of imaging features have been described in congenital CMV infection. Gestational age at the time of infection predicts the nature of lesions seen on CMV infection. As a general rule, infection during the first two trimesters causes malformations and during the third trimester it causes destruction of tissue. CT scan shows atrophy, ventricular dilatation, and parenchymal calcifications. It can cause widespread parenchymal calcifications in various locations but the subependymal and periventricular region are the most common sites. MR image is more sensitive in detection of white matter abnormalities as well as associated migrational anomalies such as lissencephaly and polymicrogyria. The white matter abnormalities include delayed myelination, and focal areas of parenchymal destruction. Cortical dysplasias are more common in congenital CMV than in toxoplasmosis.

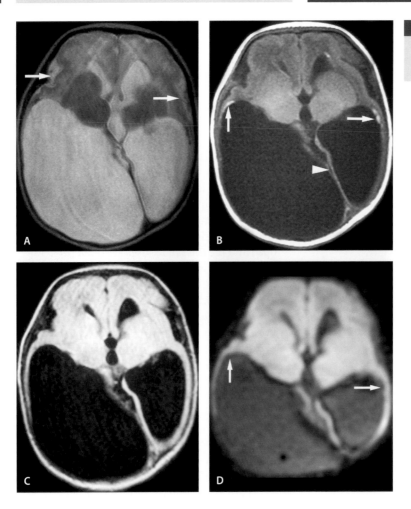

Figure 4.18

Congenital cytomegalovirus infection

Differential diagnosis of subependymal and periventricular calcifications includes toxoplasmosis (lack of cortical abnormality, more scattered calcifications), rubella (also microcephaly and cataracts), and tuberous sclerosis. The basal ganglia and cortex are the common sites of calcifications in toxoplasmosis. Tuberous sclerosis in addition to subependymal calcification (not in the newborn) shows cortical tubers and a mass lesion in the region of foramen of Monro.

Suggested Reading

Bale JF Jr, Bray PF, Bell WE (1985) Neuroradiographic abnormalities in congenital cytomegalovirus infection. Pediatr Neurol 1:42–47

Barkovich AJ, Lindan CE (1994) Congenital cytomegalovirus infection of the brain: imaging analysis and embryologic considerations. AJNR Am J Neuroradiol 15:703–715

Sugita K, Ando M, Makino M, Takanashi J, Fujimoto N, Niimi H (1991) Magnetic resonance imaging of the brain in congenital rubella virus and cytomegalovirus infections. Neuroradiology 33:239–242

Figure 4.19
Cytomegalovirus encephalitis

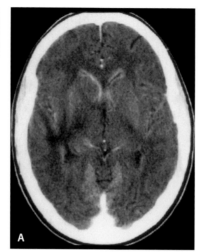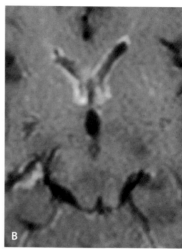

Cytomegalovirus Encephalitis

Clinical Presentation

A 20-year-old immunocompromised female presents with headache, low-grade fever and confusion.

Images (Fig. 4.19)

A. Contrast-enhanced CT scan shows diffuse ependymal enhancement
B. Contrast-enhanced T1-weighted image reveals a relatively thick periventricular enhancement around the frontal horns

Discussion

CMV is a herpes virus that can cause infection of the CNS in immunosuppressed patients such as HIV-positive and organ-transplant patients. CMV encephalitis in the immunocompromised host can have a wide variety of clinical presentations ranging from a clinically silent infection diagnosed at autopsy to fulminant progressive encephalitis resulting in death within days of presentation. The virus exists in the latent form in the general population and reactivates in the setting of immunocompromise. Although the CNS infection usually is limited to minimal encephalitis and/or ventriculitis, myelitis, polyradiculitis and retinitis are other manifestations of this disease. The majority of changes are limited to the ependymal or subependymal region, but a diffuse process can be found in the gray and white matter anywhere in the brain. The white matter is usually less involved than the gray matter.

MR imaging is most sensitive to the periventricular abnormalities seen in CMV. The T2-weighted and proton density images as well as FLAIR demonstrate a thick hyperintensity in the ependymal region sometimes extending to the surrounding white matter. Only one-third of patients demonstrate contrast enhancement. CNS lymphoma may occasionally mimic CMV and demonstrate periventricular thin enhancement. Although CMV infection of the CNS is diagnosed in up to 40% of AIDS patients' brain at autopsy, a clinical diagnosis of CMV is difficult to obtain and this disease process is under-diagnosed. Clinically the PCR test isolates viral DNA from CSF. The clinical symptoms of CMV are nonspecific and they can mimic symptoms of HIV encephalopathy. CSF typically shows neutrophilic pleocytosis, elevated protein and low glucose.

Suggested Reading

Ketonen LM, Arya S, van Epps K, et al (1997) MR findings of autopsy-proved cytomegalovirus encephalitis in AIDS. Presented at the 35th Annual Meeting of the American Society of Neuroradiology, Toronto, Canada

Miller RF, Lucas SB, Hall-Craggs MA, Brink NS, Scaravilli F, Chinn RJ, Kendall BE, Williams IG, Harrison MJ (1997) Comparison of magnetic resonance imaging with neuropathological findings in the diagnosis of HIV and CMV associated CNS disease in AIDS. J Neurol Neurosurg Psychiatry 62:346–351

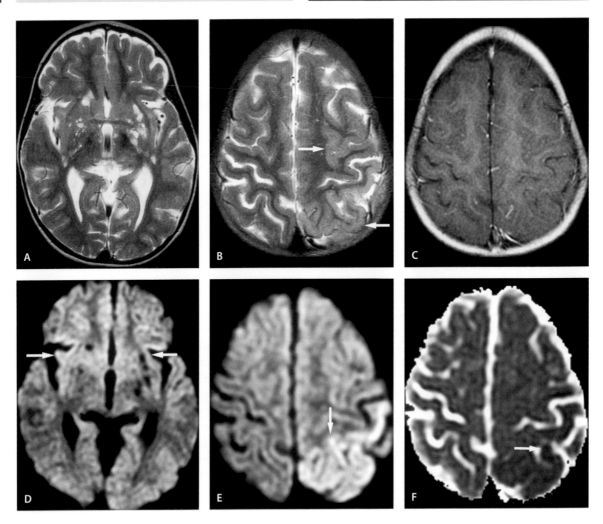

Figure 4.20

Viral encephalitis (influenza encephalopathy)

Viral Encephalitis
(Influenza Encephalopathy)

Clinical Presentation

A 3-year-old girl with influenza A experiences sudden onset of right hemiparesis and partial seizures.

Images (Fig. 4.20)

A. T2-weighted image through the basal ganglia is unremarkable
B. T2-weighted image through the centrum semiovale shows edematous and swollen gyri with hyperintensity in the left posterior frontoparietal region (*arrows*)
C. The swollen gyri do not show abnormal contrast enhancement on T1-weighted image
D. DW image through the basal ganglia shows a tiny area of increased signal (*arrows*)

E. DW image through the centrum semiovale where the swollen gyri exhibit increased signal consistent with restricted diffusion seen in cytotoxic edema (*arrow*). The same area developed focal atrophy in the follow-up images. The patient also continued to have seizures

F. ADC map of the same area as E reveals the diffusion abnormality to have decreased signal (*arrow*)

Discussion

Acute encephalitis/encephalopathy is a rare complication of influenza virus infection. It is of great clinical significance because of its high morbidity and mortality. It is presumed that influenza encephalitis results from hematogenous spread of virus and direct invasion by the virus mainly of neurons in the cortex.

MR imaging plays an important role in evaluation of the extent and characterization of the lesion. Abnormally hyperintense lesions located in the cortex and subcortical white matter are seen on T2-weighted images. Post-gadolinium images do not show enhancement. The DW image has higher sensitivity in detection of these lesions. They are seen as high-intensity lesions on DW images with a low ADC value due to cytotoxic edema.

Suggested Reading

Tokunaga Y, Kira R, Takemoto M, et al (2000) Diagnostic usefulness of diffusion weighted magnetic resonance imaging in influenza-associated acute encephalopathy or encephalitis. Brain Dev 22:451–453

Tsuchiya K, Katase S, Yoshino A, Hachiya J (2000) MRI of influenza encephalopathy in children: value of diffusion-weighted imaging. J Comput Assist Tomogr 24:303–307

Congenital Human Immunodeficiency Virus (HIV) Infection

Clinical Presentation

An 11-year-old-male with known congenital acquired immunodeficiency syndrome (AIDS) presents with seizures. The patient has received 10 days toxoplasmosis treatment for a ring-enhancing right parietal mass lesion. This and many other ring-enhancing lesions were improved, but during the therapy a new left occipital lesion appears. Patient undergoes an open brain biopsy that shows this lesion to be a primary CNS lymphoma. This disappears with radiation.

Images (Fig. 4.21)

A. Noncontrast CT scan shows diffuse atrophy and bifrontal subcortical white matter calcifications (*arrowheads*). Right posterior temporal edema is present (*arrow*)

B. Contrast-enhanced CT shows no enhancement in the frontal lobes

C. Noncontrast T1-weighted image 2 days later shows also the frontal calcifications (*arrowheads*)

D. Noncontrast T1-weighted image shows hyperintense area in the right posterior temporal region (*arrow*). This represents blood products (no calcification was seen on noncontrast CT scan, A)

E. Coronal contrast-enhanced spoiled gradient echo image reveals an enhancing lesion at the site of the blood products (seen in D)

F. Contrast-enhanced T1-weighted image through the frontal calcifications shows an improving lesion in the right parietal region (*arrow*)

G. T2-weighted image shows extensive diffuse white matter changes that spare the subcortical "U" fibers (*arrow*). This is consistent with HIV leukoencephalopathy

H. The HIV-induced leukoencephalopathy is seen also in the centrum semiovale

I. T2-weighted follow-up study 1 month later shows a growing mass lesion in the left occipital lobe (*arrow*)

J. T2-weighted image shows stable frontal lobe calcifications (*arrowheads*). The white matter changes show progression

K. Contrast-enhanced T1-weighted image shows ring-enhancing lesion in the left occipital region (*arrow*). In the brain biopsy it proved to be primary CNS lymphoma

L. T2-weighted image follow-up study nearly 7 years later shows diminished HIV-related leukoencephalopathy (compare with H). The frontal lobe calcifications are not seen. This was later confirmed on CT scan

M. DW image shows mild white matter brightness consistent with the "T2-shine through" phenomenon

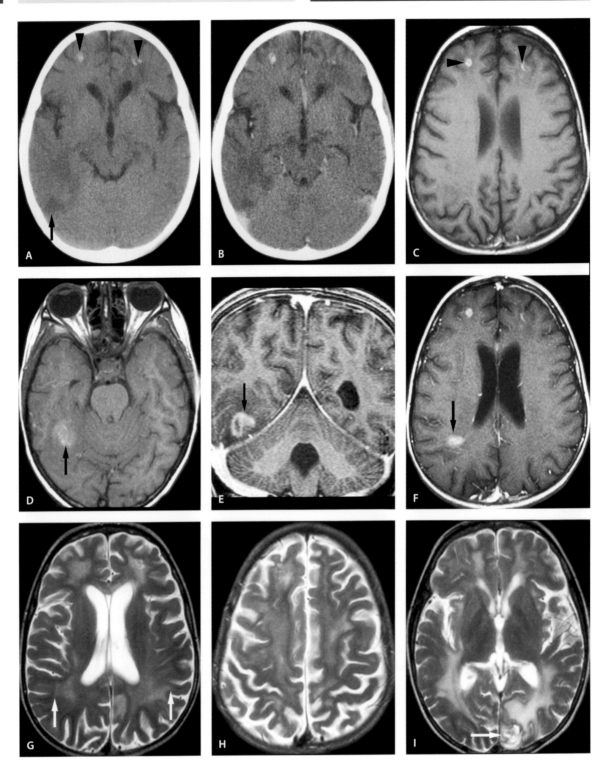

Figure 4.21 A–I

Congenital human immunodeficiency virus (HIV) infection (J–M see next page)

Figure 4.21 J–M

Congenital human immunodeficiency virus (HIV) infection

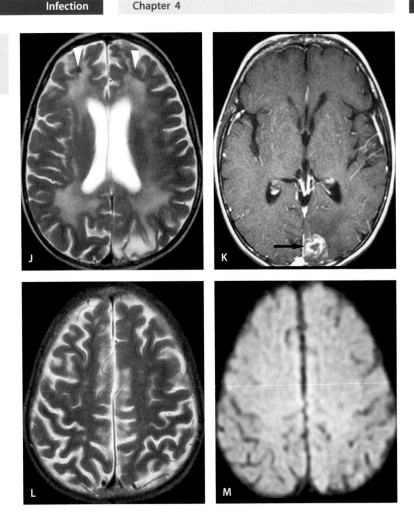

Discussion

Congenital HIV infection is also known as congenital AIDS or maternally transmitted AIDS. AIDS in the pediatric population was first reported in 1982. Since then it has become a significant congenitally transmitted infection. About 78% of pediatric HIV infection is maternally transmitted, even though fewer than 40% of HIV-positive mothers pass on the infection. The risk of infection varies with maternal plasma titers of the HIV virus. Transmission of HIV can occur in utero, intrapartum, and postpartum via breast milk. The transplacental route accounts for most pediatric AIDS cases. Infants tend to be asymptomatic at birth, then develop chronic symptoms slowly over many months. The diagnosis in the newborn may be difficult because passively transmitted maternal antibodies may be present in children for up to 15 months after birth. CNS symptoms are high in this age group. Developmental delay and micro-cephaly are the most common features. The children also show signs of movement disorders such as ataxia and spastic paraparesis. Cognitive and motor deficits are common features. In contrast to adults, infants and children rarely develop opportunistic CNS complications such as lymphoma and toxoplasmosis. Lymphoma occurs in fewer than 5% of infected children. Progressive multifocal leukoencephalopathy (PML) is the most common secondary CNS infection in pediatric AIDS patients. Atrophy is the most common imaging finding on both CT and MR imaging. On CT scan there is also decreased white matter attenuation and cerebral calcifications. Calcifications are mostly seen in the basal ganglia. Calcifications are also seen in the subcortical frontal white matter and in the cerebellum. Calcifications may be difficult to appreciate unless gradient echo sequence is obtained. MR findings include atrophy and increased T2 and FLAIR signal in the white matter.

Toxoplasmosis in HIV Infection The incidence of toxoplasmosis associated with HIV infection varies from 5% to 30% of AIDS patients. The clinical symptoms include headache, confusion, fever, and personality changes. In toxoplasmosis, approximately 70% of lesions are multiple and are most commonly located in the cerebral hemispheric white matter and subcortical gray matter, such as the thalamus and basal ganglia. Rarely, solitary lesion may also be seen. CT scanning may show them as ring-enhancing lesions. MR imaging demonstrates multiple discrete high-signal foci on T2-weighted images with nodular and peripheral enhancement. Contrast enhancement may be absent in immunocompromised patients. Edema and hemorrhages are commonly associated with these lesions.

Primary Brain Lymphoma in HIV Infection Primary brain lymphoma has seen reported in 6–20% of HIV-infected patients. It is more commonly seen in males. HIV lymphoma is more commonly multifocal. The common sites of involvement are cerebral hemispheres, periventricular regions, and the corpus callosum, with a tendency to extend along the ventricular wall. On CT scan, lymphomatous lesions may be seen as hypo- or hyperdense, nodular or ring-enhancing lesions. The lesions are usually low signal on T1-weighted and intermediate to high signal on T2-weighted MR images. Marked nodular enhancement is seen.

Toxoplasmosis is a close mimicker of lymphoma. However, the location of the lesions and the pattern of enhancement along with other imaging modalities may help in differentiating the two entities. MR spectroscopy shows remarkably high lactate/lipid peaks with absence of normal brain metabolites in patients with toxoplasmosis. Lymphoma shows high choline peak and moderate elevation of lactate/lipids. MR perfusion may show decreased cerebral blood volume in toxoplasmosis, whereas increased cerebral blood volume is seen in lymphoma. Thallium-201 SPECT may show increased uptake in lymphoma and is highly specific for differentiating these two entities when other imaging modalities are equivocal.

Progressive Multifocal Leukoencephalopathy and Leukoencephalopathy in HIV Infection HIV leukoencephalopathy is similar to PML but it is symmetric and spares the subcortical "U" fibers.

On MR angiography dilatation of the vessels of the circle of Willis is seen. Intracranial hemorrhages and infarction may complicate pediatric AIDS patients' brain imaging. MR spectroscopy shows nonspecific findings: decreased NAA, increased Cho/Cr and presence of amino acids. Delayed myelination is also seen in the developing brain.

Suggested Reading

De la Pena RC, Ketonen L, Villanueva-Meyer J (1996) Simultaneous Tl-201 and Tc-99m sestamibidi SPECT in differentiating CNS lymphoma from nontumorous conditions in AIDS patients. J Neuro-AIDS 2:33–40

De la Pena RC, Ketonen L, Villanueva-Meyer J (1998) Imaging of brain tumors in AIDS patients by means of dual-isotope thallium-201 and technetium-99m sestamibi single-photon emission tomography. Eur J Nucl Med 10:1404–1411

Laissy JP, Soyer P, Tebboune J, et al (1994) Contrast-enhanced fast MRI in differentiating brain toxoplasmosis and lymphoma in AIDS patients. J Comput Assist Tomogr 18:714–718

Patsalides AD, Wood LV, Atac GK, Sandifer E, Butman JA, Patronas NJ (2002) Cerebrovascular disease in HIV-infected pediatric patients: neuroimaging findings. Am J Roentgenol 179:999–1003

Simone IL, Federico F, Tortorella C, et al (1998) Localised 1H-MR spectroscopy for metabolic characterisation of diffuse and focal brain lesions in patients infected with HIV. J Neurol Neurosurg Psychiatry 64:516–523

Figure 4.22
Intraventricular cysticercosis

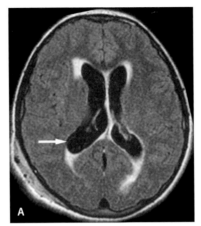 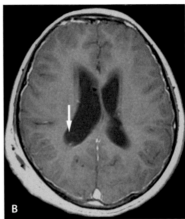

Figure 4.22
Intraventricular cysticercosis

Cysticercosis

Intraventricular Cysticercosis

Clinical Presentation

A 12-year-old girl presents with headaches.

Images (Fig. 4.22)

A. FLAIR image shows a thin-walled cyst in the occipital horn of the right lateral ventricle (*arrow*). Patient has acute hydrocephalus with transependymal CSF leak. The subcutaneous swelling is related to recent shunting

B. Contrast-enhanced T1-weighted image better demonstrates the scolex (*arrow*)

Subarachnoid Cysticercosis

Clinical Presentation

A 24-year-old Mexican female presents with headaches.

Images (Fig. 4.23)

A. FLAIR image shows asymmetric enlargement of the right ambient and quadrigeminal plate cisterns (*arrow*). Transependymal CSF leak is seen around the ventricles

B. T2-weighted image shows hydrocephalus in addition to asymmetric cisternal enlargement

C. Contrast-enhanced T1-weighted image. The cysticercal cysts within the basal cisterns are nonenhancing. No scolex is present. The cysts contain CSF-like fluid

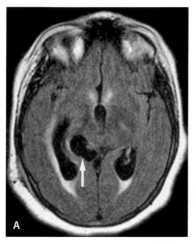
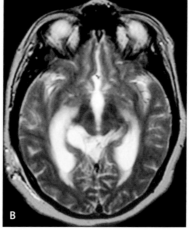
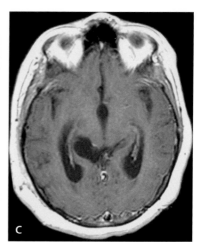

Figure 4.23

Subarachnoid cysticercosis

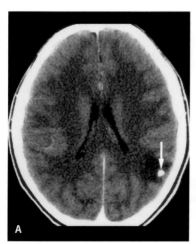
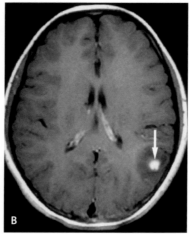

Figure 4.24

Parenchymal cysticercosis

Parenchymal Cysticercosis

Clinical Presentation

An 18-year-old Mexican male presents with first-time seizures.

Images (Fig. 4.24)

A. Contrast-enhanced CT scan shows an enhancing nodule with surrounding edema (*arrow*). This represents the colloid stage when the viable cyst dies and antigenic material leaks across the cyst wall. An inflammatory reaction leads to breakdown to the blood-brain barrier. Surrounding edema is present
B. Contrast-enhanced T1-weighted image shows the enhancing nodule and surrounding low-signal edema (*arrow*)

Figure 4.25
Calcified cysticercosis

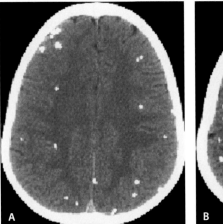 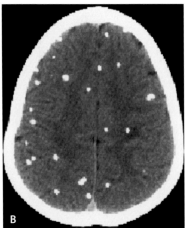

Calcified Cysticercosis

Clinical Presentation

A 17-year-old male has a long history of seizures.

Images (Fig. 4.25)

A and B: CT scans show numerous focal calcified lesions consistent with the final stage of parenchymal disease

Discussion

Neurocysticercosis is common in Asia, Central and South America, Africa and Mexico, and is being increasingly seen in North America. Ingestion of the eggs of the adult pork tapeworm, *Taenia solium*, by humans is followed by larval release in the intestine and their subsequent migration hematologically to the brain, eye, orbit, or other subcutaneous tissue. CNS involvement is seen in 60% to 90% of patients with cysticercosis. The brain parenchyma is the most commonly affected site followed by intraventricular and subarachnoid space. The parenchymal form more often has a tumoral form of presentation. Cisternal cysticerci in their racemose form can form mass lesions in the basal cisterns causing obstructive hydrocephalus or meningitis.

The natural course of cerebral cysticercosis lesions may be divided into four stages: vesicular, colloid vesicular, granular nodular and nodular calcified. MR findings vary according to stage. The vesicular stage is seen as a round CSF-like cyst with a mural nodule that represents its scolex. In the colloid vesicular stage, cyst fluid is hyperintense with ring-like enhancement. A target or bull's eye appearance may be seen in the granular nodular stage.

Suggested Reading

Bannur U, Rajshekhar V (2001) Cisternal cysticercosis: a diagnostic problem – a short report. Neurol India 49:206–208

Sheth TN, Pilon L, Keystone J, Kucharczyk W (1998) Persistent MR contrast enhancement of calcified neurocysticercosis lesions. AJNR Am J Neuroradiol 19:79–82

Zee CS, Segall HD, Boswell W, Ahmadi J, Nelson M, Colletti P (1988) MR imaging of neurocysticercosis. J Comput Assist Tomogr 12:927–934

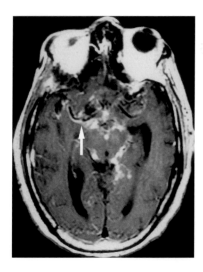

Figure 4.26

Tubercular meningitis

Tuberculosis

Tubercular Meningitis

Clinical Presentation

A 20-year-old male with a several-week history of headaches and low-grade fever.

Images (Fig. 4.26)

A. Contrast-enhanced T1-weighted image shows thick basilar meningeal enhancement. The enhancement surrounds the middle cerebral arteries (*arrow*) and can cause infarctions in the lenticulostriate arteries. Enhancement is also seen around the midbrain, optic nerves, pituitary stalk and interpeduncular fossa

Discussion

Tubercular meningitis is characterized as meningoencephalitis because it affects not only the meninges but also the parenchyma and the vasculature of the brain. Thick tuberculous exudates are formed which adhere around the interpeduncular fossa, optic nerves at the chiasma and extending over the pons and cerebellum, often into the sylvian fissures.

Post-contrast MR images demonstrate thick sheath-like enhancement of the meninges with irregular margins and exudates, especially involving the suprasellar and perimesencephalic cisterns. FLAIR images have higher sensitivity in demonstrating thick meninges. Basal meningeal enhancement and a parenchymal enhancing nodule are strongly suggestive of tuberculous lesions. CSF examination often shows strikingly low glucose levels in tubercular meningitis, narrowing the differential diagnosis.

Intracranial Tuberculoma

Clinical Presentation

A 15-year-old immigrant with new onset of seizures, headaches and malaise.

Images (Fig. 4.27)

A. Contrast-enhanced T1-weighted image demonstrates a tuberculoma in the solid granulomatous stage (*arrow*). There is an enhancing nodule with surrounding edema

Discussion

Parenchymal disease may occur with or without meningitis and usually presents as a solitary or multiple tuberculomas. Tuberculomas may vary from 1 mm to 8 cm in size. Tuberculomas can be seen throughout the cerebral hemispheres, basal ganglia, the cerebellum, and the brain stem.

MR imaging is considered superior to CT scanning in anatomic localization and characterization of such lesions. Intracranial tuberculomas are seen characteristically as hypointense on T2-weighted images and iso- to hypointense on T1-weighted images with variable perifocal edema. The hypointensity on T2-weighted images is due to caseation necrosis. These granulomas show rim enhancement on postgadolinium images. Other imaging patterns are predominantly hyperintense lesion with areas of hypointensity on T2-weighted images, and isointense to the surrounding parenchyma on T2-weighted images that may show nodular or variegated enhancement

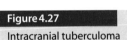

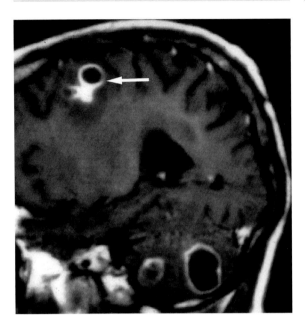

Figure 4.27

Intracranial tuberculoma

Figure 4.28

Tuberculous abscesses

on contrast administration. On MR spectroscopy there are lipid resonance peaks at 1.3 ppm, 2.02 ppm and 3.7 ppm. This spectral pattern in a hypointense T2 lesion is considered characteristic of CNS tuberculoma. The healing stage of neurocysticercosis, fungal granulomas, chronic pyogenic abscess, metastases, toxoplasmosis and some gliomas may simulate tuberculomas.

Suggested Reading

Kim TK, Chang KH, Kim CJ, Goo JM, Kook MC, Han MH (1995) Intracranial tuberculoma: comparison of MR with pathologic findings. AJNR Am J Neuroradiol 16:1903–1908

Nogami K, Nomura S, Kashiwagi S, Kato S, Yamashita K, Ito H (2000) Fluid-attenuated inversion-recovery imaging of cerebral infarction associated with tuberculous meningitis. Comput Med Imaging Graph 24:333–337

Roy J, Paul S, Mitra S, Gangopadhyay PK (2001) Diffuse meningeal involvement in tubercular meningitis. Neurol India 49:216

Shah GV (2000) Central nervous system tuberculosis: imaging manifestations. Neuroimaging Clin North Am 10:355–374

Tuberculous Abscesses

Clinical Presentation

A 20-year-old male with headaches, malaise and unsteady gait.

Images (Fig. 4.28)

A. Sagittal contrast-enhanced T1-weighted image shows multiple scattered ring-enhancing lesions. It is not uncommon to see multiloculated rings (*arrow*). They may simulate bacterial abscesses

Discussion

Although tuberculous brain abscesses are very rare, making the correct diagnosis is important from a management point of view. Recently magnetization transfer (MT) MR imaging has been used for better tissue characterization. The MT ratio is influenced by the proteins and amino acids and this is used to differentiate tuberculous abscess (no amino acids rich in lipids) from pyogenic abscess (rich in amino acids).

Suggested Reading

Gupta RK, Vatsal DK, Husain N, et al (2001) Differentiation of tuberculous from pyogenic brain abscesses with in vivo proton MR spectroscopy and magnetization transfer MR imaging. AJNR Am J Neuroradiol 22:1503–1509

Limbic Encephalitis (Paraneoplastic Limbic Encephalitis)

Clinical Presentation

A 5-year-old boy presents in the emergency room with a purple rash on his arms, fever and seizures. He had confusion before the seizures. Four days after admission a brain perfusion study with Tc 99m sodium pertechnetate confirms complete absence of cerebral blood flow.

Images (Fig. 4.29)

A. Noncontrast CT scan at the time of presentation shows vague low density in the right hippocampus (*arrow*)
B. Noncontrast CT scan 1 day later shows extensive low density involving both hippocampi that are swollen (*arrows*)
C. Contrast-enhanced CT scan reveals no abnormal enhancement in the swollen and low-density hippocampi
D. Bilateral swollen hippocampus-amygdala complexes are seen on T2-weighted image
E. Coronal FLAIR reveals additionally bilateral thalamic swelling with abnormal hyperintensity. The swollen hyperintense hippocampi are again seen
F. Contrast-enhanced T1-weighted fast image with magnetization transfer shows vague bilateral hippocampus enhancement (*arrows*)
G. Contrast-enhanced gradient echo (SPGR) image fails to demonstrate abnormal enhancement in the temporal lobes. Hippocampus swelling is again seen

Discussion

Paraneoplastic limbic encephalitis is a rare disorder characterized by personality changes, irritability, depression, memory loss and sometimes dementia. Limbic encephalitis is subacute encephalitis that predominantly involves the limbic system and is frequently associated with malignant tumors, especially oat cell carcinoma. Other tumors associated with specific paraneoplastic syndromes include female genital tract tumors with cerebellar degeneration, neuroblastoma with opsoclonus, and Hodgkin's lymphoma with demyelinating neuropathy. The limbic system (temporal lobes, insula, cingulated gyri) is the typical location.

Imaging features are nonspecific. On T2-weighted images, hyperintense abnormalities are seen in the temporal lobe. Lesions may extend to involve the inferior frontal lobes and the cingulated gyrus. Gyral enhancement is seen in more than 50% of cases. Hemorrhage is uncommon. On imaging, it is difficult to differentiate from viral encephalitis, especially from herpes encephalitis, since both demonstrate T2 hyperintensity in the same anatomic locations.

Suggested Reading

Gultekin SH, Rosenfield MR, Voltz R, Eichen J, Posner JB, Dalmau J (2000) Paraneoplastic limbic encephalitis: neurological symptoms, immunological findings and tumor association in 50 patients. Brain 123:1481–1494
Hiasa Y, Kunishige M, Mitsui T, et al (2003) Complicated paraneoplastic neurological syndromes: a report of two patients with small cell or non-small cell lung cancer. Clin Neurol Neurosurg 106:47–49
Kodama T, Numaguchi Y, Gellad FE, Dwyer BA, Kristt DA (1991) Magnetic resonance imaging of limbic encephalitis. Neuroradiology 6:520–523

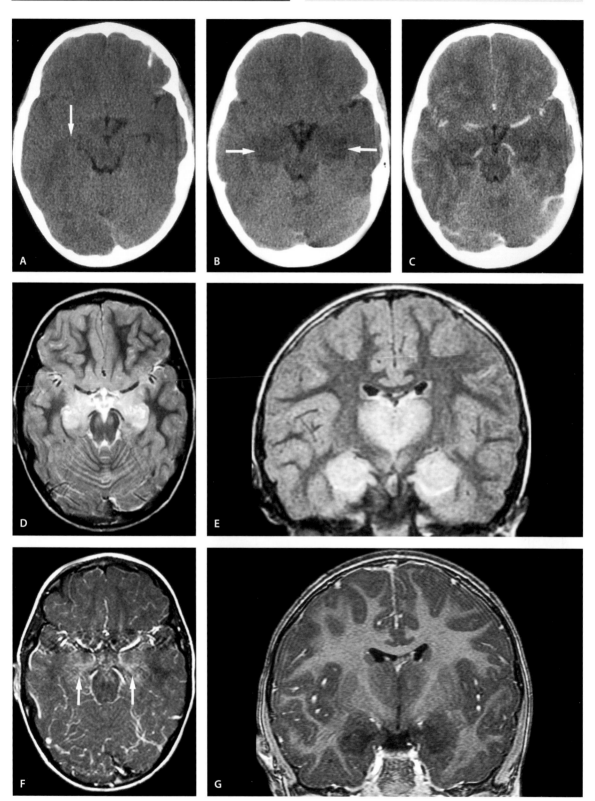

Figure 4.29

Limbic encephalitis (paraneoplastic limbic encephalitis)

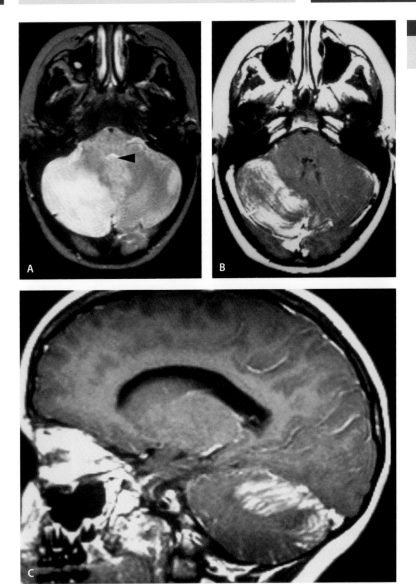

Figure 4.30

Acute cerebellitis

Acute Cerebellitis

Clinical Presentation

An 8-year-old female presents in the emergency room with nausea, headaches and ataxia.

Images (Fig. 4.30)

A. T2-weighted image shows a right cerebellar hyperintensity with mild mass effect upon the fourth ventricle (*arrowhead*)

B. Contrast-enhanced T1-weighted image shows intense enhancement in the right cerebellar hemisphere

C. Sagittal contrast-enhanced T1-weighted image confirms the cerebellar enhancement

Discussion

Acute cerebellitis is an inflammatory process involving the cerebellum. Bilateral cerebellar hemisphere involvement is the most common finding. It is a disease entity with a heterogeneous pathogenesis including many viral illnesses and paraneoplasia. It is

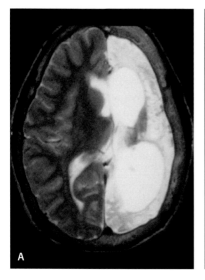
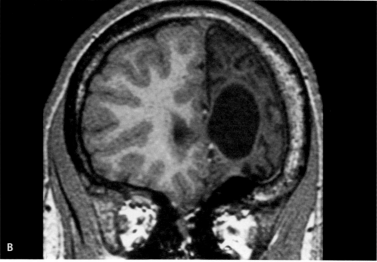

Figure 4.31

Rasmussen's encephalitis

mainly considered to be of viral etiology, although it may be a variant of acute disseminated encephalomyelitis (ADEM). Many childhood illnesses can produce a cerebellar inflammation and edema including measles, mumps, pertussis, and Epstein-Barr virus and varicella-zoster virus infections. Cerebellitis may occur hours to weeks after a viral illness. Paraneoplastic phenomena can also lead to cerebellar inflammation.

The most characteristic finding on CT and MR imaging is diffuse cortical swelling of the cerebellum, often complicated by hydrocephalus or tonsillar herniation. CT scan demonstrates low density of the cerebellar hemisphere with displacement of the fourth ventricle and prepontine cistern. This leads to various degrees of hydrocephalus. MR image reveals prolongation of T1-weighted image and T2-weighted image relaxation time in the involved area. Parenchymal enhancement is present in variable amounts. Meningeal enhancement may also be present. The syndrome is rarely fatal and typically cerebellar atrophy is a late consequence of the disease.

Suggested Reading

De Bruecker Y, Claus F, Demaerel P, et al (2004) MRI findings in acute cerebellitis. Eur Radiol Feb 13 [Epub ahead of print]

Jabbour P, Samaha E, Abi Lahoud G (2003) Hemicerebellitis mimicking a tumour on MRI. Childs Nerv Syst 2:122–125

Sawaishi Y, Takada G (2002) Acute cerebellitis. Cerebellum 1:223–228

Rasmussen's Encephalitis

Clinical Presentation

A 12-year-old male with a several-year history of intractable seizures.

Images (Fig. 4.31)

A. T2-weighted image shows significant left hemiatrophy with hyperintensity in the gray and white matter and basal ganglia. The diploic space is thicker on the left. This is indicative of a chronic process and hemiatrophy

B. Coronal SPGR image confirms the hemiatrophy and thickened calvaria

Discussion

Rasmussen's encephalitis is a progressive childhood disease characterized by unilateral brain dysfunction, intractable focal seizures, progressive hemiplegia, cognitive decline, and inflammatory histopathology. The onset is usually between the ages of 14 months and 14 years, but can occur in adults. Viral infections and antibodies to the glutamate receptor have been implicated in the physiopathology of this illness. It is rarely fatal.

CT and MR imaging may be apparently normal at or soon after the initial onset of seizures. Focal or hemispheric cortical atrophy develops eventually. Cortical atrophy most commonly affects the temporal and frontal lobes and is progressive in nature. Increased T2 signal may also be seen in the white matter and basal ganglia. DW image shows high ADC values in the diseased parenchyma as compared to normal cerebral parenchyma. This is indicative of high molecular motion in the disintegrated brain tissue with active demyelination and glial proliferation associated with chronic inflammation. MR spectroscopy demonstrates decreased NAA peaks. Positron emission tomography reveals hypometabolism in diseased brain parenchyma. Surgical hemispherectomy of the affected hemisphere is the only known treatment.

Suggested Reading

Sener RN (2002) Diffusion MRI in Rasmussen's encephalitis, herpes simplex encephalitis, and bacterial meningoencephalitis. Comput Med Imaging Graph 26:327–332

Sener RN (2003) Diffusion MRI and spectroscopy in Rasmussen's encephalitis. Eur Radiol 13:2186–2191

Topcu M, Turanli G, Aynaci FM, et al (1999) Rasmussen encephalitis in childhood. Childs Nerv Syst 15:395–403

Posterior Fossa Tumors

Introduction

The central nervous system is the most common location for solid neoplasms in children. The classification and locations of pediatric brain tumors and treatment options have been well reviewed in the literature. Approximately half of all intracranial neoplasms in children are found within the posterior fossa. Children from 4 to 11 years of age have more infratentorial neoplasms than children under the age of 3 years.

For practical purpose, the posterior fossa tumors can be divided into the following anatomic locations: (1) cerebellar and/or fourth ventricle tumors, (2) brain stem neoplasms and (3) extra-axial neoplasms. More than 80% of posterior fossa tumors arise within the fourth ventricle and cerebellar hemisphere. The most common cerebellar and fourth ventricle tumors are medulloblastoma (primitive neuroectodermal tumor, PNET), astrocytoma and ependymoma. Subarachnoid metastatic seeding from the primary medulloblastoma is seen in one-third of the cases making it necessary to include spinal canal examination with contrast enhancement into the MRI protocol of medulloblastomas, some pineal tumors and atypical teratoid/rhabdoid tumors.

Three-dimensional imaging capability, detailed anatomic information and lack of bone artifacts commonly seen in CT scanning make the posterior fossa MR imaging more reliable than CT. CT, however, is more sensitive than standard MRI in detecting small foci of calcification. Gradient-echo imaging improves the visualization of calcium on MRI. The results are not, however, specific since blood can exhibit similar signal pattern. Occasionally also there is overlap in the CT appearance and density of blood and calcium.

Diffusion-Weighted Imaging (DW imaging)

The signal intensity of neoplasms on DW images is variable. In general, high-grade tumors tend to show hyperintensity on DW images with decreased apparent diffusion coefficient (ADC). The cause of decreased ADC in high-grade brain tumors might be hypercellularity, total nuclear area and tumor grade. Therefore, hypercellular tumors such as high-grade glioma, lymphoma and PNET are hyperintense on DW images with decreased ADC. Other tumors have normal or increased ADC depending on the tumor grade and cellularity.

The value of DW imaging for the delineation of peritumoral invasion in primary brain tumors is controversial. Some authors have suggested that ADC is useful to determine the extent of tumor invasion, but most of the recent studies have failed to show peritumoral infiltration on DW images and ADC maps.

MR Spectroscopy

In many cases information obtained from standard MRI and/or CT scanning is enough to give correct information of tumor type and whether it is benign or malignant. Exceptions exist and tumors can mimic each other. MR spectroscopy (MRS) enables the reader to assess the biology and certain metabolites of various tissues in a noninvasive way. This metabolic information obtained from MRS can be used to complement the MR and CT information to give an additional dimension to predict the tumor aggressiveness. The MRS appearance of normal gray and white matter at a given age is predictable. A control spectrum from the normal-appearing corresponding brain area serves an internal control, especially in young children with developing brain. Age-associated brain maturation of young pediatric brain (from birth to 2 years) and normal MRS appearance has been well reviewed in the literature.

The best tumor marker for pediatric brain tumors in MRS is choline (Cho) peak which is easily visualized in both long and short echo-time studies. In the pediatric population malignant transformation of low-grade brain tumor is uncommon. Marked change especially in the Cho peak is a cause of concern since stable disease gives consistent spectra over time. Although it has been hypothesized that malignant tumors have a high metabolic rate, there has been no direct correlation between hypermetabolism detected by PET studies and elevated lactate in MRS. Elevated lactate has been documented in mixed glioma: ependymoma-astrocytoma, ganglioglioma and teratoma. On the other hand in some PNET no lactate was seen. Elevated lactate suggests either oxygen deprivation or a defect in cancer cell metabolism. It is not uncommon to see a lipid signal that may prevent the detection of lactate since they both resonate at 1.3 ppm.

As a general rule, contrast-enhanced MRI scans in a child with brain tumor has a higher diagnostic value than MRS. Since MRS is usually obtained following the contrast injection, the reader must be aware of potential sources of error. The presence of low molecular weight gadolinium contrast which accumulates in enhancing tumor can cause broadening of the MR spectra in strongly enhancing tumors. The Cho peak may be even decreased more than 15% in MRS if done following contrast enhancement.

Tumor imaging and MRS are also discussed in chapter 6.

Suggested Reading

Alger JR, Frank JA, Bizzi A, et al (1990) Metabolism of human gliomas: assessment with H-1 MR spectroscopy and F-18 fluorodeoxyglucose PET. Radiology 177:633–641

Bulakbasi N, Kocaoglu M, Ors F, Tayfun C, Ucoz T (2003) Combination of single-voxel proton MR spectroscopy and apparent diffusion coefficient calculation in the evaluation of common brain tumors. AJNR Am J Neuroradiol 24:225–233

Castillo M, Smith JK, Kwock L, Wilber K (2001) Apparent diffusion coefficients in the evaluation of high-grade cerebral gliomas. AJNR Am J Neuroradiol 22:60–64

Crist WM, Kun LE (1991) Common solid tumors of childhood. N Engl J Med 324:461–471

Di Chiro G, de la Paz RL, Brooks RA, et al (1982) Glucose utilization of the cerebral gliomas measured by [18F]fluorodeoxyglucose and positron emission tomography. Neurology 32:1323–1329

Farwell JR, Dohrmann GJ, Flannery JT (1977) Central nervous system tumors in children. Cancer 40:3123–3132

Gauvain KM, McKinstry RC, Mukherjee P, et al (2001) Evaluating pediatric brain tumor cellularity with diffusion-tensor imaging. AJR Am J Roentgenol 177:449–454

Guo AC, Cummings TJ, Dash RC, Provenzale JM (2002) Lymphomas and high-grade astrocytomas: comparison of water diffusibility and histologic characteristics. Radiology 224:177–183

Klisch J, Husstedt H, Hennings S, von Velthoven V, Pagenstecher A, Schumacher M (2000) Supratentorial primitive neuroectodermal tumours: diffusion-weighted MRI. Neuroradiology 42:393–398

Kono K, Inoue Y, Nakayama K, et al (2001) The role of diffusion-weighted imaging in patients with brain tumors. AJNR Am J Neuroradiol 22:1081–1088

Kotsenas AL, Roth TC, Manness WK, Faerber EN (1999) Abnormal diffusion-weighted MRI in medulloblastoma: does it reflect small cell histology? Pediatr Radiol 29:524–526

Kreis R, Ernst T, Ross BD (1993) Development of the human brain: in vivo quantification of metabolite and water content with proton magnetic resonance spectroscopy. Magn Reson Med 30:424

Pollack IF (1994) Brain tumors in children. N Engl J Med 331:1500–1507

Sijens PE, van den Bent MJ, Nowak PJCM, et al (1997) ¹H chemical shift imaging reveals loss of brain tumor choline signal after administration of Gd-contrast. Magn Reson Med 37:222–225

Stadnik TW, Chaskis C, Michotte A, et al (2001) Diffusion-weighted MR imaging of intracerebral masses: comparison with conventional MR imaging and histologic findings. AJNR Am J Neuroradiol 22:969–976

Stadnik TW, Demaerel P, Luypaert RR, et al (2003) Imaging tutorial: differential diagnosis of bright lesions on diffusion-weighted MR images. Radiographics 23:E7–7

Sugahara T, Korogi Y, Kochi M, et al (1999) Usefulness of diffusion-weighted MRI with echo-planar technique in the evaluation of cellularity in gliomas. J Magn Reson Imaging 9:53–60

Taylor JS, Reddick WE, Kingsley PB, et al (1995) Proton MRS after gadolinium contrast agent. Programs and abstracts of the Society of Magnetic Resonance Third Scientific Meeting – European Society for Magnetic Resonance in Medicine and Biology 12th annual meeting 1995. Nice Acropolis, Nice, France, p 1854

Tien RD, Felsberg GJ, Friedman H, Brown M, MacFall J (1994) MR imaging of high-grade cerebral gliomas: value of diffusion-weighted echoplanar pulse sequences. AJR Am J Roentgenol 162:671–677

Van der Kamp MS, van der Grond J, van Rijen PC, et al (1990) Age-dependent changes in localized proton and phosphorus MR spectroscopy of the brain. Radiology 176:509

Vezina LG (1997) Diagnostic imaging in neuro-oncology. Pediatr Clin North Am 44:701–719

Wang Z, Sutton LN, Cnaan A, et al (1995) Proton MR spectroscopy of pediatric cerebellar tumors AJNR Am J Neuroradiol 16:1821–1833

Figure 5.1 A–C

Solid medulloblastoma

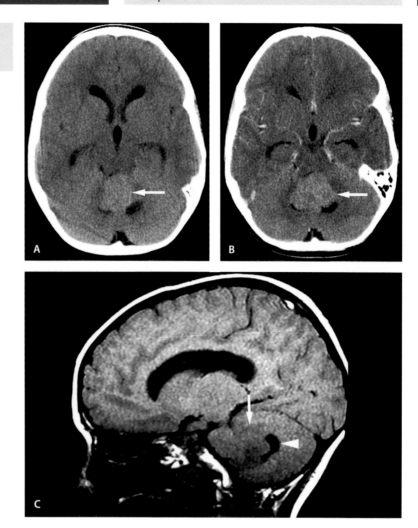

Medulloblastoma

Solid Medulloblastoma

Clinical Presentation

A 9-year-old male with headaches, nausea and vomiting.

Images (Fig. 5.1)

A and B. Noncontrast (A) and contrast-enhanced (B) CT scans show slightly hyperdense vermian mass (*arrow*) with mild, but homogeneous enhancement (B). The mass produces hydrocephalus

C and D. Sagittal (C) and axial (D) noncontrast T1-weighted image shows slightly hypointense mass (*arrows*) in the inferior vermis. The fourth ventricle is displaced posteriorly (*arrowheads*)

E. T2-weighted image shows the mass to be hyperintense (*arrow*). There is a mass effect upon the fourth ventricle and pons

F. Contrast-enhanced sagittal T1-weighted image shows intense and homogeneous enhancement in the mass (*arrow*)

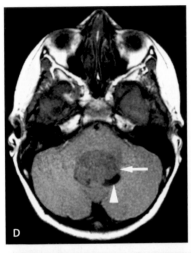
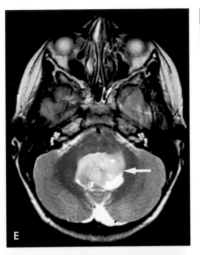

Figure 5.1 D–F

Solid medulloblastoma

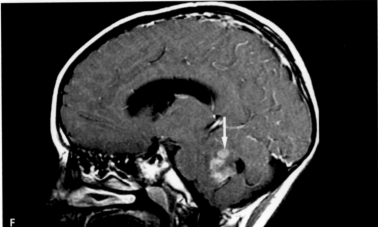

Hemorrhagic/Necrotic Medulloblastoma

Clinical Presentation

A 9-year-old female with persistent nausea and vomiting and headaches.

Images (Fig. 5.2)

A and B.
  Sagittal (A) and axial (B) T1-weighted images through the posterior fossa show a mixed right paramidline mass (*arrows*) with peritumoral edema and hemorrhage. Hydrocephalus is present

C. T2-weighted image shows heterogeneous signal indicating blood products (*arrowheads*), mass effect and marked peritumoral edema

D. FLAIR image separates well the tumor mass (*arrow*), blood products (*arrowhead*) and peritumoral edema (*small arrowheads*)

E. Contrast-enhanced T1-weighted image shows intense enhancement within the tumor

F. Gradient echo image shows better the hemorrhagic area (*arrowhead*)

G. DW image shows mainly hypointensity due to blood products (*arrowhead*). A small nonhemorrhagic tumor area shows hyperintensity (*arrow*). Note that vasogenic edema is not visualized on the DW image; it is best seen in the T2-weighted and FLAIR images

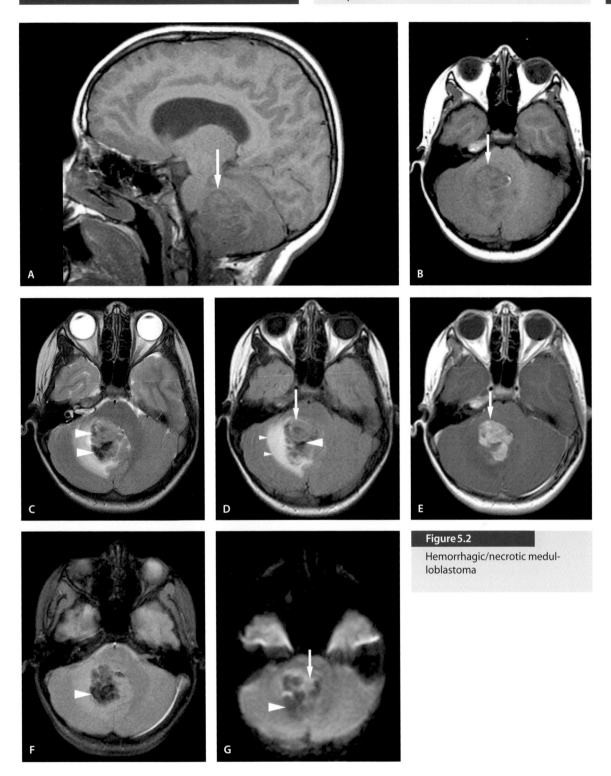

Figure 5.2

Hemorrhagic/necrotic medulloblastoma

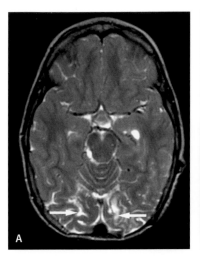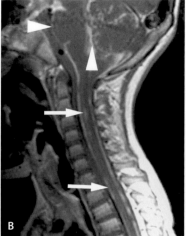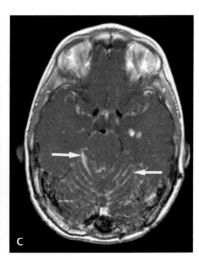

Figure 5.3

Medulloblastoma with CSF seeding

Medulloblastoma with CSF Seeding

Clinical Presentation

A 9-year-old male with persistent nausea and vomiting. Patient has known medulloblastoma operated earlier in the same year.

Images (Fig. 5.3)

A. T2-weighted image shows edematous meninges in the occipital lobes (*arrows*) and superior vermis
B. Sagittal T1-weighted contrast-enhanced image shows meningeal enhancement ("sugar coating") in the surface of the pons (*arrowheads*) and cerebellum. Meningeal enhancement and multiple enhancing nodules along the spinal cord (*arrows*) are also present
C. Contrast-enhanced T1-weighted image through the posterior fossa and temporal lobes shows intense but irregular meningeal enhancement (*arrows*) consistent with CSF seeding ("malignant meningitis") of the known medulloblastoma

Discussion

Medulloblastomas are malignant PNET tumors that account for 25% of all intracranial neoplasms in infants and children. They are the most common posterior fossa tumor in children. Most tumors occur in the first 10 years of life. They are most commonly seen involving the cerebellar vermis and they protrude into the fourth ventricle. They may have focal areas of necrosis and hemorrhage. Medulloblastomas are the most common tumor to disseminate along the CSF pathways (see case no. 3). Approximately 40% of patients demonstrate CSF seeding or solid CNS metastasis at the time of initial diagnosis. On CT, they are seen as an iso- to hyperdense mass with uniform enhancement. Calcification occurs in 10 to 20% of cases. MR appearances are variable. They are usually hypointense on T1-weighted and heterogeneous on T2-weighted images. The heterogeneity in the T2-weighted image is secondary to calcification, cysts, necrosis, hemorrhage and vascular flow voids. Disseminated medulloblastoma is predominantly seen in leptomeningeal area but rarely may involve vertebral marrow. Metastatic or recurrent medulloblastoma may or may not enhance leading to a potential underestimation of the disease process. Enhancement is marked and variable in the primary tumor. Contrast-enhanced MR imaging is the modality of choice for detection of disseminated disease in the pial margins of the spinal cord and along other CSF pathways ("sugar coating" and "malignant or neoplastic meningitis"). This neoplastic meningitis can be the sole presentation of the neoplasm without a detectable mass lesion.

Suggested Reading

Jennings M, Slatkin N, D'Angelo M, et al (1993) Neoplastic meningitis as the sole presentation of an occult CNS primitive neuroectodermal tumor. J Child Neurol 8:306–312

Kleihues P, Burger PC, Scheithauer BW (1993) Histological classification of CNS tumors. In: Sobin LH (ed) Histological typing of tumors of the central nervous system, 2nd edn. Springer, Berlin Heidelberg New York, pp 1–105

Mayers SP, Kemp SS, Tarr RW (1992) MR imaging features of medulloblastomas. AJNR Am J Neuroradiol 158:859–865

Meyers SP, Wildenhain SL, Chang JK, et al (2000) Postoperative evaluation for disseminated medulloblastoma involving the spine: contrast-enhanced MR findings, CSF cytologic analysis, timing of disease occurrence, and patient outcomes. AJNR Am J Neuroradiol 21:1757–1765

Tortori-Donati P, Fondelli MP, Rossi A, et al (1995) Medulloblastoma in children: CT and MRI findings. Neuroradiology 38:352–359

Cerebellar Pilocytic Astrocytoma

Mostly Solid Cerebellar Pilocytic Astrocytoma

Clinical Presentation

A 3-year-old female with vomiting and headache.

Images (Fig. 5.4)

A. T1-weighted image shows a hypointense lesion in the superior vermis (*arrow*)

B. T2-weighted image shows a heterogeneous, but mainly hyperintense lesion in the vermis consistent with cystic and solid parts of the tumor (*arrow*)

C. Contrast-enhanced T1-weighted image shows enhancement of the nodule (*arrow*)

D. DW image shows an iso- to hypointense lesion in the vermis (*arrow*)

E. Single voxel MRS with TE 144 ms of the mural nodule shows mildly decreased N-acetyl aspartate and increased Cho peaks with a small lactate peak

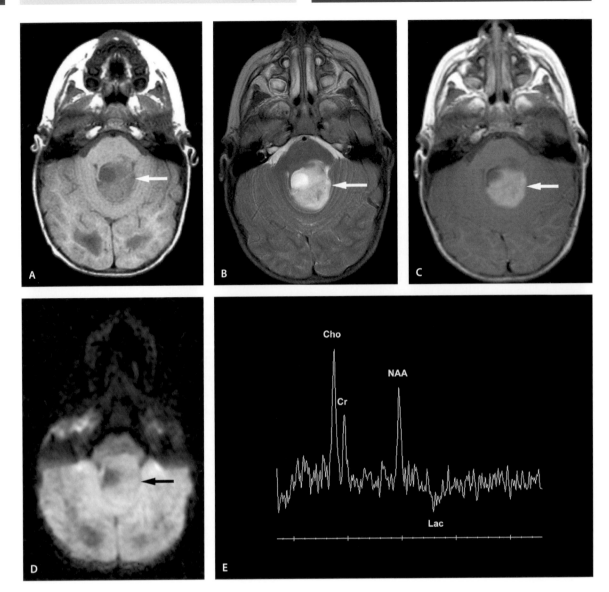

Figure 5.4

Mostly solid cerebellar pilocytic astrocytoma

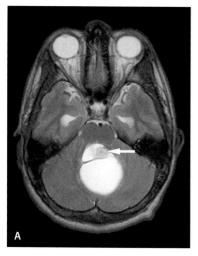 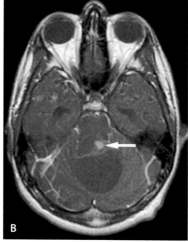 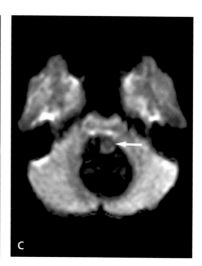

Figure 5.5

Cystic cerebellar pilocytic astrocytoma with mural nodule

Cystic Cerebellar Pilocytic Astrocytoma with Mural Nodule

Clinical Presentation

A 14-year-old male with headache.

Images (Fig. 5.5)

A. T2-weighted image shows a hyperintense mass in the cerebellum with a mural nodule in the tumor (*arrow*)
B. Contrast-enhanced T1-weighted image shows enhancement in the nodule (*arrow*)
C. DW image shows marked hypointense cystic component with mild hypointensity in the nodule (*arrow*)

Discussion

Cerebellar astrocytoma is the second most common posterior fossa tumor in children. About 75% of cerebellar astrocytomas are benign juvenile pilocytic astrocytomas (JPA) and the rest are fibrillary, diffuse astrocytomas. The peak incidence of JPA is in the first decade of life and in the fibrillary form later in childhood or in young adulthood.

Because of the benign nature and slow growth of the JPA the tumor is usually large at presentation. Hydrocephalus is a common presenting symptom. JPA may arise from vermis or hemisphere. Calcification is an infrequent finding. Nearly 50% of tumors are cystic with an enhancing mural nodule. The mural nodule is the tumor and the cyst wall does not include tumor cells. About 40% of tumors are solid with cystic or necrotic centers and the rest are solid mass lesions.

On CT the cyst is usually of higher density than the CSF owing to its higher protein content. On T1- and T2-weighted images the cyst signal is higher than that of the CSF partially for the same reason, and partially because of lack of CSF flow. The mural nodule enhances with gadolinium. The solid tumors show usually heterogeneous enhancement.

Despite the benign histology of pilocytic astrocytomas, a lactate peak has been reported to be commonly present in these tumors. Elevated lactate is commonly a marker of necrosis or ischemia but an altered metabolic pathway is also suspected as in pilocytic astrocytomas. Since increased lipids are seen in necrosis and malignant lesions, the lack of it suggests that increased lactate is related to another mechanism than necrosis and malignancy as seen in this case. Another feature of JPA that also mimics a malignant behavior is increased glucose utilization at FDG PET study. These paradoxical features make the role of MR imaging even more important in estimation of the tumor recurrence.

Suggested Reading

Felix R, Schorner W, Laniado M, et al (1985) Brain tumors: MR imaging with gadolinium-DTPA. Radiology 156:681–688

Fulham MJ, Melisi JW, Nishimiya J, Dwyer AJ, di Chiro G (1993) Neuroimaging of juvenile pilocytic astrocytomas: an enigma. Radiology 189:221–225

Hwang J-H, Egnaczyk GF, Ballard E, Dunn RS, Holland SK, Ball WS (1998) Proton MR spectroscopic characteristic of pediatric pilocytic astrocytomas. AJNR Am J Neuroradiol 19:535–540

Ependymoma

Clinical Presentation

A 32-month-old female with vomiting and ataxia.

Images

Initial Study (Fig. 5.6 A–D)

A. Noncontrast CT shows a slightly hyperdense mass in the tentorial incisura (*arrow*). There is hydrocephalus
B. T1-weighted image shows hypointense tumor in the tentorial incisura (*arrow*). Hydrocephalus with transependymal CSF leak is present
C. The tumor is isointense to gray matter on T2-weighted image (*arrow*)
D. Contrast-enhanced T1-weighted image shows homogeneous enhancement

Follow-up MRI at the Age of 14 Years (Fig. 5.6 E–J)

E. Sagittal T1-weighted image shows a large hemorrhagic mass (*arrows*) compressing the brainstem and midline structures
F. T2-weighted image shows a large mixed signal lesion that involves the major part of the central brain (*arrow*). The hyperintense signal in the center of the lesion is consistent with necrosis (*arrowhead*). Enlarged and displaced ventricles are seen
G. Contrast-enhanced T1-weighted image shows an intense enhancement (*arrow*) with nonenhancing necrotic areas (*arrowhead*)
H. Contrast-enhanced coronal spoiled gradient recalled echo (SPGR) image shows best the full extent of the tumor
I. DW image shows heterogeneous intensity in the solid component of the tumor (*arrows*). The necrotic portion shows hypointensity (*arrowhead*)
J. ADC map shows heterogeneous intensity in the tumor. Some parts of the solid component show mild hypo- to isointensity which might represent hypercellularity (*arrows*). The necrotic component shows hyperintensity representing increased diffusibility (*arrowhead*).

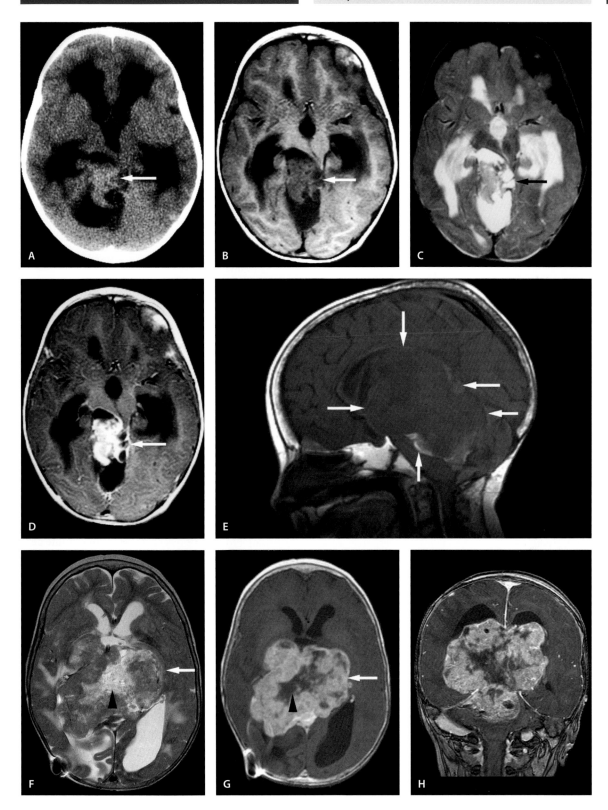

Figure 5.6 A–H

Ependymoma

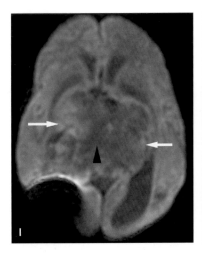
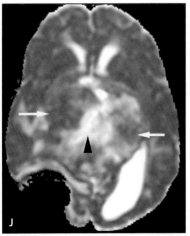

Figure 5.6 I, J
Ependymoma

Discussion

Ependymomas account for 10 % of all pediatric brain tumors and are the third most common fourth ventricular neoplasm in children. The peak incidence of infratentorial ependymomas is 5 years of age. Approximately 70 % of ependymomas are infratentorial. They arise in the epithelial lining of the fourth ventricle and extend into the lateral recesses and through the foramina of Luschka into the cerebellopontine angle cisterns. Posteroinferior extension through the foramen of Magendie into the cisterna magna is also common. Metastasis occurs along the CSF pathways and it is almost always intraspinal. On CT, the ependymomas appear as an iso- to hyperdense intraventricular mass with multifocal calcification and moderate enhancement. On MRI, they are seen as a heterogeneously hypointense mass on T1-weighted and an iso- to hypointense mass on T2-weighted images. Foci of high signal are seen representing necrotic or cystic tissue and low-signal areas as calcification and hemorrhage. Heterogeneous enhancement is seen after gadolinium administration.

Suggested Reading

Lefton DR, Pinto RS, Martin SW (1998) MRI features of intracranial and spinal ependymomas. Pediatr Neurosurg 28:97–105

Osborn AG, Rauschning W (1994) Brain tumors and tumor-like masses – classifications and differential diagnosis. In: Osborn AG (ed) Diagnostic neuroradiology. Mosby, St Louis

Brain Stem Glioma

Clinical Presentation

An 8-year-old female presents with headaches and hydrocephalus.

Images (Fig. 5.7)

A. T2-weighted image shows a hyperintense lesion in the pons with pons edema and expansion (*arrow*). The basilar artery is encased by the lesion (*arrowhead*). The fourth ventricle is distorted

B. T1-weighted image shows a hypointense lesion with ill-defined borders (*arrow*)

C. Contrast-enhanced T1-weighted image shows no appreciable enhancement

D. DW image shows isointensity of the lesion (*arrow*)

Figure 5.7

Brain stem glioma

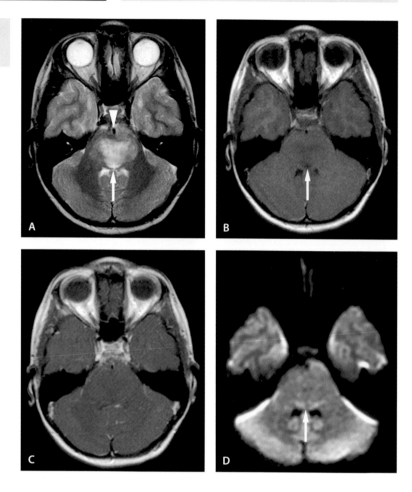

Discussion

Brain stem tumors usually arise within the pons and less frequently in the medulla or midbrain. Pontine gliomas represent about 30 % of posterior fossa tumors in children. Symptoms of hydrocephalus and cranial nerve neuropathy are common at presentation. The peak incidence is usually before the age of 10 years. The brain stem gliomas consist of slow-growing fibrillary or pilocytic astrocytomas and less commonly anaplastic astrocytomas and glioblastomas. The most common tumors (80 %) are diffuse fibrillary astrocytomas. A number of fibrillary astrocytomas present with necrosis and hemorrhagic foci that are uncommon in pilocytic astrocytomas. The typical appearance is enlarged pons with obliteration of the adjacent cisterns and compression on the fourth ventricle causing hydrocephalus. Encasement of the basilar artery is not an uncommon finding. On CT scan the lesions are predominantly hypodense.

Following contrast injections half of the tumors enhance minimally. More than half of the tumors demonstrate exophytic extension to the cerebellopontine angle cistern. MRI is clearly superior to CT in detecting pons gliomas. On noncontrast MR images the lesions are hypointense on T1-weighted images and hyperintense on FLAIR and T2-weighted images. Following contrast injection, gadolinium enhancement is better appreciated on T1-weighted image than CT enhancement.

Suggested Reading

Barkovich AJ, Edwards MSB (1995) Brain tumors in childhood. In: Barkovitch AJ (ed) Pediatric neuroimaging. Raven, New York, p 321

Guo AC, Cummings TJ, Dash RC, Provenzale JM (2002) Lymphomas and high grade astrocytomas: comparison of water diffusibility and histologic characteristics. Radiology 224:177–183

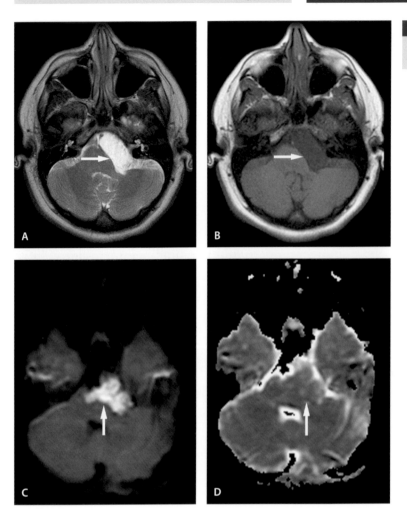

Figure 5.8
Epidermoid tumor

Epidermoid Tumor

Clinical Presentation

A 23-year-old female with long history of headache and known cerebellopontine angle mass.

Images (Fig. 5.8)

A. T2-weighted image shows a hyperintense mass in the left cerebellopontine angle (*arrow*)
B. T1-weighted image shows a hypointense mass (*arrow*)
C. DW image shows hyperintensity in the mass (*arrow*)
D. ADC of this mass is similar to that of brain parenchyma (*arrow*)

Figure 5.9

Arachnoid cyst

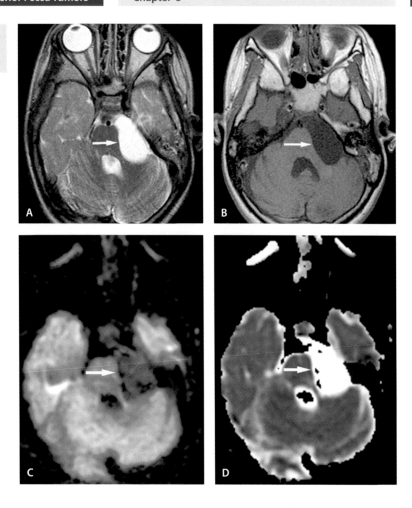

Arachnoid Cyst

Clinical Presentation

A 9-year-old female with developmental delay.

Images (Fig. 5.9)

A. T2-weighted image shows a hyperintense mass in the left cerebellopontine angle (*arrow*)
B. T1-weighted image shows the hypointense mass (*arrow*)
C. DW image shows hypointensity in the mass (*arrow*)
D. ADC map shows marked hyperintensity (*arrow*) similar to that of the CSF

Discussion

Epidermoid tumors are benign neoplasms of ectodermal origin with stratified squamous epithelium and keratinaceous debris. These lesions are typically located away from the midline and are common in the cerebellopontine angle. The findings of CT and T1- and T2-weighted MR imaging are similar to those for arachnoid cyst or CSF. FLAIR images, constructive interference steady-state (CISS) images and DW images can be used to make the distinction between epidermoid tumors and arachnoid cysts. DW images show typical hyperintensity in epidermoid tumors. ADC of epidermoid tumors is reported to be lower than that of CSF and equal to or higher than that of brain parenchyma. Therefore, the hyperintensity of epidermoid tumors on DW images is primarily caused by a T2 shine-through effect.

Suggested Reading

Bergui M, Zhong J, Bradae GB, Sales S (2001) Diffusion-weighted images of intracranial cyst-like lesions. Neuroradiology 43:824–829

Chen S, Ikawa F, Kurisu K, Arita K, Takaba J, Kanou Y (2001) Quantitative MR evaluation of intracranial epidermoid tumors by fast fluid-attenuated inversion recovery imaging and echo-planar diffusion-weighted imaging. AJNR Am J Neuroradiol 22:1089–1096

Maeda M, Kawamura Y, Tamagawa Y (1992) Intravoxel incoherent motion (IVIM) MRI in intracranial, extraaxial tumors and cysts. J Comput Assist Tomogr 16:514–518

Tsuruda JS, Chew WM, Moseley ME, Norman D (1990) Diffusion-weighted MR imaging of the brain: value of differentiating between extraaxial cysts and epidermoid tumors. AJNR Am J Neuroradiol 11:925–931

Von Hippel-Lindau Disease (VHL)

Clinical Presentation

A 20-year-old male with family history of VHL disease has been followed for years for enhancing cerebellar and cord lesions.

Images (Fig. 5.10)

A. T2-weighted image shows left cerebellar edema (*arrow*) and right paramedullary nodule (*arrowhead*)

B. FLAIR image shows two high-signal areas, one in the left cerebellar hemisphere (*arrow*) and the other in the right paramedullary area (*arrowhead*)

C. T1-weighted image with gadolinium shows intense enhancement of these lesions

D. Coronal contrast-enhanced SPGR image shows intense enhancing left cerebellar hemangioblastoma (*arrow*)

E. Coronal contrast-enhanced SPGR image shows exophytic growth of the medullary lesion

F. Coronal contrast-enhanced SPGR image through the cervical cord shows an enhancing mass in the cord (*arrow*)

G. DW image shows hypointensity in the left cerebellar hemisphere and paramedullary lesions (*arrow*)

Discussion

Hemangioblastomas are benign (WHO grade I) tumors that occur in the cerebellum, brain stem and spinal cord. They are the most common tumors in VHL disease, affecting 60–80% of all patients. The responsible gene in VHL disease has been mapped to the short arm of chromosome 3.

In addition to CNS lesions, other manifestations include retinal angioma, renal cell carcinoma, adrenal pheochromocytoma, as well as benign cysts in the lungs, liver, kidneys, and pancreas. Compared with sporadic cases of hemangioblastomas, the tumors in VHL disease develop at an earlier age and are often multifocal. Multiple hemangioblastomas occur in up to 20% of patients with VHL disease.

On CT, hemangioblastomas may mimic astrocytomas, with a large cystic mass and an enhancing mural nodule. They can also be solid tumors. The cystic portion of the mass is nonneoplastic and does not enhance. The main differential diagnosis is pilocytic astrocytoma which typically occurs in a younger age group. On MR imaging, the cystic component is typically slightly hyperintense to the CSF signal unless associated with hemorrhage. The mural nodule shows moderate to marked enhancement. The solid tumors are also intense enhancing lesions.

Suggested Reading

Elster AD, Arthur DW (1988) intracranial hemangioblastomas: CT and MR findings. J Comput Assist Tomogr 12:736–739

Slater A, Moore NR, Huson SM (2003) The natural history of cerebellar hemangioblastomas in von Hippel-Lindau disease. AJNR Am J Neuroradiol 24:1570–1574

Yamashita J, Handa H, Kim C, Kim S (1982) Familial occurrence of cerebellar hemangioblastomas; analysis of five families. Neurosurgery 11:761–763

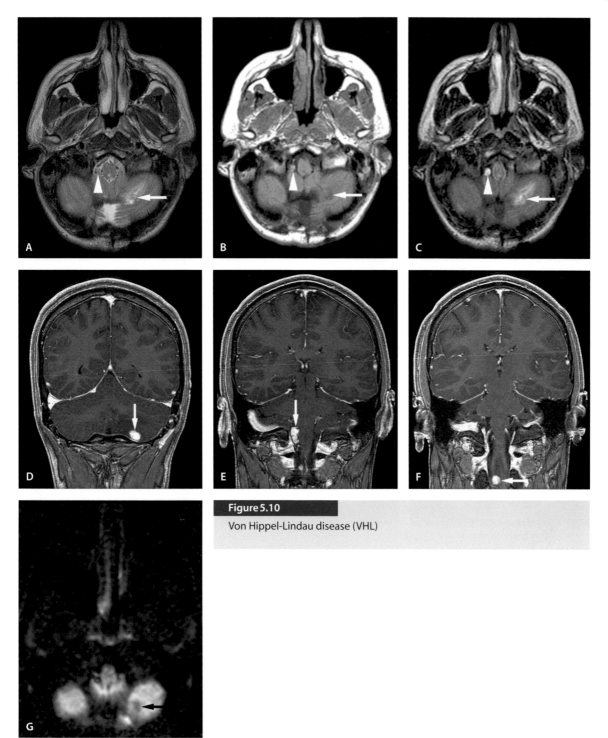

Figure 5.10

Von Hippel-Lindau disease (VHL)

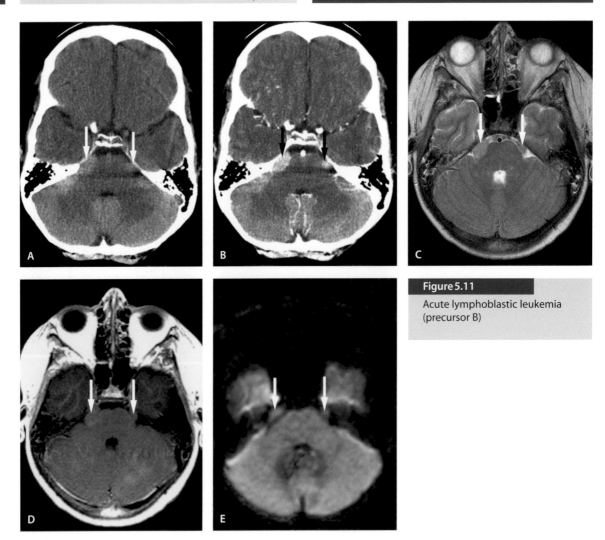

Figure 5.11
Acute lymphoblastic leukemia
(precursor B)

Acute Lymphoblastic Leukemia (Precursor B)

Clinical Presentation

A 15-year-old male with mental status changes.

Images (Fig. 5.11)

A. Noncontrast CT shows hyperdense masses in both cerebellopontine angles (*arrows*)
B. Contrast-enhanced CT shows homogeneous enhancement in these lesions (*arrows*)
C. T2-weighted image shows mild hyperintensity (*arrows*)
D. Contrast-enhanced T1-weighted image shows minimal enhancement
E. DW image shows isointensity (*arrows*)

Discussion

Granulocytic sarcoma is a rare extramedullary collection of granulocytic cells, also known as chloroma. It is seen in 3% to 8% of all patients with acute myelogenous leukemia, and other myeloproliferative disorders. They can be seen as parenchymal and meningeal lesions and hemorrhage may occur. Typically, granulocytic sarcomas are isodense or hyperdense to brain on noncontrast CT. T2-weighted images show iso- to hyperintensity and T1-weighted images show hypo- to isointensity with variable enhancement. In this case, the differential diagnoses include other cerebellopontine angle tumors, such as acoustic neuroma. To our knowledge, no case series study of DW imaging and MR spectroscopic findings has been reported.

Suggested Reading

Barnett MJ, Zussman WV (1986) Granulocytic sarcoma of the brain: a case report and review of the literature. Radiology 160:223–225

Pui MH, Fletcher BD, Langston JW (1994) Granulocytic sarcoma in childhood leukemia: imaging features. Radiology 190:698–702

Vazquez E, Lucaya J, Castellote A (2002) Neuroimaging in pediatric leukemia and lymphoma: differential diagnosis. Radiographics 22:1411–1428

Chordoma

Clinical Presentation

An 18-year-old female with history of surgery and radiation for clivus chordoma. Now the patient has swallowing difficulties.

Images (Fig. 5.12)

A. Sagittal T1-weighted image shows a large tumor centered at the clivus (*arrow*). The mass is isointense to the brain tissue. The medulla and upper cord are pushed posteriorly (*arrowheads*). Radiation changes are seen in C2 and C3 vertebral bodies that appear hyperintense due to fatty replacement of the bone marrow

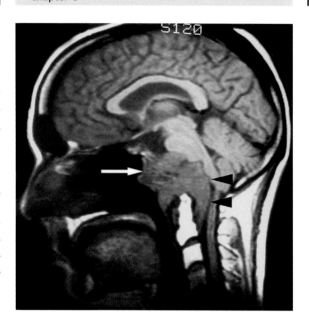

Figure 5.12
Chordoma

Discussion

Chordomas are locally aggressive tumors of the notochordal region. Chordomas are distinctly uncommon neoplasm in the first two decades of life. Chordomas commonly arise in the sacrococcygeal (50–60%) or sphenooccipital regions (25–40%). The vertebral column may rarely be involved.

On CT scan, chordoma typically appears as a well-circumscribed, expansile soft-tissue mass with extensive bone destruction. Calcification is seen in 50–70% of cases. On T1-weighted images, chordomas are seen as intermediate to low intensity and are easily recognized within the high intensity fat of the clivus. On T2-weighted images, they characteristically demonstrate very high signal intensity. Chordomas show moderate to marked heterogeneous enhancement. The multiplanar capability of MR is particularly useful for surgical planning. After treatment tumors may recur at the primary site or may form nodal or distant metastases. Metastasis at the primary site is the more common form of treatment failure. Another treatment failure may be seen along the surgical pathway. The distant metastases are reported to occur at the lungs, lymph nodes, skin, liver and bone.

Suggested Reading

Fischbein NJ, Kaplan MJ, Holliday RA, Dillon WP (2000) Recurrence of clival chordoma along the surgical pathway. AJNR Am J Neuroradiol 21:578–583

Handa J, Suzuki F, Nioka H, Koyama T (1987) Clivus chordoma in childhood. Surg Neurol 28:58–62

Supratentorial Brain Tumors

Introduction

The central nervous system (CNS) is the most common site for solid tumors in children. Of all intracranial tumors 15–20% occur in childhood. CNS malignancy in the pediatric age group is the second most common form of malignancy after hematological malignancies.

Studies before the introduction of cross-sectional imaging showed infratentorial tumors to be more common than supratentorial. However, the new imaging techniques have changed this concept and brain tumors are clearly evenly divided between the supra- and infratentorial compartments. Supratentorial tumors are more common in neonates and children under the age of 3 years, whereas infratentorial tumors are more common in children from 4 to 11 years of age.

In a pathologically proven material of 269 pediatric brain tumors (Texas Children's Hospital, Houston) over a 10-year period the most common supratentorial tumor were gliomas and gangliogliomas followed by primitive neuroectodermal tumors (PNET) and craniopharyngiomas.

The location of supratentorial brain tumors can aid in the differential diagnosis. Intraaxial hemispheric tumors include tumors of glial origin – astrocytoma, oligodendroglioma, ependymoma and pleomorphic xanthoastrocytoma (PXA) – and rare metastases. Neoplastic lesions of the basal ganglia and thalamus include gliomas and lymphomas. Extraaxial tumors arise in the sellar and parasellar, pineal and intraventricular regions. Parasellar neoplasms or mass lesions include craniopharyngioma, germ-cell tumors, tumors of maldevelopment (epidermoid, dermoid, teratoma), tumors of optic chiasma and hypothalamus and pituitary neoplasms. Pineal region masses include germ-cell tumors and pineal tumors. Intraventricular neoplasms originate often from the choroid plexus (papilloma and choroid plexus carcinoma) or subependymal layer (ependymoma, giant cell astrocytoma, PNET, central neurocytoma). Meningiomas and teratomas can occur in the region as well.

Imaging studies such as CT and MR imaging play an important role in the diagnosis and anatomic location of intracranial tumors. The imaging tests provide information about the morphology and pathology of mass lesions. There have been numerous histopathological classifications of primary brain tumors since that of Bailey and Cushing in 1926. Current tumor classification is based on the predominant cell type and graded based on the highest evidence of malignancy in the tissue sample. There is, however, an inherent problem with this system. If the sampling volume is small such as may occur in stereotactic biopsies, scattered foci or more malignant cells may escape attention. This leads to underestimation of tumor grade. Many brain tumors in children are relatively benign and can be successfully treated. This is contrary to commonly seen adult gliomas for which survival figures are much worse and malignant transformation of low-grade gliomas is a frequent and expected occurrence.

CT and MR studies are complimentary tests. The advantage of MRI is its ability to scan the brain in three planes without bone-related artifacts. Gadolinium-enhanced MRI is superior to nonenhanced MRI or CT. However, CT is more sensitive than MRI in detecting small foci of calcification or subarachnoid bleed. Gradient-echo images improve the ability of MRI to demonstrate calcification or blood products. Although the gradient-echo image improves the detection of calcium and blood, they both may exhibit similar signal characteristics. Most tumors demonstrate low signal on T1-weighted images and are hyperintense in spin-echo T2-weighted images and FLAIR sequence. Increased signal on T1-weighted images is seen in neoplasms with chronic blood (methemoglobin), fat, high protein concentration or melanin. Flow-related enhancement of the vessels appear as high signal on T1-weighted images as well. Decreased signal on T2-weighted images is usually related to blood products of various ages (deoxy-hemoglobin, intracellular methemoglobin, hemosiderin), calcification, fibrocollagenous stroma of the tumor, high protein concentration and flow voids in vasculature. Dense cellularity with limited cytoplasm can appear as low signal on T2-weighted images.

Tumor enhancement seen in both CT and MR imaging often helps to find the anatomic location of the lesion in addition to characterizing the tumor. The tumor enhancement implies a disturbance in the blood-brain barrier, a large blood pool or tumor arising in the structure without the blood-brain barrier. The tumor calcification can be dystrophic or part of the interstitial matrix of the lesion. The tumor may contain cystic regions that are smooth and well-marginated and containing fluid. The fluid can simulate cerebrospinal fluid or have variant concentrations of protein, cholesterol or paramagnetic ions or blood products. Necrosis is due to ischemia in the tumor when it outgrows its blood supply. The necrotic cavity is typically irregular in appearance, and has a concentric irregular wall with uneven enhancement.

DW Imaging

Diffusion weighted imaging with ADC map and exponential image have been increasingly used, not only in ischemia diagnosis, but also in the diagnosis of neoplastic lesions, regardless of the controversial opinions of its usefulness in tumor diagnosis. For more details of this subject the reader is referred to chapter 5.

MR Spectroscopy

In addition to the traditional anatomic CT and MR imaging, analysis of certain metabolites in the tumor tissue can facilitate the differential diagnosis and provide information on a tumor's biological characteristics and response to treatment. The basics of MR spectroscopy and various imaging techniques have been well reviewed in the literature. Tumor recurrence and change in biological degree of malignancy may also be seen with MR spectroscopy. The MR spectroscopic imaging method analyzes certain metabolites either in the signal voxel region or in multiple voxel areas. Multiple voxel studies in which gradient-based phase encoding is used to encode two of the spatial dimensions generate spectra from a large number of voxels within a slab of tissue. Since the MR spectroscopy metabolite pattern of a normal brain at a given age is known and predictable, deviation of the normal metabolites can give additional information on the tumor composition, grade and change of grade over time or response to treatment. In evaluating young children's MR spectroscopy pattern, the normal brain development must be taken into account. The spectroscopy changes are particularly significant during rapid brain development and maturation from birth to 2 years of age.

Proton MR spectroscopy differentiates normal brain from abnormal tissue easily. In short- and long-echo time MR spectroscopy techniques the most obvious peak is that of an N-acetyl aspartate (NAA) that is a marker of mature neuron density and viability and is therefore decreased in all tumors in which healthy neurons are substitute with malignant cells. During rapid brain development (birth to 2 years), the NAA levels rises fourfold. The NAA peak continues to increase slowly with age into adolescence.

Choline (Cho) is one of the most important peaks when analyzing brain tumors. It reflects the metabolism of cellular membrane turnover. It is increased in all processes leading to hypercellularity. It is not specific for neoplastic lesions and increased Cho peaks are also seen in many other processes. The Cho peak is increased in all primary and secondary brain tumors, and there is evidence that higher choline/creatine ratios are found in highly malignant tumors. It may not be used solely for the purpose of grading the tumor. Elevated Cho is also been seen in the young developing brain, demyelinating disorders involving remyelination such as multiple sclerosis and in acute disseminated encephalomyelitis. Although an increased Cho peak indicates cell membrane proliferation, there is no direct relationship between it and the rate of tumor growth. Some slow-growing tumors, such as meningiomas may be rich in Cho and some highly malignant primary brain tumors with considerable necrosis may show decreased Cho.

Under normal conditions lactate is not found in the brain. The presence of lactate indicates that the normal oxidative respiration of the tissue has been altered and carbohydrates are being metabolized by a nonoxidative pathway. This situation occurs in metabolically highly active and cellular lesions that outgrow their blood supply. It is thought that the presence of lactate may indicate a high degree of malignancy. Lipids resonate at similar frequencies to lactate. Lipids are generally found in tumors that contain necrosis and are considered to be an indicator of high-grade malignancy as well.

Suggested Reading

Barker PB, Glickson JD, Bryan RN (1993) In vivo magnetic resonance of human brain tumors. Top Magn Reson Imaging 5:32–45

Barkovich AJ, Edwards MSB (1990) Brain tumors of childhood. In: Barkovich AJ (ed) Pediatric neuroimaging. Raven, New York, pp 149–204

Castillo M, Kwock L, Mukherst SK (1996) Clinical application of proton MR spectroscopy. AJNR Am J Neuroradiol 17: 1–15

Farwell JR, Dohrmann GJ, Flannery JT (1977) Central nervous system tumors in children. Cancer 40:3123–3232

Fitz CR, Rao KCVG (1987) Primary tumors in children. In: Lee SH, Rao KCVG (eds) Cranial computed tomography and MRI. McGraw Hill, New York, pp 365–412

Haddad SF, Menezes AH, Bell WE, et al (1991) Brain tumors occurring before 1 year of age: a retrospective review of 22 cases in an 11-year period (1977–1987). Neurosurgery 29: 8–13

Mercuri S, Russo A, Palma L (1981) Hemispheric supratentorial astrocytomas in children: long term results in 29 cases. J Neurosurg 55:170–173

Moonen CTW, van Zijl PCM, Frank JA, et al (1990) Functional magnetic resonance imaging in medicine and physiology. Science 250:53–61

Naidich TUP, Zimmerman RA (1984) Primary brain tumors in children. Semin Roentgenol 14:100–114

Pfleger MJ, Gerson LP (1993) Supertentorial tumors in children. Neuroimaging Clin North Am 3:671–687

Radkowski MA, Naidich TP, Tomita T, et al (1988) Neonatal brain tumors: CT and MR findings. J Comput Assist Tomogr 12:10–20

Salibi N, Brown MA (1998) Clinical MR spectroscopy. Wiley-Liss, New York

Tomita T, McLone G (1985) Brain tumors during the first twenty-four months of life. Neurosurgery 17:913–919

Glioblastoma Multiforme (GBM)

Clinical Presentation

A 14-year-old female with headaches, diplopia and first seizure of life.

Images (Fig. 6.1)

A. T1-weighetd image shows heterogeneous, mainly hypointense mass (*arrow*) in the left occipitotemporal lobe
B. T2-weighted image shows hyperintense mass (*arrow*) with surrounding edema
C. Contrast-enhanced T1-weighted image shows ring-like enhancement (*arrow*)
D. Coronal contrast-enhanced SPGR image shows enhancement in the periphery (*arrow*) and solid portion of the tumor (*arrowhead*)
E. DW image shows hypointensity in the lesion representing increased diffusibility in the cystic/necrotic portion (*arrow*)

Discussion

Glioblastoma multiforme (GBM) has become synonymous with high-grade astrocytoma. The gliomas are graded based on the most aggressive tumor cell type. As the name implies, these tumors are extremely heterogeneous, often being composed of several different cell populations. Mitoses are frequent. The hallmarks of GBM are microscopic and gross necrosis as well as neovascularity. Many GBM arise within a preexisting lower grade diffuse astrocytoma. They are usually solitary ring enhancing lesions with extensive surrounding vasogenic edema. The rich neovascularity in these tumors is composed of vessels that are freely permeable without a blood-brain barrier. Correlation between imaging and pathology can be lacking, when a tumor with foci of GBM is largely composed of lower grade tissue, thus imaging findings are mainly related to this lower grade tumor. To date no imaging technique can determine the exact lesion boundary. It is a well-known fact that tumor cells extend beyond the enhancing tumor. The most commonly used imaging techniques such as contrast-enhanced CT and MR imaging, MR spectroscopy, CT and MR perfusion study, and diffusion

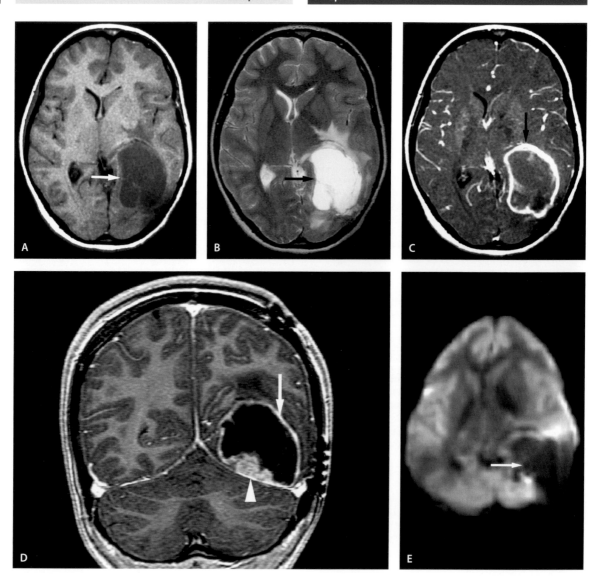

Figure 6.1

Glioblastoma multiforme (GBM)

and metabolic studies (PET) identify only the main bulk of the tumor.

Of all glioblastomas, approximately 3% occur in children. The overall average age of diagnosis is 10 years; however, a biphasic age distribution has been recorded at 4–5 years and 1l–12 years of age. About 90% of childhood GBM occur in the cerebral hemispheres. In children the most common location is within the frontal lobe followed by the parietal lobe, in contrast to adults where frontal lobe tumors are followed in frequency by temporal lobe tumors. Symptoms are non-specific and dependent on the tumor location. They usually include headache, vomiting, paralysis and seizures. MRI appearance of the lesion is usually that of an irregular ring with heterogeneous but strong enhancement. GBM rarely calcify. Hemorrhage and necrosis are similar in children and adults. GBM are diffusely infiltrating and often involve the corpus callosum. Although CSF spread is not a common finding, it can happen.

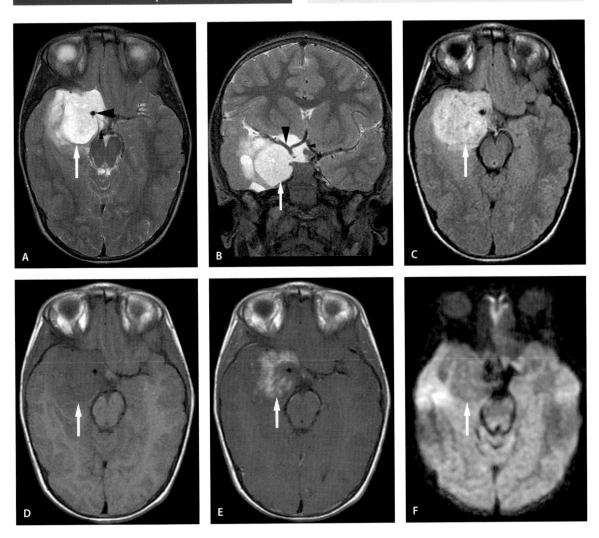

Figure 6.2

Juvenile pilocytic astrocytoma

Suggested Reading

Dohrmann GJ, Farwell JR, Flannery JT (1976) Glioblastoma multiforme in children. J Neurosurg 44:442–448

Juvenile Pilocytic Astrocytoma (JPA)

Clinical Presentation

A 5-year-old female with new onset of seizures.

Images (Fig. 6.2)

A and B. Axial (A) and coronal (B) T2-weighted images demonstrate a large solid high signal mass in the right temporal lobe (*arrows*). The lesion is surrounded by a minimal amount of edema. The right middle cerebral artery is partially encased by the tumor (*arrowheads*). The middle cerebellar artery is displaced upwards on the surface of the lesion. The tumor occupies partially the right side of the suprasellar cistern (*small arrowheads*)

C. FLAIR image shows a solid hyperintense lesion (*arrow*)

D. T1-weighted image demonstrates hypointensity of the lesion (*arrow*)

E. Contrast-enhanced T1-weighted image demonstrates enhancement in the central part of the lesion (*arrow*)

F. DW image shows mild hypointensity of the tumor (*arrow*)

Discussion

Pilocytic astrocytomas are the most common tumor in children and occur typically in the cerebellum, hypothalamus and optic nerves. They occur also in the hemisphere. The peak age of incidence is 7 to 8 years, that is slightly higher than for brain stem or cerebellum astrocytomas. The supratentorial pilocytic astrocytomas are either cystic or multicystic with a mural nodule (55%) or solid mass (45%). The solid portion may sometimes calcify but hemorrhage is rare. MRI usually shows a well-defined solid or cystic mass that is hypointense on T1-weighted image, demonstrates dense enhancement and is hyperintense on T2-weighted and FLAIR image.

Pilocytic astrocytomas are associated with an excellent outcome. In spite of that, PET studies have shown high glucose utilization indicating that also some benign tumor can be metabolically active. In the hypothalamus and in brain stem the clinical course tends to be less favorable. These tumors rarely undergo anaplastic change. The pilocytic astrocytomas present a unique feature: despite their benign nature and histology MR spectroscopy presents a lactate peak without necrosis. A high Cho peak has also been reported.

Suggested Reading

Felix R, Schorner W, Laniado M, et al (1985) Brain tumors: MR imaging with gadolinium-DTPA. Radiology 156:681–688

Fulham MJ, Melisi JW, Nishimiya J, Dwyer AJ, di Chiro G (1993) Neuroimaging of juvenile pilocytic astrocytomas: an enigma. Radiology 189:221–225

Hwang J-H, Egnaczyk GF, Ballard E, Dunn RS, Holland SK, Ball WS (1998) Proton MR spectroscopic characteristic of pediatric pilocytic astrocytomas. AJNR Am J Neuroradiol 19:535–540

Mixed Pleomorphic Xanthoastrocytoma (PXA) and Ganglioglioma

Clinical Presentation

A 13-year-old female with complex partial seizures.

Images (Fig. 6.3)

A. Sagittal precontrast T1-weighted image demonstrates a temporal lobe mass involving the superior and medial temporal gyrus (*arrow*)

B. and C.
Axial (B) and coronal (C) T2-weighted images demonstrate a mixed signal lesion without surrounding edema in the medial temporal lobe (*arrows*)

D. Coronal FLAIR image demonstrates mildly swollen medial temporal lobe with signal abnormality (*arrow*)

E. Contrast-enhanced T1-weighted magnetization transfer image demonstrates minimal enhancement on the lesion (*arrow*)

F. DW image demonstrates isointensity of the lesion (*arrow*)

Discussion

PXA is one of the new tumor categories from 1993 WHO revision. This tumor is a bridge between the low-grade circumscribed astrocytoma with a stable histology and infiltrating diffuse astrocytoma that over time will advance in grade. Because of this malignant potential it is never better than grade II in the tumor classification. Most patients present with seizures. PXA arises from subpial astrocytes in the hemisphere. Microscopically the tumor is pleomorphic. Variable differentiation into neuronal and ganglion cells has been reported. Because of this differentiation some researchers suggest that there is a relationship between PXA and other developmental neoplasms including dysembryoplastic neuroepithelial tumor (DNET) and ganglioglioma. The radiological image is rarely diagnostic, even though it is suggestive. PXA shares many imaging features with DNET and ganglioglioma: they are slow-growing and can cause remodeling in the inner table of the skull. In addition to being a cortical lesion with a mass effect, they are cystic. PXA often mimics pilocytic as-

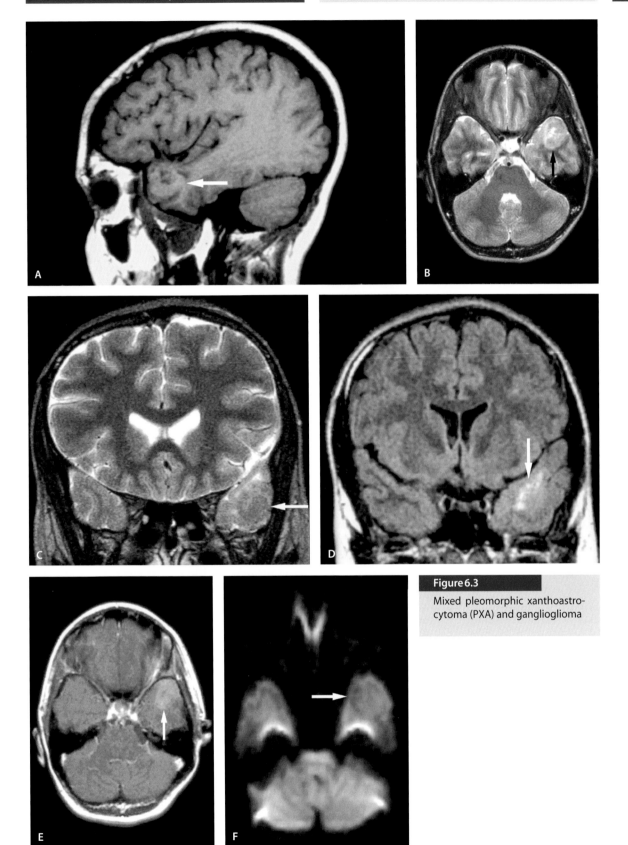

Figure 6.3

Mixed pleomorphic xanthoastro-cytoma (PXA) and ganglioglioma

trocytoma with a cyst with a mural nodule. The mural nodule is usually in the superficial part of the cystic lesion.

Suggested Reading

Kepes JJ (1993) Pleomorphic xanthoastrocytoma: the birth of a diagnosis and a concept. Brain Pathol 3:269–274

Tonn JC, Paulus W, Warmuth-Metz M, et al (1997) Pleomorphic xanthoastrocytoma: report of six cases with special consideration of diagnostic and therapeutic pitfalls. Surg Neurol 47:162–169

Oligodendroglioma

Clinical Presentation

A 17-year-old male with headaches.

Images

Initial Study (Fig. 6.4 A–H)

A. Sagittal T1-weighted image shows a hypointense mass in the left frontal lobe (*arrow*)

B. T1-weighted image shows a hypointense mass in the left frontal lobe (*arrow*)

C. T2-weighted image shows hyperintense mass in the left frontal lobe (*arrow*)

D. Coronal FLAIR image shows hyperintense mass in the left frontal lobe (*arrow*)

E. Contrast-enhanced T1-weighted image shows no significant enhancement (*arrow*)

F. DW image shows heterogeneous hyperintensity (*arrow*)

G. ADC map also shows heterogeneous hyperintensity (*arrow*)

H. MR spectroscopy (TE 144 ms) shows a slightly increased Cho peak with a small lactate peak

Follow-up Study 16 Months Later (Fig. 6.4 I–O)

I. Sagittal T1-weighted image shows a hypointense mass in the left frontal lobe (*arrow*), which is increased in size

J. T1-weighted image shows a hypointense mass in the left frontal lobe (*arrow*), which is increased in size

K. T2-weighted image shows hyperintense mass in the left frontal lobe (*arrow*), which is increased in size

L. Contrast-enhanced T1-weighted image shows no significant enhancement (*arrow*)

M. DW image shows heterogeneous hyperintensity (*arrow*)

N. ADC map shows hyperintensity (*arrow*)

O. MR spectroscopy (TE 144 ms) shows a markedly increased Cho peak with a lactate peak that is more prominent than in the previous study

Discussion

Oligodendrogliomas are glial tumors that arise from oligodendrocytes. Oligodendrogliomas are uncommon tumors in the pediatric population. They are more commonly seen in young adults. Imaging appearances depend upon the histological characteristics. Oligodendrogliomas include a mixed population of cells, commonly astrocytes. Pure oligodendrogliomas (without mixed cell elements) have less calcification, contrast enhancement and edema than adult (mixed-cell) lesions. In addition, very slow growth or no growth is more often seen in childhood tumors. In the mixed-cell lesions there is often subtle distinction between oligodendroglioma and astrocytoma. On imaging, oligodendrogliomas are typically well defined, peripheral, hemispheric, white-matter lesions extending to the cortex. They have iso- or decreased attenuation on noncontrast-enhanced CT scan, with areas of nodular or clumped calcification (40–90%). Areas of cystic degeneration or hemorrhage may also be present. On MRI, a heterogeneous iso- to hypointense signal on T1-weighted images and a hyperintense signal on T2-weighted images is seen with moderate heterogeneous enhancement. Differential diagnosis includes ganglioglioma, low-grade astrocytoma, DNET, and neurocytoma.

Figure 6.4 A–G ▶

Oligodendroglioma (H–O see next pages)

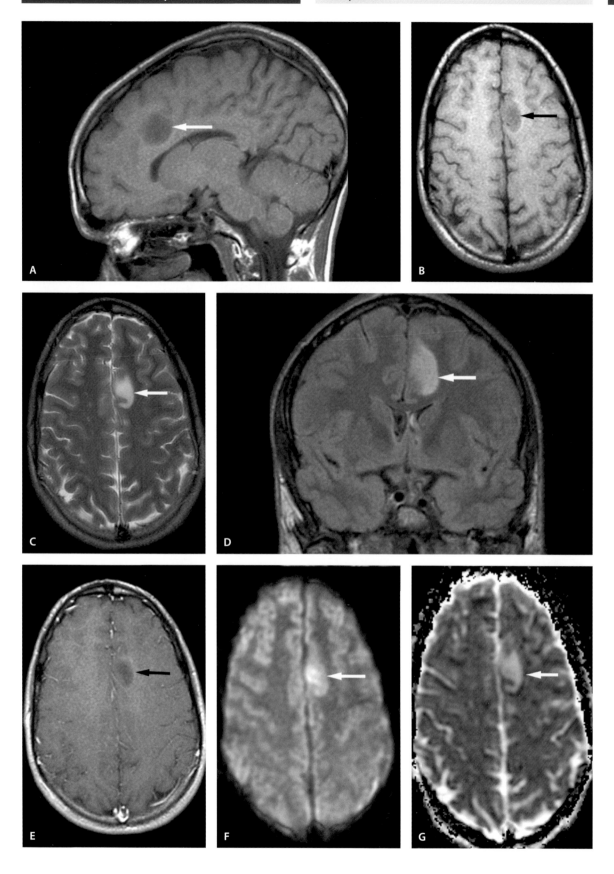

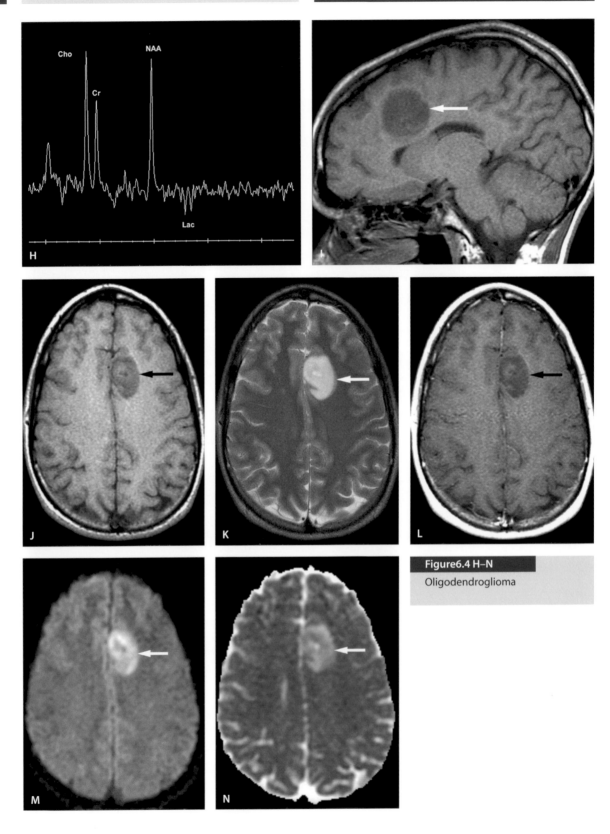

Figure6.4 H–N
Oligodendroglioma

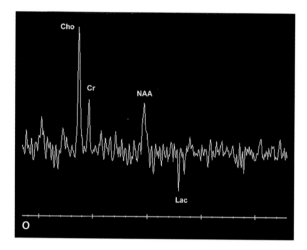

Figure 6.4 O

Oligodendroglioma

Suggested Reading

Engelhard HH, Stelea A, Mundt A (2003) Oligodendroglioma and anaplastic oligodendroglioma: clinical features, treatment, and prognosis. Surg Neurol 60:443–456

Tice H, Barnes PD, Goumnerova L, Scott RM, Tarbell NJ (1993) Pediatric and adolescent oligodendrogliomas. AJNR Am J Neuroradiol 14:1293–1300

Ependymoma

Clinical Presentation

A 4-month-old female with increased head size.

Images (Fig. 6.5)

A. Noncontrast CT scan demonstrates a large right temporal lobe multicystic and solid mass (*arrow*) with medial calcification (*arrowhead*). Low-density surrounding edema is seen. Left temporal horn is trapped and dilated. Hydrocephalus is present

B. T2-weighted image shows a large cystic and solid tumor (*arrow*) with medial hypointense calcification (*arrowhead*). Hydrocephalus is present. The cyst fluid has a higher signal than the CSF, consistent with a higher protein content and/or blood

C. T1-weighted image shows the large hyperintense cyst (*arrow*) and mixed signal in the dilated temporal horn

D. Contrast-enhanced coronal SPGR image shows irregular enhancement in the periphery of the cystic tumor (*arrows*)

E. Three-dimensional time-of-flight MR angiography without contrast enhancement. Collapsed image. It shows displacement and stretching of the right middle cerebral artery. Tumor vessels are supplied by the posterior cerebral artery (*arrow*) and middle cerebral artery. Hyperintense cyst is seen

F. Phase-contrast angiography (velocity encoding 60 cm/s) shows displaced and abnormal tumor vessels (*arrow*). The cyst is not visualized in this sequence

Discussion

Ependymomas derive from neoplastic transformation of the ependyma. Infratentorial tumors occur more frequently in children and supratentorial tumors in adults. Ependymomas are usually ventricular tumors but extraventricular nests of ependymal cells may lead to the hemispheric ependymomas. Ependymomas are malignant tumors that are classified as WHO grade II or III. Supratentorial tumors have less tendency than the infratentorial tumors to seed through CSF pathways. The imaging appearance is that of a large mass with significant surrounding edema. The margins of the tumor are well defined. Cysts are a typical feature of hemispheric ependymoma, and they are usually large cysts. Half of the tumors calcify. Although hydrocephalus is the classic presentation in infratentorial ependymomas, it is less often present in hemispheric tumors. Intratumoral hemorrhage is uncommon. The MRI signal is variable and depends on the presence of the cystic and solid parts and calcification.

Suggested Reading

Coulon RA, Till K (1977) Intracranial ependymomas in children: a review of 43 cases. Childs Brain 3:154–168

Lyons MK, Kelly PJ (1991) Posterior fossa ependymomas: report of 30 cases and review of the literature. Neurosurgery 28:659–665

Spoto GP, Press GA, Hesselink JR, et al (1990) Intracranial ependymoma and sub-ependymoma: MR manifestations. AJNR Am J Neuroradiol 11:83–91

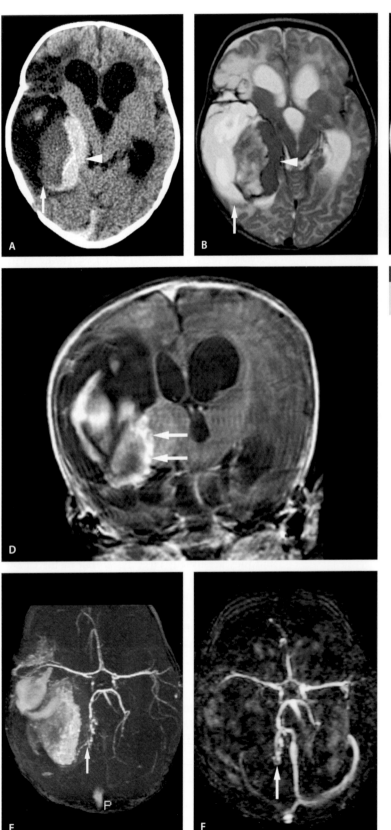

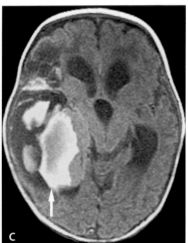

Figure 6.5

Ependymoma

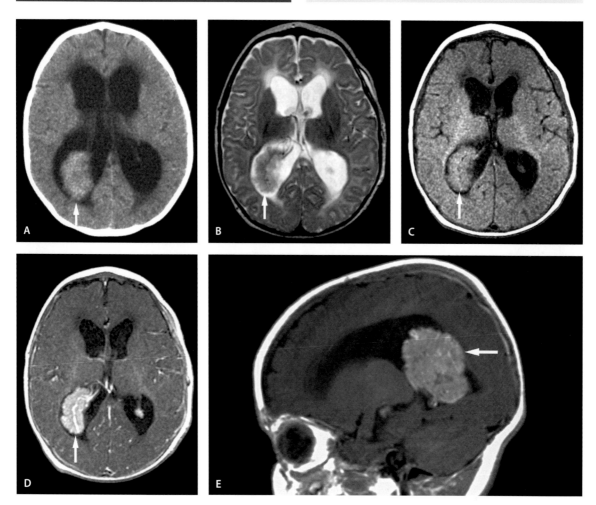

Choroid plexus papillomas

Choroid Plexus Papilloma in the Trigone

Clinical Presentation

A 3-month-old female with hydrocephalus.

Images (Fig. 6.6)

A. Noncontrast CT scan shows slightly hyperdense intraventricular tumor in the right trigone (*arrow*)
B. T2-weighted image shows the intraventricular tumor (*arrow*) and hydrocephalus
C. Axial noncontrast T1-weighed image shows isointense intraventricular mass (*arrow*)
D. Axial contrast-enhanced T1-weighted image shows homogeneous enhancement (*arrow*)
E. Sagittal contrast-enhanced T1-weighted image demonstrates the classic trigone location of the choroid plexus papilloma (*arrow*).

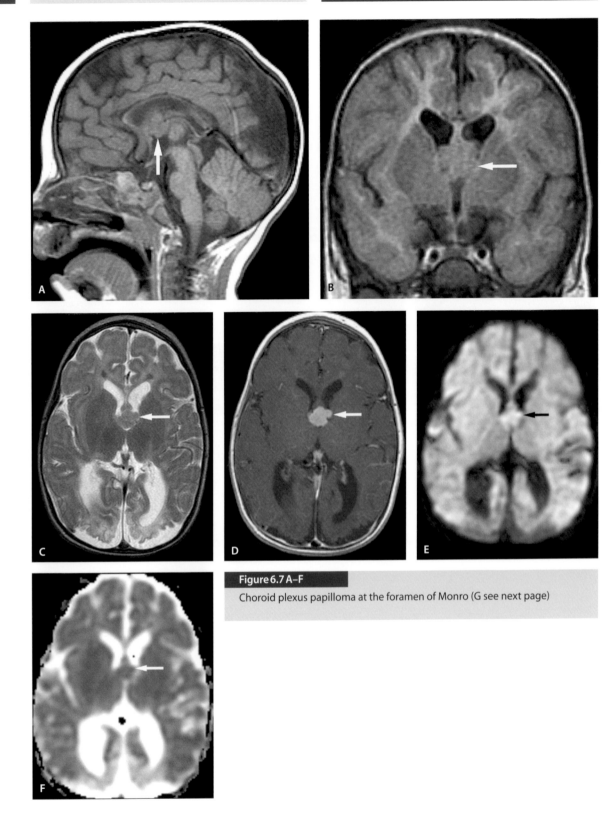

Figure 6.7 A–F

Choroid plexus papilloma at the foramen of Monro (G see next page)

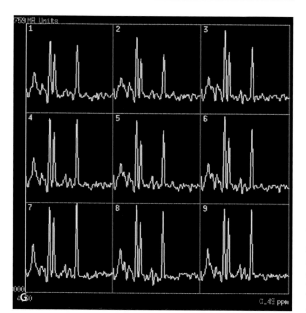

Figure 6.7 G

Choroid plexus papilloma at the foramen of Monro

Choroid Plexus Papilloma at the Foramen of Monro

Clinical Presentation

A 10-month-old female with seizures.

Images (Fig. 6.7)

A. Sagittal T1-weighted image demonstrates an isointense mass near the foramen of Monro (*arrow*)

B. Coronal FLAIR image shows isointense mass between the frontal horns at the region of the foramen of Monro (*arrow*)

C. The mass is slightly hyperintense on T2-weighted image (*arrow*)

D. Contrast-enhanced T1-weighted image shows homogeneous enhancement (*arrow*)

E. The mass is slightly hyperintense on DW image (*arrow*)

F. ADC map demonstrates isointensity of the mass (*arrow*)

G. Multivoxel MR spectroscopy (TE 144 ms). Voxels no. 2 and no. 5 placed on the tumor show a mild increase in the Cho peak. The NAA peak shows contamination from the surrounding brain

Discussion

Choroid plexus papillomas represent 1.5 to 6.4% of all pediatric CNS neoplasms. These tumors usually occur in first decade of life and have a male preponderance. They are most commonly located in the lateral ventricle, followed by the fourth and third ventricles and, rarely, in the cerebellopontine angle. In children, the most common location is the atrium of the lateral ventricle. The majority of children have hydrocephalus and the generally accepted explanation is overproduction of CSF by the tumor. An additional explanation may be decreased resorption due to the proteinaceous material secreted by the tumor. Histologically they resemble normal choroid plexus. They have a malignant counterpart that behaves aggressively and invades the parenchyma. On CT scan, papillomas are seen as well-marginated, lobulated or smooth masses, with homogeneous iso- or increased attenuation secondary to calcification or hemorrhage with marked enhancement. On MRI, papillomas are typically iso- to hypointense on T1-weighted images and iso- to slightly hyper- or hypointense to brain parenchyma on T2-weighted images depending on the presence of blood products, calcium and vascularity. Post-contrast images show marked enhancement. The tumor can seed along the CSF pathways.

Suggested Reading

Erman T, Gocer AI, Erdogan S, Tuna M, Ildan F, Zorludemir S (2003) Choroid plexus papilloma of bilateral lateral ventricle. Acta Neurochir (Wien) 145:139–143

Jelinek J, Smirniotopoulos JG, Parisi JE, Kanzer M (1990) Lateral ventricular neoplasms of the brain: differential diagnosis based on clinical, CT, and MR findings. AJR Am J Roentgenol 155:365–372

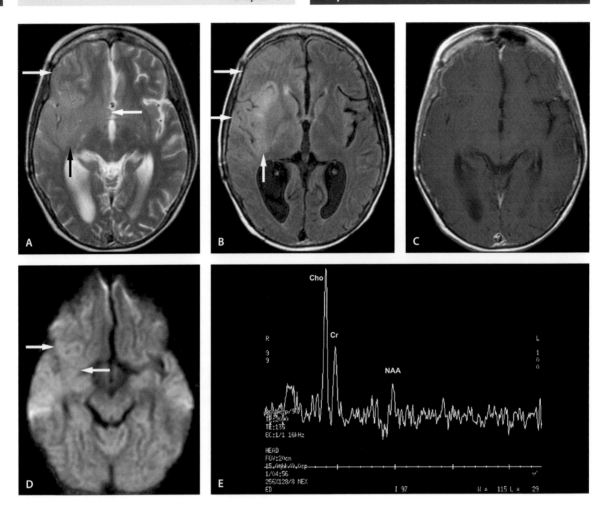

Figure 6.8

Gliomatosis cerebri

Gliomatosis Cerebri

Clinical Presentation

A 17-year-old male with complex partial seizures refractory to medication. The first presentation and biopsy were at the age of 12 years.

Images (Fig. 6.8)

A and B. There is a large and irregular hyperintense lesion on T2-weighted (A) and FLAIR (B) images in the right temporal and frontal lobe (*arrows*). There is a minimal mass effect upon the cortical sulci and sylvian fissure

C. Contrast-enhanced T1-weighted image shows no significant parenchymal enhancement

D. DW image shows mild hyperintensity due to T2 shine-through effect in the right cerebral hemisphere (*arrows*)

E. Single voxel MR spectroscopy (TE 135 ms) demonstrates a significantly decreased NAA peak with an increased Cho peak. No lactate peak is present

Discussion

Gliomatosis cerebri is a rare tumor considered to be an extreme form of diffusely infiltrating glioma. WHO has not recognized gliomatosis cerebri as a distinct entity. It is characterized by diffuse glial overgrowth in the cerebral hemisphere, but can extend to the midbrain, pons and spinal cord. The criteria for diagnosis include involvement of at least two areas of brain. Clinically patients with gliomatosis cerebri present with nonspecific symptoms, which are often disproportionately mild relative to the extent of the lesion.

Gliomatosis can be difficult to appreciate on CT scan. It does not calcify or bleed. On MR images, the lesion is hyperintense on T2-weighted and FLAIR images with negligible or minimal enhancement. On MR spectroscopy there is a variable decrease in the NAA peak and an increase in the Cho peak. Areas with elevated Cho levels have been shown to correlate with the malignancy. The Cho level of gliomatosis cerebri (a fibrillary astrocytoma which is typically a grade II lesion) has been shown to be near the top of the high-grade malignant range. This observation corresponds with the biological behavior of this tumor regardless of its histopathology.

Suggested Reading

Bendszus M, Warmuth-Metz M, Klein R, et al (2001) MR spectroscopy in gliomatosis cerebri. AJNR Am J Neuroradiol 21:375–380

Rust P, Ashkan K, Ball C, Stapleton S, Marsh H (2001) Gliomatosis cerebri: pitfalls in diagnosis. J Clin Neurosci 8:361–363

Tedeschi G, Lundbom N, Raman R, et al (1997) Increased choline signal coinciding with malignant degeneration of cerebral gliomas: a serial proton magnetic resonance spectroscopy imaging study. J Neurosurg 87:516–524

Ganglioglioma

Clinical Presentation

A 12-year-old female with seizures.

Images (Fig. 6.9)

A. Axial T2-weighted image shows a well-outlined hyperintense lesion in the right occipital lobe (*arrow*)
B. Contrast-enhanced T1-weighted image shows heterogeneous enhancement with indistinct borders (*arrow*)
C. DW image shows heterogeneous, mild hyperintensity in the lesion (*arrow*)
D. ADC map shows hyperintensity of the lesion (*arrow*)

Discussion

Gangliogliomas comprise between 1% and 8% of primary brain tumors in the pediatric age group. These tumors are composed of neoplastic ganglion and glial cells in variable proportions. These tumors are benign and typically slow-growing. The most common location in the brain is the temporal lobe, followed by the occipital and frontal lobes. Seizure is the commonest presenting symptom. MR spectroscopy reflects the benign nature and shows a mildly increased Cho peak with a somewhat decreased NAA peak.

The imaging appearances are varied, but the typical appearance on CT scan is a mass of decreased attenuation (solid or cystic) with variable calcification and enhancement in approximately 50% of cases. If the tumor is located near the calvarium it can remodel the inner table. MRI may show variable signal ranging from hypo- to hyperintense to brain on both T1- and T2-weighted sequences with enhancement after contrast administration. The differential diagnosis includes low-grade astrocytoma, pleomorphic xanthoastrocytoma, oligodendroglioma, and arachnoid or porencephalic cyst.

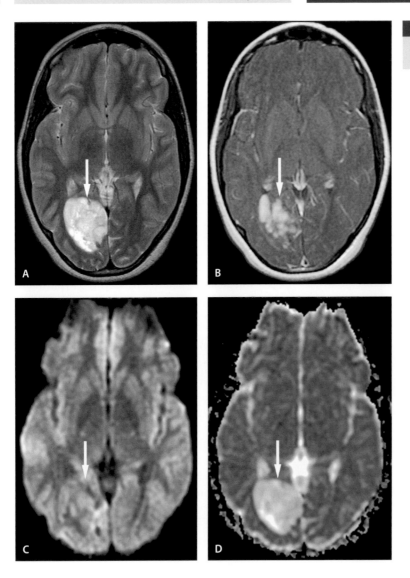

Figure 6.9
Ganglioglioma

Suggested Reading

Provenzale JM, Ali U, Barborial DP, Kallmes DF, Delong DM, McLendon RE (2000) Comparison of patient age with MR imaging features of gangliogliomas. AJR Am J Roentgenol 174:859–862

Smith NM, Carli MM, Hanieh A, Clark B, Boume AJ, Byard RW (1992) Gangliogliomas in childhood. Childs Nerv Syst 8:258–262

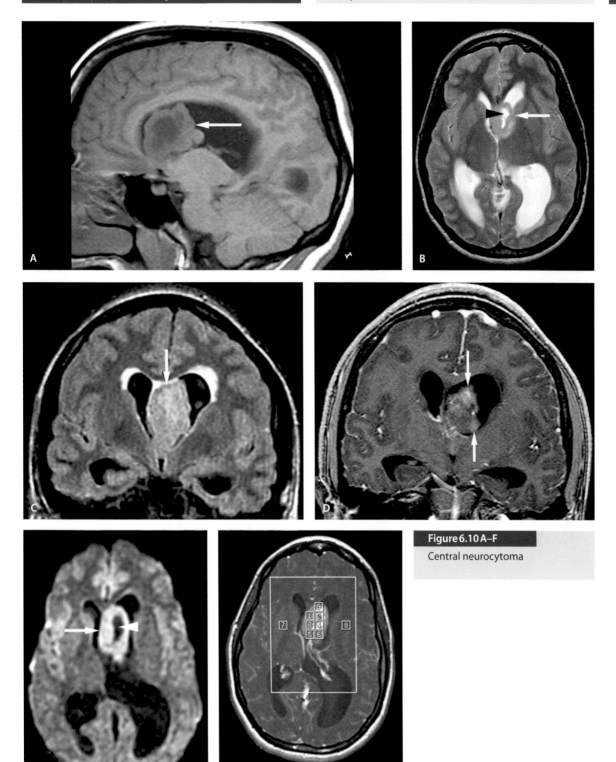

Figure 6.10 A–F

Central neurocytoma

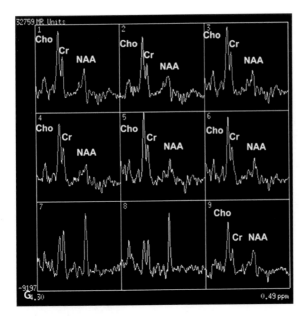

Figure 6.10 G

Central neurocytoma

Central Neurocytoma

Clinical Presentation

A 22-year-old female presenting with papilla edema and headaches.

Images (Fig. 6.10)

A. Sagittal T1-weighted image demonstrates a hypointense intraventricular tumor (*arrow*)
B. T2-weighted image demonstrates a lesion adjacent to the septum pellucidum (*arrow*). It also demonstrates the cystic/necrotic nature of the lesion (*arrowhead*). Hydrocephalus is present
C. Coronal FLAIR image also demonstrates the signal to be near isointense to the cortical gray matter (*arrow*)
D. Coronal contrast-enhanced SPGR image demonstrates heterogeneous enhancement (*arrows*)
E. DW image demonstrates increased signal (*arrow*) in the tumor with central decreased signal intensity (*arrowhead*) in the cystic/necrotic part of the tumor

F. and G.
   Multivoxel proton MR spectroscopy (TE 144 ms). F demonstrates the location of the voxels. Voxels labeled 1–6 and 9 are through the tumor. They all demonstrate an increased Cho peak with a significantly decreased NAA peak without a lactate peak (G)

Discussion

Central neurocytoma is a recently defined tumor of neuronal origin that occurs within the ventricles. The age range of presentation is from 15 to 50 years. It is typically a tumor of young adults with rare cases reported in young children. Neurocytomas are generally slow-growing and are considered low-grade malignant tumors. They are classified as WHO grade II. Ventricle wall, fornix, anterior roof of the third ventricle and septum pellucidum are the primary locations of this tumor that is nearly always intraventricular. Some tumors contain scattered calcifications. On CT scan there is a visible amount of focal calcifications and cystic areas. Contrast enhancement and hydrocephalus are usually present at the time of discovery of the lesion. On MRI the lesion is heterogeneous. Areas of hypointensity on the T1- and T2-weighted images are most likely related to the foci of calcification, and areas of hyperintensity on T2-weighted images probably relate to areas of cystic necrosis. Gadolinium enhancement is heterogeneous. The calcification is difficult to appreciate in the MR image unless gradient echo imaging is used. Sometimes tubular flow voids are seen inside the lesion. These are related to intratumoral vessels.

Suggested Reading

Figarella-Branger D, Pellisier JF, Daumas-Duport C, et al (1992) Central neurocytomas. Am J Surg Pathol 16:97–109

Jelinek J, Smirniotopoulos JG, Parisi JE, et al (1990) Lateral ventricular neoplasms of the brain: differential diagnosis based on clinical, CT and MR findings. AJR Am J Roentgenol 155:365–372

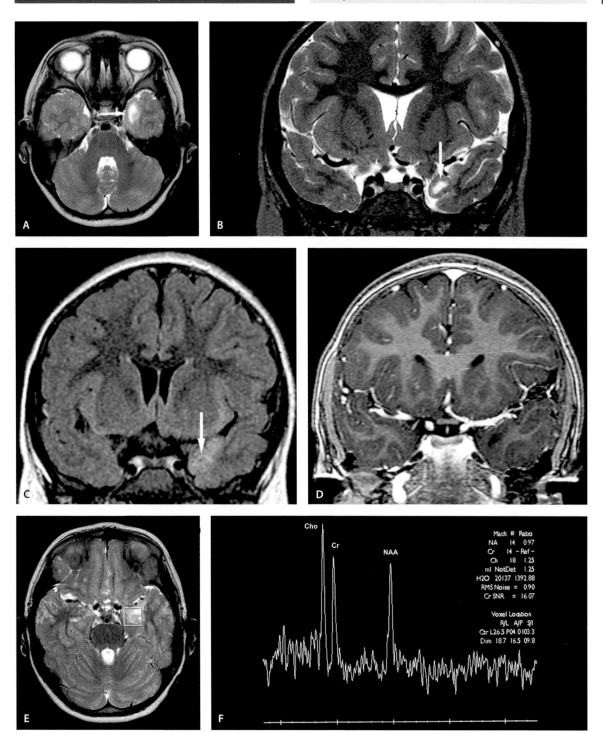

Figure 6.11

Dysembryoplastic neuroepithelial tumor (DNET)

Dysembryoplastic Neuroepithelial Tumor (DNET)

Clinical Presentation

A 5-year-old male with prolonged focal seizures.

Images (Fig. 6.11)

A. and B.
Coronal (A) and axial (B) T2-weighted images show a hyperintense lesion in the left parahippocampal gyrus (*arrows*). A mild cortex expansion is present
C. FLAIR image also demonstrates the hyperintense lesion in the left parahippocampal gyrus (*arrow*)
D. Contrast-enhanced coronal SPGR image shows no abnormal enhancement
E. and F.
MR Spectroscopy (TE 135 ms). T2-weighted image (E) demonstrates the voxel placement. The Cho peak is slightly increased with a mildly decreased NAA peak. No abnormal metabolites are seen. Some artifacts from the skull base are present

Discussion

DNET is one of the newly described entities accepted into the 1993 WHO revision. It arises from secondary germinal layers. DNETs are typically located in the temporal or frontal lobes, often with a cortical location. Due to its cortical location the most common presentation is seizures. There is a megagyric variety with expansion of the cortex and a multinodular form. CT scan usually demonstrates a well-defined hypodense mass with occasional focal contrast enhancement. The slow growth and cortical location may lead to scalloped remodeling of the inner table of the skull. MRI shows hypointensity on T1-weighted images and hyperintensity on T2-weighted images, with variable enhancement. The lesion typically contains multiple cysts. The differential diagnosis includes low-grade glioma and ganglioglioma and even PXA.

Suggested Reading

Kimura S, Kobayashi T, Hara M (1996) A case of dysembryoplastic neuroepithelial tumor of the parietal lobe with characteristic magnetic resonance imaging. Acta Paediatr Jpn 38:168–171

Kuroiwa T, Bergey GK, Rothman MI, et al (1995) Radiologic appearance of the dysembryoplastic neuroepithelial tumor. Radiology 197:233–238

Ostertun B, Wolf HK, Campos MG, Matus C, Solymosi L, Elger CE, Schramm J, Schild HH (1996) Dysplastic neuroepithelial tumors: MR and CT evaluation. AJNR Am J Neuroradiol 17:419–430

Germinoma of the Pineal Region

Clinical Presentation

A 27-year-old male with headaches.

Images (Fig. 6.12)

A. T2-weighted image shows two hyperintense tumors (*arrows*), one in the pineal and the other in the suprasellar region. The pineal tumor is surrounded by edema
B. Sagittal T1-weighted image shows the tumors to be isointense to gray matter (*arrows*)
C. Contrast-enhanced T1-weighted image shows intense enhancement in both tumors (*arrows*)
D. Sagittal contrast-enhanced T1-weighted image shows intense but slightly inhomogeneous enhancement of the lesions (*arrows*)

Discussion

Germ-cell tumors are the most common tumors in the pineal region, although there are 17 different histological types of tumors in this region. Germinoma accounts for two-thirds of germ-cell tumors and 40–50% of all pineal region masses. The pineal germinoma is histologically identical to the parasellar germinoma and they share the same imaging findings. The germinomas are commonly seen between 10 and 30 years of age with a male preponderance. On noncontrast CT scan, germ-cell tumors are typically homogeneous with attenuation slightly higher than that of gray matter. On MRI, these masses show isointense signal to gray matter on both T1- and T2-

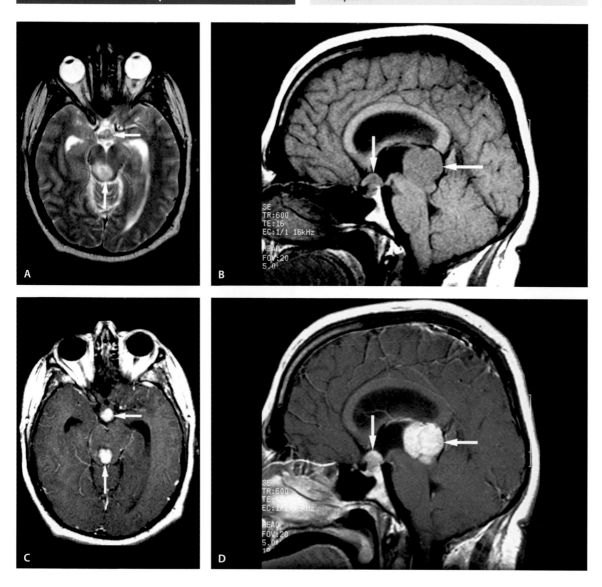

Figure 6.12

Germinoma of the pineal region

weighted sequences. Marked homogeneous enhancement is seen on both CT scan and MR imaging. Occasionally cystic areas may also be present. Calcification of the pineal gland should be considered abnormal and suspicious for tumor in children younger than 5 years.

Suggested Reading

Jaing TH, Wang HS, Hung IJ, et al (2002) Intracranial germ cell tumors: a retrospective study of 44 children. Pediatr Neurol 26:369–373

Liang L, Korogi Y, Sugahara T, et al (2002) MRI of intracranial germ-cell tumors. Neuroradiology 44:382–388

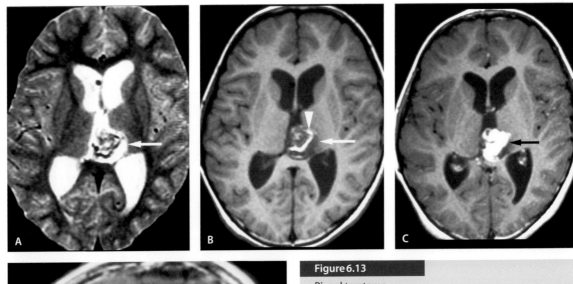

Figure 6.13
Pineal teratoma

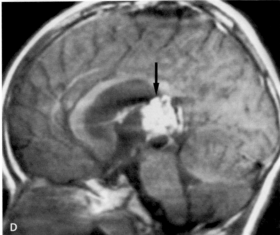

Pineal Teratoma

Clinical Presentation

Young male with headaches.

Images (Fig. 6.13)

A. T2-weighted image shows mixed signal intensity (*arrow*) in the tumor. Mild hydrocephalus is present

B. T1-weighted image shows mixed signal intensity tumor (*arrow*) with bright fat in the tumor (*arrowhead*)

C and D. Axial (C) and sagittal (D) contrast-enhanced T1-weighted images show intense but inhomogeneous enhancement (*arrows*)

Discussion

Teratoma is the second most common tumor in the pineal region accounting for 15% of all masses in the pineal area and 2% of pediatric CNS neoplasms. The peak incidence is in first two decades of life with a strong male preponderance. Imaging findings vary depending upon the histology of these tumors. All three germ-cell layers are found in this tumor type. Histologically the lesion may be classified as benign or malignant. The malignant tumor can produce elevated serum or CSF levels of alpha-fetoprotein and beta-human chorionic gonadotropin. Teratomas are very heterogeneous masses with a variable attenuation value due to the presence of fat, calcification, soft tissue, and CSF. The presence of fat favors a benign nature of the mass. Chemical meningitis may occur secondary to rupture of these tumors. The tumor may enhance somewhat or not at all. The tumor is also heterogeneous on MRI secondary to calcification and fat. The MRI appearance of teratoma is usually specific.

Suggested Reading

Cho BK, Wang KC, Nam DH, et al (1998) Pineal tumors: experience with 48 cases over 10 years. Childs Nerv Syst 14:53–58

Jaing TH, Wang HS, Hung IJ, et al (2002) Intracranial germ cell tumors: a retrospective study of 44 children. Pediatr Neurol 26:369–373

Pineoblastoma

Clinical Presentation

A 10-year-old male with sixth nerve palsy and papilledema.

Images (Fig. 6.14)

A. Noncontrast CT scan shows hyperdense tumor in the pineal region (*arrow*). Shunted hydrocephalus is seen

B. T2-weighted image shows slightly heterogeneous tumor (*arrow*) with areas isointense to white and gray matter

C. T1-weighted image shows peripheral hyperintensity, representing hemorrhagic areas (*arrowheads*)

D. Sagittal contrast-enhanced T1-weighted image shows heterogeneous enhancement in the mass (*arrow*)

Discussion

Pineal parenchymal tumors are extremely rare accounting for 0.3% of primary brain tumors. They can be divided into pineocytomas (45%), pineoblastomas (45%), and pineal parenchymal tumors with intermediate differentiation (10%).

Pineoblastoma is a highly malignant tumor occurring typically in the first decade of life. There is a male preponderance. They have a tendency to invade the adjacent brain and disseminate to the CSF. They arise from small pineoblasts and are histologically similar to medulloblastoma and neuroblastoma. Imaging findings are not specific. Pineoblastomas appear as lobulated, homogeneous tumors that are larger and less-frequently calcified than pineocytomas. They are also accompanied by a more severe degree of hydrocephalus. Cystic changes are less-often seen as compared to pineocytomas.

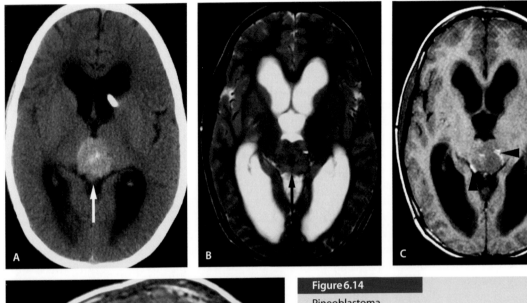

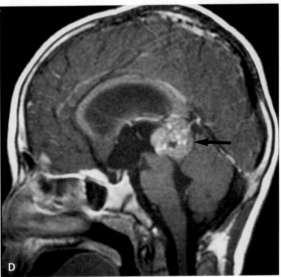

Figure 6.14

Pineoblastoma

Suggested Reading

Nakamura M, Saeki N, Iwadate Y, Sunami K, Osato K, Yamaura A (2000) Neuroradiological characteristics of pineocytoma and pineoblastoma. Neuroradiology 42:509–514

Sugiyama K, Arita K, Okamura T, Yamasaki F, et al (2002) Detection of a pineoblastoma with large central cyst in a young child. Childs Nerv Syst 18:157–160

Pineal Embryonal Carcinoma

Clinical Presentation

A 16-year-old male with visual symptoms and headaches.

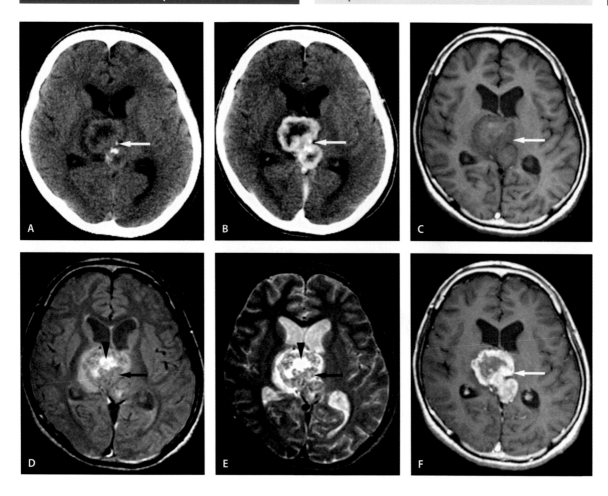

Figure 6.15

Pineal embryonal carcinoma

Images (Fig. 6.15)

A and B. Noncontrast (A) and contrast-enhanced (B) CT scans demonstrate irregular ring enhancing tumor in the pineal region (*arrows*)

C. T1-weighted image shows a heterogeneous pineal region tumor that is mainly isointense to gray matter (*arrow*)

D and E. Proton density image (D) and T2-weighted image (E) show heterogeneous low signal in the solid part of the tumor (*arrows*) with increased signal in central necrosis (*arrowheads*). Peripheral edema is seen

F. Contrast-enhanced T1-weighted image shows intense enhancement, but irregular enhancement in the solid parts of the tumor (*arrow*)

Discussion

Embryonic cell carcinoma is a highly malignant form of germ cell tumor. These tumors share the same imaging findings with other malignant tumors in this area, such as choriocarcinoma and endodermal sinus tumors (yolk sac tumor). Embryonic cell carcinoma and teratoma secrete alpha-fetoprotein and beta-human chorionic gonadotropin.

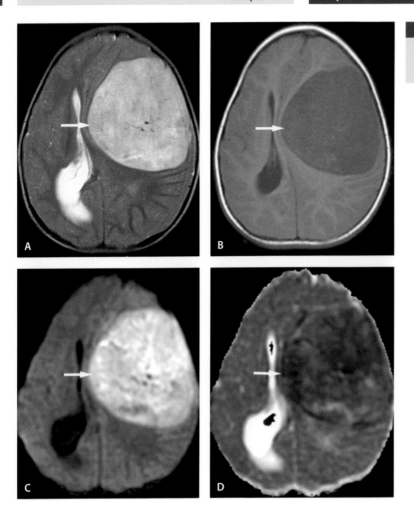

Suggested Reading

Cho JU, Kim DS, Chung SS, et al (1998) Pineal tumors: experience with 48 cases over 10 years. Childs Nerv Syst 14:53–58

Zee CS, Segall H, Apuzzo M, et al (1991) MR imaging of pineal region neoplasms. J Comput Assist Tomogr 15:56–63

Primitive Neuroectodermal Tumor (PNET)

Clinical Presentation

A 20-month-old female with lethargy and nausea.

Images (Fig. 6.16)

A. T2-weighed image demonstrates a well-outlined mainly hyperintense lesion in the left frontal lobe (*arrow*). There is a significant mass effect upon the ventricles and midline structures
B. T1-weighted image shows a mainly hypointense lesion with some isointense areas (*arrow*)
C. DW image shows hyperintensity (*arrow*)
D. ADC map shows heterogeneous hypointensity which may indicate hypercellularity (*arrow*)

Discussion

PNETs are the most common primary malignant CNS tumors in children. They are a group of malignant, primarily undifferentiated tumors that occur within the cerebral hemispheres and include primitive tumors with common neuroepithelial precursors in the brainstem, cerebellum, and spinal cord and extra- CNS locations. They have the tendency to demonstrate subarachnoid dissemination. Screening of the entire neuraxis is recommended. The peak incidence is up to 5 years of age. On CT scans, PNETs are seen as a hyperdense mass with variable enhancement. Calcification, calvarial asymmetry and bone erosion may occasionally be seen. On MRI, they are hypointense on T1-weighted images and iso- to hyperintense on T2-weighted images with variable heterogeneous enhancement. DW imaging shows restricted diffusion which may be due to densely packed cellular material with scanty interstitial tissue.

Suggested Reading

Klisch J, Husstedt H, Hennings S, von Velthoven V, Pagenstecher A, Schumacher M (2000) Supratentorial primitive neuroectodermal tumors: diffusion-weighted MRI. Neuroradiology 42:393–398

Tortori-Donati P, Fondelli MP, Rossi A, et al (1996) Medulloblastoma in children: CT and MRI findings. Neuroradiology 38:352–359

Atypical Teratoid Rhabdoid Tumor

Clinical Presentation

A 4-year-old female with chromosome abnormality (ring chromosome 22), developmental delay, nausea and vomiting.

Images (Fig. 6.17)

A. Noncontrast CT scan following shunt shows large mixed density tumor (*arrow*) in the pineal region with hemorrhagic foci. Pneumocephalus is present following shunting

B. T2-weighted image before shunting shows a large mixed signal intensity lesion in the pineal region (*arrow*). Hydrocephalus with transependymal CSF leak is present. A prominent vascular structure (flow voids) is seen inside the lesion (*arrowhead*). Dark signal hemorrhagic foci are also present

C. Noncontrast T1-weighted image shows a mixed signal intensity lesion, mainly isointense to the gray matter (*arrow*)

D. Contrast-enhanced T1-weighted image demonstrates mixed enhancement in the lesion, mainly anteriorly (*arrow*)

E. Sagittal contrast-enhanced T1-weighted image shows pineal lesion with mixed enhancement, mainly in the anterior superior part of the lesion (*arrow*)

Discussion

Primary atypical teratoid/rhabdoid tumor of the CNS is a recently described embryonal tumor with characteristic large rhabdoid cells. It is a highly malignant neoplasm with a poor prognosis. Over the past 10 years it has been noticed that this atypical teratoid/rhabdoid tumor, with histological features somewhat similar to, but biological features dramatically different from, those of medulloblastoma-PNET, has been misdiagnosed as medulloblastoma. Radiologically it is indistinguishable from medulloblastoma, but these two tumors may be separated on histologic, molecular and cytogenetic grounds. These tumors occur mainly in young children. They are equally often seen in brain and cerebellum but may involve the pineal gland. Imaging features are nonspecific, but similar to those of medulloblastoma-

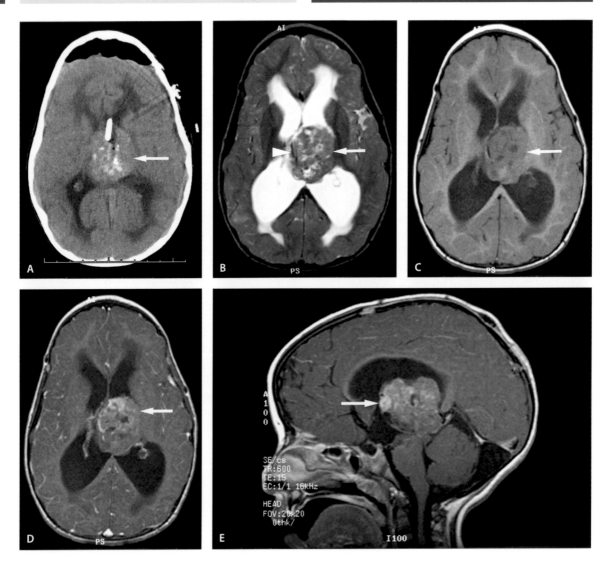

Figure 6.17

Atypical teratoid rhabdoid tumor

PNET. There is increased density on noncontrast CT scan and heterogeneous enhancement. On MR images, there is decreased signal intensity on T1-weighted images and iso- or decreased intensity on T2-weighted images. The enhancement pattern is heterogeneous on MR images. Cysts and hemorrhage are common. Since these tumors seed through the CSF space, examination of the whole spinal axis is needed to evaluate the extent of the disease. These tumors are associated with a poor prognosis.

Suggested Reading

Fenton LZ, Foreman NK (2003) Atypical teratoid/rhabdoid tumor of the central nervous system in children: an atypical series and review. Pediatr Radiol 33:554–558

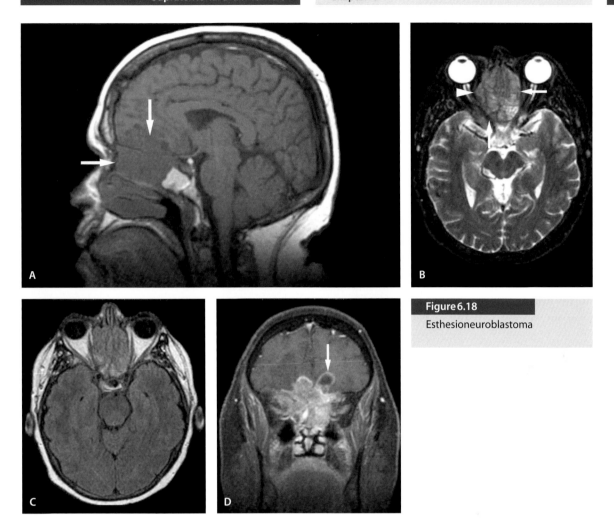

Figure 6.18

Esthesioneuroblastoma

Esthesioneuroblastoma

Clinical Presentation

An 18-year-old male with nasal stuffiness and anosmia.

Images (Fig. 6.18)

A. Sagittal T1-weighted image shows a large mass lesion in the midline (*arrows*). The lesion is isointense to brain tissue
B. T2-weighted image shows mildly hypointense mass lesion (*arrow*) that has expanded and remodeled the nasal cavity and extends to the right orbit (*arrowhead*)

C. The tumor is mildly hyperintense on FLAIR image
D. Coronal contrast-enhanced T1-weighted image shows extension through the cribriform plate into the anterior cranial fossa. The expansile mass fills the sphenoid sinus, the upper nasal cavity, ethmoid air cells and extends to the right orbit. There is a typical cystic area in the intracranial margin (*arrow*) that is suggestive of esthesioneuroblastoma

Discussion

Esthesioneuroblastoma is a rare malignant slow-growing neurogenic tumor that originates in the olfactory neuroepithelium in the olfactory plate or upper nasal cavity. It can also originate in the cribriform plate, middle turbinates and adjacent paranasal sinuses. As the symptoms and signs are nonspecific, patients usually present with advanced disease. Although the tumors are most common in adults, they also occur in children with a first peak incidence in the second decade. There is a male predominance. Intracranial extension occurs in 25 % of cases. Metastatic disease occurs in 20 % of patients primarily to cervical lymph nodes, liver, lung or bone. Esthesioneuroblastoma can induce severe bone remodeling and rarely hyperostosis of the adjacent bone. There is bone destruction when it extends into the anterior cranial fossa.

CT scan shows a homogeneous soft tissue mass with relatively uniform enhancement. On MR images, signal intensity on T1- and T2-weighted images is more heterogeneous with a variable amount of enhancement. Although MRI is most useful in delineating the extent of the tumor, the signal intensity characteristics overlap with those of many tumors.

Suggested Reading

Derdeyn CP, Moran CJ, Wippold FJ II, et al (1994) MRI of esthesioneuroblastoma. J Comput Assist Tomogr 18:16–21

Regenbogen VS, Zinreich SJ, Kim KS, et al (1988) Hyperostotic esthesioneuroblastoma: CT and MR findings. J Comput Assist Tomogr 12:52–56

Schuster JJ, Phillips CD, Levine PA (1994) MR of esthesioneuroblastoma (olfactory neuroblastoma) and appearance after cranial facial resection. AJNR Am J Neuroradiol 15:1169–1177

Youssem DM, Hayden RE, Doty RL (1993) Olfactory neuroblastoma. AJNR Am J Neuroradiol 14:1167–1171

Trigeminal Neurofibroma

Clinical Presentation

A 4-year-old male with left "eye pressure" and visual symptoms.

Images (Fig. 6.19)

A. Contrast-enhanced CT scan shows asymmetry in the cavernous sinus enhancement with fewer enhancements on the left (*arrow*). The cisternal part of the fifth cranial nerve is thickened (*arrowhead*). Erosion of the left side of the clivus and enlarged left superior orbital fissure are also seen

B. Coronal inversion recovery image shows a heterogeneous mass in the left cavernous sinus (*arrow*). The mass grows through the foramen ovale that is enlarged

C. and D.
Coronal (C) and axial (D) fat-suppressed contrast-enhanced T1-weighted images show enhancement along the enlarged trigeminal nerve in the left cavernous sinus, orbital apex, foramen ovale and the infratemporal fossa (*arrows*)

Discussion

Primary nerve sheath tumors of the trigeminal nerve include schwannomas and neurofibromas. Schwannomas (also termed neurinomas or neurilemmomas) of the trigeminal nerve are uncommon, accounting for 0.07 % to 0.36 % of intracranial tumors and 0.8 % to 8 % of intracranial schwannomas. They are associated with neurofibromatosis type 2 (NF-2). They can occur at any age, but predominate during the third and fourth decades.

Sporadic cases of trigeminal schwannomas in children have been reported. Family history of neurofibromatosis is usually positive. Lesions arising from the cisternal segment of the trigeminal nerve account for 20 % of trigeminal schwannomas, those arising in Meckel's cave for 50 %, tumors affecting both segments (dumb-bell) for 25 %, and the remaining 5 % arise from distal intracranial branches and extend intracranially. Primary nerve-sheath tumors of the trigeminal nerve present with a variety of symptoms and signs depending upon the location of the lesion.

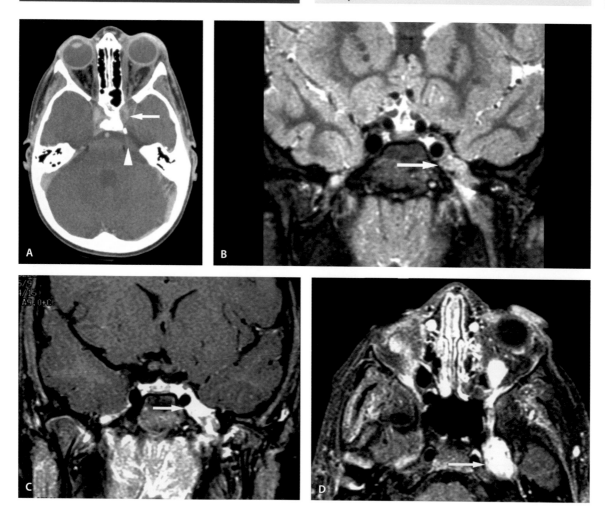

Figure 6.19

Trigeminal neurofibroma

On MRI, they usually appear as well-delineated masses iso- or hypointense to gray matter on T1-weighted sequences and iso- or hyperintense on T2-weighted sequences. Enhancement is strong and heterogeneous. Large schwannomas may show heterogeneous signal due to cystic degeneration or hemorrhage.

Suggested Reading

Mojoie CB, Hulsmans FJ, Castelijns JA, Sie LH, et al (1999) Primary nerve-sheath tumors of the trigeminal nerve: clinical and MRI findings. Neuroradiology 41:100–108

Nager GT (1984) Neurinomas of the trigeminal nerve. Am J Otolaryngol 5:301–333

Ross DL, Tew JM Jr, Benton C, Eisentrout C (1984) Trigeminal schwannoma in a child. Neurosurgery 15:108–110

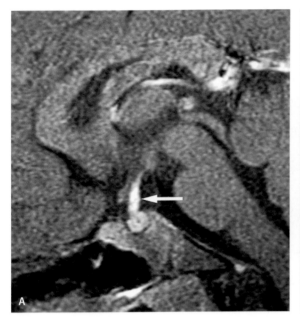 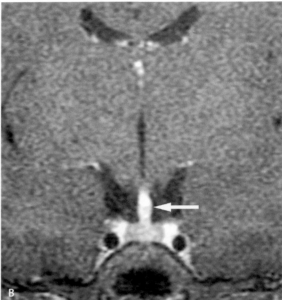

Figure 6.20

Eosinophilic granuloma

Eosinophilic Granuloma

Clinical Presentation

A 6-year-old male with polyuria and polydipsia.

Images (Fig. 6.20)

A and B. Sagittal (A) and coronal (B) contrast-enhanced T1-weighted images show diffuse enlargement of the pituitary stalk with homogeneous enhancement (*arrows*)

Discussion

Eosinophilic granulomatosis or Langerhans cell histiocytosis is a group of diseases characterized by proliferation of histiocytes. The granulomatous lesions may occur in the hypothalamus and pituitary stalk. On CT and MR images there is thickening of the pituitary stalk with significant and usually homogeneous enhancement.

Suggested Reading

Rosenfield NS, Abrahams J, Komp D (1990) Brain MRI in patients with Langerhans cell histiocytosis: findings and enhancement with Gd-DTPA. Pediatr Radiol 20:433–436

Craniopharyngioma

Clinical Presentation

A 7-year-old female with headache, vomiting and papilla edema.

Images (Fig. 6.21)

A. Contrast-enhanced CT scan shows a lobulated hyperdense mass in the suprasellar region (*arrow*). Posteriorly the mass extends to the pons and cerebellopontine angle on the left
B. Sagittal noncontrast T1-weighted image shows a hyperintense, multiloculated suprasellar cystic and solid mass with posterior fossa extension

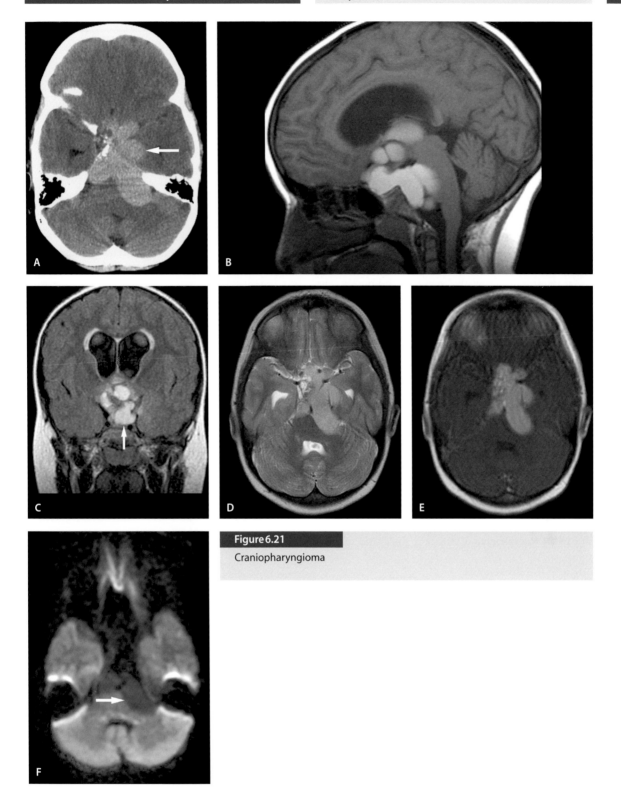

Figure 6.21

Craniopharyngioma

C. Coronal FLAIR image shows extension to the pituitary fossa (*arrow*)

D. T2-weighted image shows lobulated hyperintense mass with suprasellar and parasellar extension. The tumor extends to the posterior fossa

E. Contrast-enhanced T1-weighted image shows no significant enhancement

F. DW image shows hypointensity of the lesion due to the unrestricted diffusion (*arrow*)

Discussion

Craniopharyngiomas are benign tumors accounting for 6–9 % of pediatric intracranial tumors and are typically located in the suprasellar region. It is the most common suprasellar mass in childhood. The symptoms are related to compression of adjacent structures such as optic pathways and the pituitary and hypothalamic regions. On CT, they are seen as a heterogeneous mass with cystic and solid areas that show enhancement. Calcification is the hallmark of craniopharyngioma, which helps differentiate it from other suprasellar tumors that rarely calcify. About 80 % of childhood craniopharyngiomas demonstrate calcification. MRI is superior to CT in determining the extent and its relationship to the surrounding structures. MRI also helps in identifying intratumoral cystic areas with greater sensitivity. A unique MRI feature is produced by machine oil content of the cyst that appears hyperintense in both T1- and T2-weighted images. DW images show hypointensity due to the unrestricted diffusion in the cystic component.

Suggested Reading

Sener RN, Dzelzite S, Migals A (2002) Huge craniopharyngioma: diffusion MRI and contrast-enhanced FLAIR imaging. Comput Med Imaging Graph 26:199–203

Tsuda M, Takahashi S, Higano S, Kurihara N, Ikeda H, Sakamoto K (1997) CT and MR imaging of craniopharyngioma. Eur Radiol 7:464–469

Pituitary Adenoma

Pituitary Macroadenoma

Clinical Presentation

A 14-year-old girl with irregular menstruation and galactorrhea.

Images (Fig. 6.22)

A. Sagittal contrast-enhanced T1-weighted image shows enlargement of the pituitary gland and peripheral enhancement of the tumor (*arrow*)

B. Coronal T2-weighted image shows the hyperintense tumor (*arrow*) on the left with the normal gland pushed to the right. The normal gland is isointense to white matter (*arrowhead*)

C. and D.
Coronal precontrast (C) and postcontrast (D) fat-suppressed T1-weighted images. The tumor is visualized as a nonenhancing area (*arrows*) with the normal enhancing gland displaced to right (*arrowheads*)

E. DW image shows hypointensity (*arrow*) in the lesion.

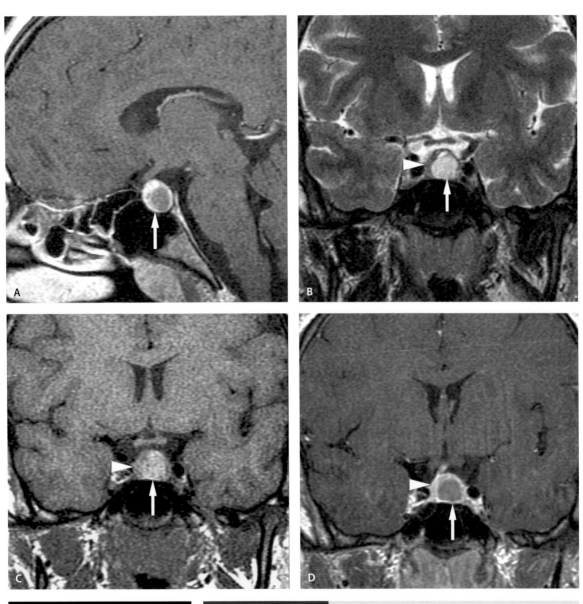

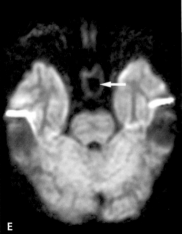

Figure 6.22

Pituitary macroadenoma

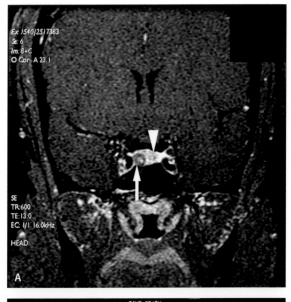

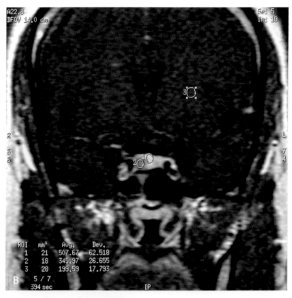

Figure 6.23

Pituitary microadenoma (prolactinoma)

Pituitary Microadenoma (Prolactinoma)

Clinical Presentation

A 17-year-old female with increased prolactin levels.

Images (Fig. 6.23)

A. Coronal postcontrast T1-weighted fat-suppressed image shows normal enhancing pituitary gland on the left (*arrowhead*). Less-enhancing tumor is seen on the right side of pituitary fossa representing microadenoma (*arrow*)

B. Dynamic contrast-enhanced MR image shows the regions of interest of the time-enhancement curves (*1* normal gland, *2* microadenoma, *3* normal brain parenchyma)

C. Time-enhancement curves show delayed enhancement in the microadenoma (*1* normal gland, *2* microadenoma, *3* normal brain parenchyma)

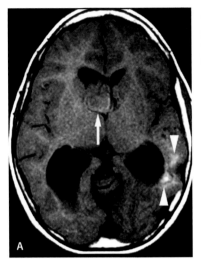
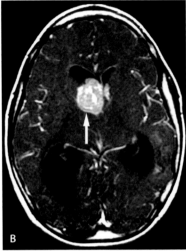
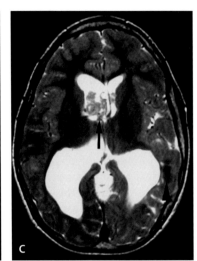

Figure 6.24

Subependymal giant cell astrocytoma (SEGA)

Discussion

Pituitary adenomas are uncommon in childhood and adolescence. They represent about 3% of all supratentorial tumors diagnosed in children. The major clinical presentations include headache, visual field defects, and endocrine symptoms. Prepubertal children are most likely to have an ACTH-secreting adenoma, whereas pubertal and postpubertal children are most likely to have prolactinoma.

On CT/MR imaging, the adenomas are seen as a hypodense/hypointense lesion compared to normal pituitary with intense homogeneous late enhancement. Heterogeneous signal may be seen if associated with hemorrhage, necrosis or cyst formation.

Suggested Reading

Mindermann T, Wilson CB (1995) Pediatric pituitary adenomas. Neurosurgery 36:259–268

Nishio S, Morioka T, Suzuki S, Takeshita I, Fukui M, Iwaki T (2001) Pituitary tumors in adolescence: clinical behaviour and neuroimaging features of seven cases. J Clin Neurosci 8:231–234

Subependymal Giant Cell Astrocytoma (SEGA)

Clinical Presentation

A 12-year-old girl with known tuberous sclerosis (TS). Now patient presents with headaches.

Images (Fig. 6.24)

A. T1-weighted image shows a sharply marginated mass in the region of right foramen of Monro (*arrow*). Associated asymmetric enlargement of the right lateral ventricle is seen. Left temporal parenchymal TS changes are seen (*arrowheads*)
B. Contrast-enhanced T1-weighted image demonstrates a large, lobulated mass with intense and homogeneous enhancement
C. T2-weighted image shows a mixed signal lesion in the right lateral ventricle in the region of foramen of Monro (*arrow*). Asymmetric lateral ventricle enlargement is again seen. The left parenchymal TS change with calcification is vaguely seen (*arrowhead*)

Discussion

SEGA is the most common cerebral neoplasm in TS. Still, it is an uncommon tumor accounting for only 1.4% of pediatric brain neoplasms in a large series. Most of them occur in the first and second decade of life, with a mean age of 11 years. The neoplasm is characterized by slow growth and benign biological behavior corresponding to WHO grade I lesion. SEGA lies practically always adjacent to the lateral ventricle near the foramen of Monro and is associated clinically with TS. This tumor has characteristics of both neuronal and astrocytic origin. Although the origin of this tumor lies outside the ventricle itself, it grows into the lateral ventricle. With progressive growth, obstruction of the CSF at the foramen Monro will occur. The symptoms are usually related to increased intracranial pressure, as in this case, or seizures. The lesion is isodense on CT scan and often has calcification. The imaging hallmark of this tumor is usually a sharply marginated and uniformly enhancing lesion on both CT and MR images. This marked contrast enhancement separates SEGA from other tumors that do not show significant enhancement. Demonstration of interval growth should be present before the diagnosis of SEGA is considered.

Suggested Reading

Hahn JS, Bejar R, Gladson CL (1991) Neonatal subependymal giant cell astrocytoma associated with tuberous sclerosis: MRI, CT and ultrasound correlation. Neurology 41:124–128

Sinson G, Sutton L, Yachnis A, Duhaine A, Schut I (1994) Subependymal giant cell astrocytomas in children. Pediatr Neurosurg 20:233–239

Atypical Meningioma

Clinical Presentation

A 14-year-old male with headache and morning vomiting for 6 weeks. Patient has a history of acute lymphoblastic leukemia diagnosed 10 years previously and treated with chemotherapy and cranial radiotherapy. Histologically the lesion was an atypical meningioma.

Images (Fig. 6.25)

A. Noncontrast CT shows well-defined heterogeneous but mainly isointense mass in the left parietal lobe
B. Contrast-enhanced CT shows intense, heterogeneous enhancement. Small necrotic areas are seen
C. Sagittal T1-weighted image shows a dural-based well-defined heterogeneous mass in the left parietal lobe
D. Coronal FLAIR image shows well-defined heterogeneous, mainly high signal mass in the left parietal lobe
E. The mass is high signal on the T2-weighted image
F. Contrast-enhanced T1-weighted image shows intense contrast enhancement
G. DW image shows heterogeneous hyperintensity
H. MR spectroscopy (single voxel, TE 144 ms) shows absence of NAA and Cr peaks with the presence of lactate peak
I. MR spectroscopy (single voxel, TE 30 ms) shows a small NAA and Cr peaks with the presence of lactate peak. The small NAA peak is likely contamination from surrounding brain

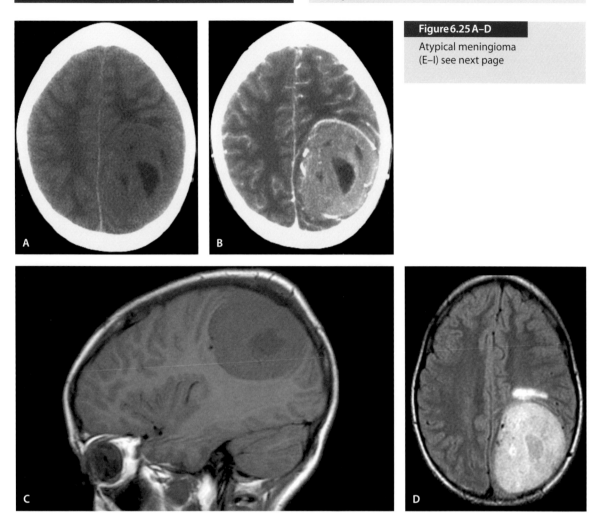

Figure 6.25 A–D
Atypical meningioma
(E–I) see next page

Discussion

Meningioma is a rare entity in childhood. Possible etiological factors in childhood meningioma include neurofibromatosis, radiation, and congenital and familial factors. Meningioma in children may develop anywhere within the cranium. However, locations considered to be rare in adults are more common in children and include ventricles, posterior fossa, orbits, deep sylvian fissures and brain parenchyma. Dural attachment is not a common sign.

Radiologically, typical features include iso- to hyperdense mass with homogeneous enhancement. However, atypical features of meningioma may be seen in 6–7% of cases. Atypical features on CT suggest malignant meningeal tumor, such as meningeal sarcoma, melanoma, or meningeal primitive neuroectodermal tumor. Tumor calcification and cystic changes are more frequent in childhood meningioma. Pathologically, meningothelial meningiomas constitute the major subtype followed by fibroblastic and transitional. The sclerosing type is commonly seen in children which is associated with marked calcification.

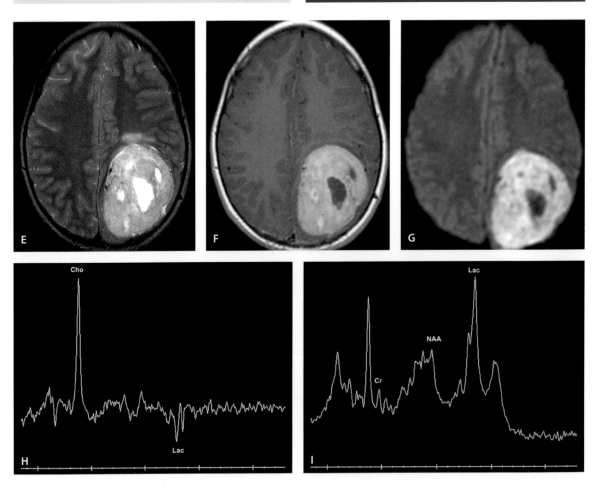

Figure 6.25 E–I

Atypical meningioma

Suggested Reading

Chan RC, Thompson GB (1984) Intracranial meningiomas in childhood. Surg Neurol 21:319–322

Hope JK, Armstrong DA, Babyn PS, Humphreys RR, Harwood-Nash DC, Chuang SH, Marks PV (1992) Primary meningeal tumors in children: correlation of clinical and CT findings with histologic type and prognosis. AJNR Am J Neuroradiol 13:1353–1364

Johnson TE, Weatherhead RG, Nasr AM, Siqueira EB (1993) Ectopic (extradural) meningioma of the orbit: a report of two cases in children. J Pediatr Ophthalmol Strabismus 30:43–47

Sheikh BY, Siqueira E, Dayel F (1996) Meningioma in children: a report of nine cases and a review of the literature. Surg Neurol 45:328–335

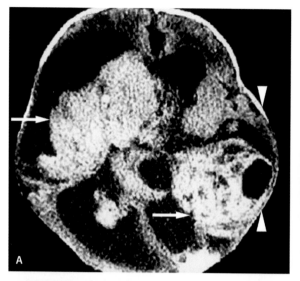

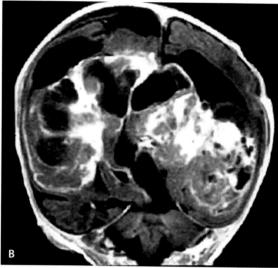

Figure 6.26

Congenital teratoma

Congenital Brain Tumors

Congenital Teratoma

Clinical Presentation

A new born with increased head circumference and failure to thrive.

Images (Fig. 6.26)

A. Noncontrast CT scan shows a large mixed density mass that involves the major part of the brain. Tumor mass is seen in both hemispheres (*arrows*) with associated hydrocephalus. The mass has produced a significant mass effect upon the midline structures and also bulging of the bone on the left (*arrowheads*)

B. Coronal contrast-enhanced T1-weighted image separates the enhancing tumor from the normal appearing brain and distorted ventricles

C. Sagittal T1-weighetd image shows the compression of the mid-brain and brain stem (*arrows*) by the tumor mass.

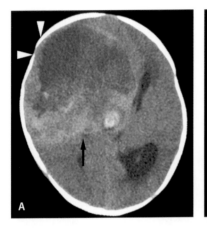 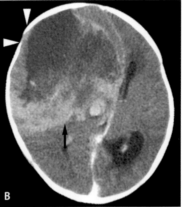

Figure 6.27

Congenital glioblastoma multiforme

Congenital Glioblastoma Multiforme

Clinical Presentation

A 2-month-old male with nystagmus and bulging fontanels. Only CT scan is available. Note the close resemblance to congenital teratoma in the previous case (A).

Images (Fig. 6.27)

A. Noncontrast CT shows a large right frontal mixed density neoplasm (*arrow*) with cystic and hemorrhagic or calcified foci. The mass has produced significant mass effect upon the midline structures and also bulging of the bone (*arrowheads*)
B. Contrast-enhanced CT shows irregular enhancement

Discussion

Congenital or neonatal brain tumors (diagnoses in infants within 60 days after birth) are rare. Two-thirds of them locate supratentorially. In a series of 45 cases the most common histology was a tumor composed of primitive, poorly differentiated tissue: teratoma and PNET. The main CT imaging feature regardless of the histology is that of a large heterogeneous mass with associated hydrocephalus. Coarse calcification is a common feature in teratomas. Prognosis is poor in these tumors. The extent and location of many congenital brain tumors make complete resection impossible. Also the radiation treatment of childhood brain tumors is complicated because postradi-

ation injury on the developing nervous tissue is often devastating although radiation would be the most effective treatment.

Suggested Reading

Buetow PC, Smirniotopoulos JG, Done S (1990) Congenital brain tumors: a review of 45 cases. AJNR Am J Neuroradiol 11:793–799

Orbital Juvenile Pilocytic Astrocytoma (JPA)

Clinical Presentation

A 2-year-old female with exophthalmos and decreased visual acuity.

Images (Fig. 6.28)

A. and B.
   Sagittal (A) and axial (B) T1-weighted noncontrast image demonstrates an oval left optic nerve mass (*arrows*)
C. T2-weighted image demonstrates a large nearly homogeneous mass within the left orbit consistent with an optic nerve glioma (*arrow*). Marked proptosis of the left globe is present
D. Contrast-enhanced T1-weighted image demonstrates intense and near homogeneous enhancement of the tumor (*arrow*)

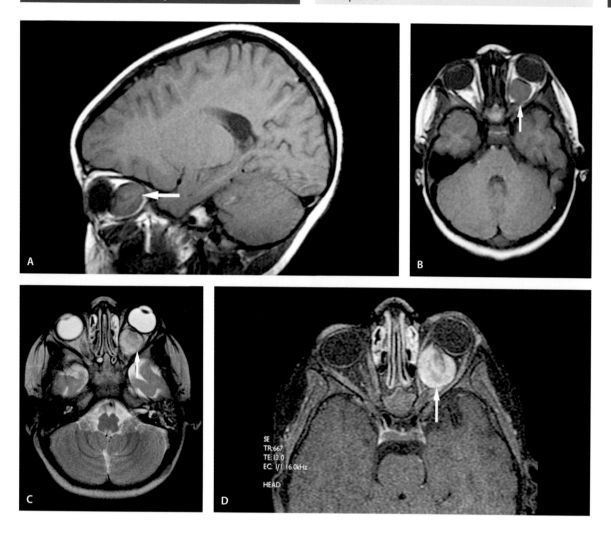

Figure 6.28

Orbital juvenile pilocytic astrocytoma (JPA)

Discussion

The peak incidence of optic nerve gliomas is 2 to 8 years of age. The presenting symptoms are usually proptosis and decreased visual acuity. Other presenting symptoms may be nystagmus and strabismus. There is a high association (up to 50%) with neurofibromatosis type 1 (NF1). Optic nerve glioma may be limited to the orbit or extend into the intracranial cavity. The tumor can also extend into the globe with intraocular seeding. On pathological examination the tumor resembles juvenile pilocytic astrocytoma.

Suggested Reading

Bilgric S, Erbengi A, Tinaztepe B (1989) Optic glioma of childhood: clinical histopathological and histochemical observations. Br J Ophthalmol 73:832–837

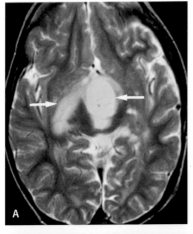
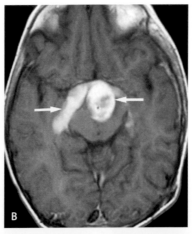

Figure 6.29

Optic pathway glioma

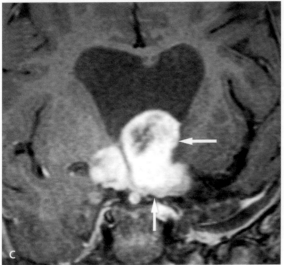
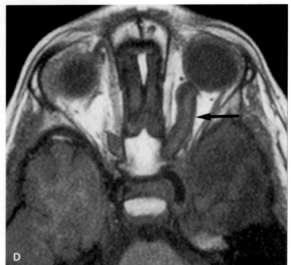

Optic Pathway Glioma

Clinical Presentation

A 9-year-old male with decreased visual acuity.

Images (Fig. 6.29)

A. T2-weighted image shows enlarged proximal optic tract on right with abnormal signal in the optic tract, chiasm and hypothalamus (*arrows*)
B. Axial contrast-enhanced T1-weighted image demonstrates intense enhancement of the lesion (*arrows*)

C. Coronal contrast-enhanced T1-weighted image demonstrates intense enhancement of the hypothalamus and optic chiasm (*arrows*)
D. T1-weighted orbital image shows enlargement of the left optic nerve (*arrow*)

Discussion

Optic pathway gliomas can arise anywhere along the optic pathway. Over 50 % of all optic pathway gliomas involve the chiasm or hypothalamus. Optic chiasm and hypothalamic glioma can be considered a single entity because it is often difficult to distinguish clearly the site of origin. Approximately 60 % are pilocytic astrocytomas and the rest are diffuse fibrillary astrocytomas. Most optic pathway gliomas occur in the first decade of life. They are the most common intracranial tumor in patients with neurofibromatosis type (NF-1). Approximately 15–40% of patients with NF-1 develop optic chiasm hypothalamic glioma whereas 10–70% of patients with optic pathway gliomas have NF-1. Patients with chiasmatic and hypothalamic gliomas at presentation often have visual symptoms in addition to hydrocephalus. Usually the tumors are quite large at presentation. The contrast enhancement is variable. About half of these lesions demonstrate enhancement. Larger tumors may have cystic degeneration. Hemorrhage and calcification are uncommon. Optic chiasm tumors may spread along the optic radiations as this case shows.

Suggested Reading

Alshail E, Rutka JT, Becker LE, et al (1997) Optic chiasmatic-hypothalamic glioma. Brain Pathol 7:799–806

Massry GG, Morgan CF, Chung SM (1997) Evidence of optic pathway gliomas after previously negative neuroimaging. Ophthalmology 104:930–935

Hypothalamic Hamartoma (Hamartoma of Tuber Cinereum)

Clinical Presentation

A 13-year-old female with a 2-year history of gelastic seizures.

Images (Fig. 6.30)

A. Sagittal T1-weighted midline image reveals a large mass in the region of the hypothalamus/tuber cinereum (*arrow*) that is isointense to gray matter
B. Coronal FLAIR shows increased signal intensity (*arrow*). Note the lack of mass effect
C. T2-weighted image shows mass effect on the mamillary bodies (*arrowheads*). The lesion is isointense to the gray matter also on T2-weighted image (*arrows*)
D. The lesion is isointense to the gray matter on DW image (*arrow*)
E. Short TE spectra of the hypothalamic mass. The myoinositol peak (*mI*) is elevated and the NAA peak lower than the corresponding peaks in reference structures

Discussion

Hypothalamic hamartomas (synonym: diencephalic hamartomas) are rare tumors, which usually effect pubertal development (precocious puberty, acromegaly, or both). Other findings include seizures, especially gelastic seizures, intellectual impairment and behavioral disturbances. Intrahypothalamic hamartomas have more tendency to cause seizures than parahypothalamic hamartomas. The classic appearance on MRI is a noncalcified and nonenhancing lesion that is homogeneously isointense to gray matter on T1-weighted images and isointense or slightly hyperintense on T2-weighted images. These findings are fairly characteristic and helpful in differentiating the hypothalamic hamartoma from the more commonly suprasellar craniopharyngioma and hypothalamic/optic chiasma glioma seen in children. Patients with Pallister-Hal syndrome have also hypothalamic hamartoma in addition to polydactyly, bifid epiglottis, renal anomalies, imperforate anus and pituitary dysplasia. This lesion is considered to be due to disturbed embryogenesis between gestational days 33 and 41. It can be classified as a neuronal migration anomaly. Two classifications have been created dividing then either into parahypothalamic hamartomas and intrahypothalamic hamartomas or pedunculated and sessile.

NAA peak has been shown to be present in hypothalamic hamartomas. Elevated myoinositol with decreased NAA peaks in these lesions have been described.

Suggested Reading

Arita K, Ikowa F, Kurisu K, et al (1999) The relationship between magnetic resonance imaging findings and a clinical manifestation of hypothalamic hamartoma. J Neurosurg 91:212–220

Boyko OB, Curnes JT, Oakes WJ, Burger PC (1991) Hamartomas of the tuber cinereum: CT, MR and pathologic findings. AJNR Am J Neuroradiol 12:309–314

Martin DD, Seeger W, Ranke MB, Grodd W (2003) MR imaging and spectroscopy of the tuber cinereum hamartoma in a patient with growth hormone deficiency and hypogonadotropic hypogonadism. AJNR Am J Neuroradiol 24:1177–1180

Tasch E, Cendes F, Li LM, Dubeau F, et al (1998) Hypothalamic hamartomas and gelastic epilepsy: a spectroscopic study. Neurology 51:1046–1050

Valdueza JM, Cristante L, Dammann O, et al (1994) Hypothalamic hamartomas: with special reference to gelastic epilepsy and surgery. Neurosurgery 34:949–958

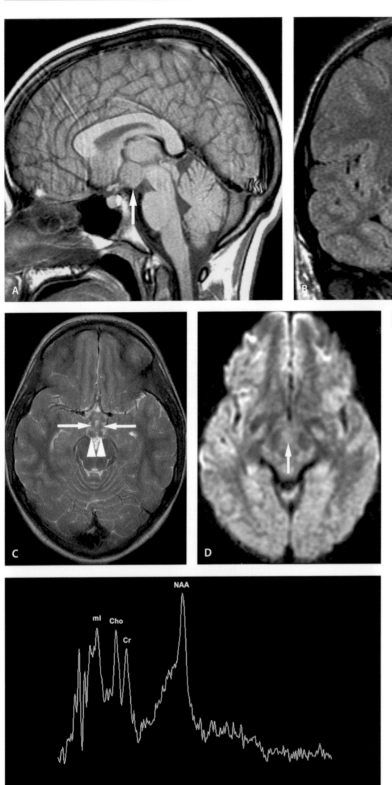

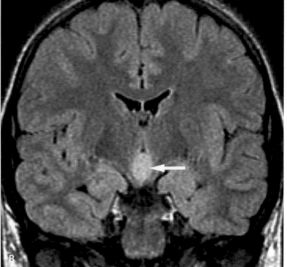

Figure 6.30

Hypothalamic hamartoma
(hamartoma of tuber cinereum)

Chapter 7

Brain Damage

In collaboration with Lawrence Buadu

Introduction

MR imaging is the most sensitive clinical tool to detect brain abnormalities caused by different types of damage while neuropathological evaluation remains most specific. MR imaging is not optimal to determine the etiology of brain damage, but it has certainly broadened our perspective on many traumatic brain injuries. One single etiology often results in multiple different types of brain injury depending on the patient's age at the time of the injury and the duration of the injury. Brain injury includes a broad spectrum of conditions such as hypoxic ischemic encephalopathy (HIE, or anoxic ischemic encephalopathy, AIE), accidental brain trauma, but also nonaccidental brain trauma (child abuse). Besides direct trauma, metabolic and cerebrovascular alterations can also cause brain damage.

Newer neuroimaging modalities such as diffusion, perfusion and spectroscopy are natural components of today's neuroradiology practice. This has necessitated the expansion of competence from the traditional anatomical knowledge to a broad understanding of the underlying physiology and pathophysiology.

In the critically ill neonate, hypoxia, anoxia and ischemia all contribute to the brain damage and the imaging findings. When the neonatal brain is exposed to severe hypoxia, anoxia or ischemia, the developing brain undergoes a number of metabolic and structural changes, which can be monitored by MR imaging and MR spectroscopy. MR spectroscopy is capable of measuring metabolites in this damaging cascade, such as excess release of excitatory neurotransmitters (glutamine and glutamate) at synaptic junctions leading to neurotoxicity. Excess lactate can also be measured. In an older child's brain the decline of N-acetylaspartate (NAA) has been associated with anoxia. NAA, however, is not a good marker in a very young brain since it is normally quite low in infants and young children and therefore a decline cannot be reliably visualized. In older children a decrease in NAA provides a good landmark for brain damage. Lactate can be significantly increased early in the anoxic event, but it is not a persistent finding even with severe brain injury.

Vascular autoregulation in the preterm child is different from that in a term child or an older child. Also the vascular arrangement in the preterm infant (<34 weeks) is different from that in the term infant. The concept of "diving reflex" in which hypoxia or anoxia results in rearrangement of the blood from less vital body structures to the more vital structures such as the brain and specifically to the basal ganglia and brain stem. This will help to minimize damage to these structures. In preterm children the autoregulation reflexes are immature or absent, and any significant drop in systemic pressure will result in decreased perfusion of the brain. This may lead to deep white matter damage. Periventricular leukomalacia (PVL) results from ischemic damage of periventricular white matter and it is often seen in preterm infants but not in term infants. In preterm infants germinal matrix hemorrhages and venous infarctions leading to hemorrhage are also seen. In term infants HIE may lead to multicystic leukomalacia of various degrees of severity.

Early ischemia is difficult to detect in MR images since the normal neonatal brain demonstrates T2 hyperintensity due to lack of myelination in this stage of development. However, diffusion imaging detects early hypoxic and ischemic events leading to cytotoxic edema and later to volume loss. Cerebrovascular occlusion with stroke in the neonate is more prevalent than previously recognized. In the preterm infant, most CNS ischemic injuries result in PVL. Brain infarctions with or without hemorrhage can occur in the term infant following HEI but also as a complication of sepsis or hypercoagulable state.

Though CT remains the main modality in assessing the patient with acute head trauma, MR imaging adds a new dimension to the diagnosis. In the suspected cases of nonaccidental trauma, MR imaging is

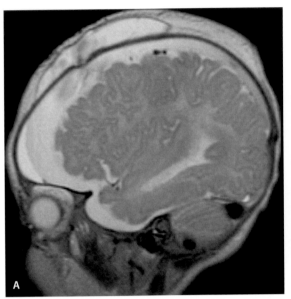 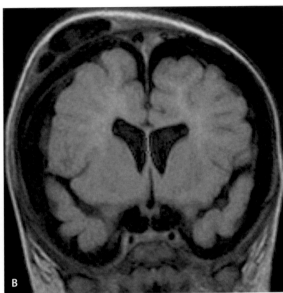

Figure 7.1

Scalp injury (subgaleal hemorrhage)

a sensitive modality not only in the evaluation of the presence of the trauma but also in the estimation of the timing of the trauma, the patient's prognosis and the extent of the trauma. However, one should remember that interpretation on pediatric neuroimaging studies always requires clinical correlation.

Nonaccidental Trauma

Scalp Injury (Subgaleal Hemorrhage)

Clinical Presentation

A 3-month-old child presenting with decreased responsiveness and suspected nonaccidental head injury.

Images (Fig. 7.1)

A. Sagittal T2-weighted image demonstrates scalp soft tissue swelling consistent with subgaleal hemorrhage
B. In addition to the low signal scalp hematoma, bilateral subdural low signal collections are also demonstrated on coronal FLAIR image. These could represent chronic subdural hematomas or hygromas

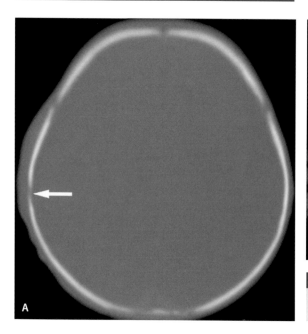

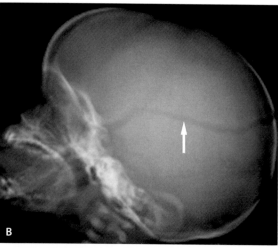

Figure 7.2
Skull fracture

Skull Fracture

Clinical Presentation

A 2-month-old female status after a recent fall.

Images (Fig. 7.2)

A. CT scan shows a right parietal skull fracture with overlying soft tissue swelling (*arrow*)
B. The fracture is seen to better advantage on the lateral plain skull radiograph (*arrow*)

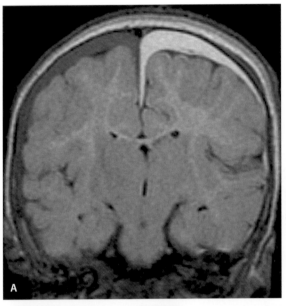

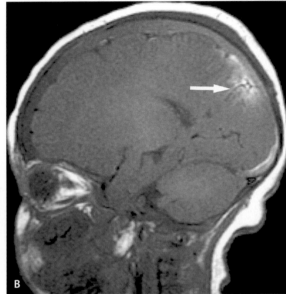

Figure 7.3
Subdural hemorrhage

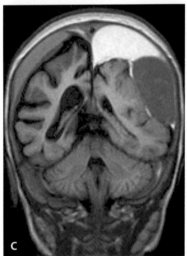

Subdural Hemorrhage

Clinical Presentation

A 2-month-old admitted with seizures. Ophthalmologic examination revealed retinal hemorrhages.

Images (Fig. 7.3)

A. Coronal FLAIR image shows bilateral subdural hemorrhages in different stages of temporal evolution. Although not conclusive, it suggests repetitive trauma
B. The finding of hemorrhagic contusion in the left parieto-occipital region (*arrow*) on sagittal T1-weighted image further raises the suspicion for nonaccidental head injury
C. Follow-up coronal FLAIR image several months later after reportedly minor trauma shows significant brain atrophy confirming severe brain injury at initial presentation

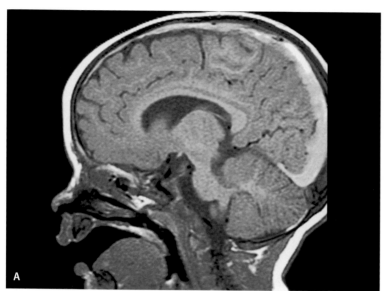
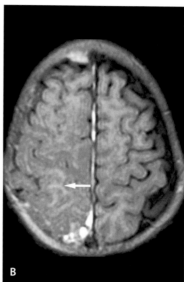

Figure 7.4

Subarachnoid and subdural hemorrhage

Subarachnoid and Subdural Hemorrhage

Clinical Presentation

A 9-month-old male with suspected nonaccidental head injury and retinal hemorrhages.

Images (Fig. 7.4)

A. Sagittal T1-weighted image shows a right subdural hematoma

B. FLAIR image shows subarachnoid hemorrhage (*arrow*) in the right parietal region

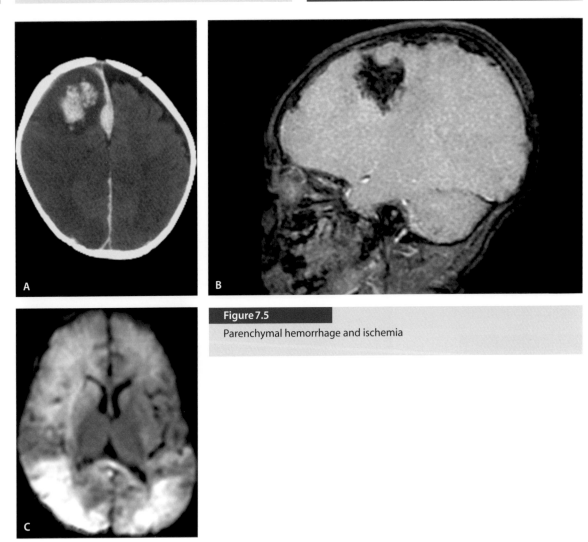

Figure 7.5

Parenchymal hemorrhage and ischemia

Parenchymal Hemorrhage and Ischemia

Clinical Presentation

A 5-month-old female presenting with altered mental status.

Images (Fig. 7.5)

A. CT scan shows focal hemorrhagic contusion in the right frontal lobe
B. Sagittal gradient-echo image confirms the presence of parenchymal hemorrhage in the right frontal lobe
C. DW image shows widespread areas of ischemia indicating severe traumatic brain injury

Figure 7.6

Diffuse axonal injury

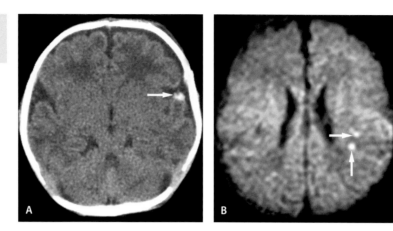

Diffuse Axonal Injury (DAI)

Clinical Presentation

A 14-day-old female with new onset of focal seizures.

Images (Fig. 7.6)

A. CT scan shows focal hemorrhage over the left temporal tip (*arrow*)

B. DW image reveals two punctuate foci of restricted diffusion (*arrows*) in the left parietal region most consistent with axonal injury

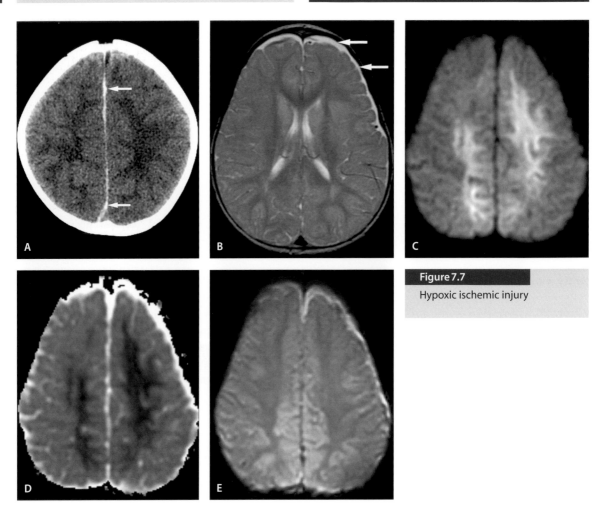

Figure 7.7

Hypoxic ischemic injury

Hypoxic Ischemic Injury

Clinical Presentation

A 14-month-old female who initially presented with vomiting and possible seizure after falling down a flight of stairs.

Images (Fig. 7.7)

A. CT scan was unremarkable except for a small subdural hemorrhage along the interhemispheric falx (*arrows*)

B. T2-weighted image confirms the presence of subdural hemorrhages (*arrows*) but is otherwise unremarkable

C. DW image demonstrates areas of restricted diffusion in both cerebral hemispheres indicating hypoxic ischemic injury

D. ADC map confirms the presence of ischemic injury. The hyperintense areas on DW image are hypointense on the ADC map consistent with cytotoxic edema

E. The acute subdural hematoma is seen as a high signal lesion in the gradient echo image. It is better seen on T2-weighted image

Figure 7.8
Infarct

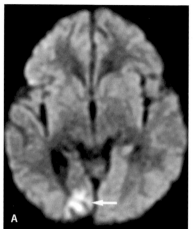
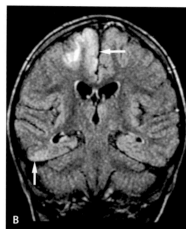

Infarct

Clinical Presentation

A 2-year-old female who initially presented with recent seizures, resolving left hemiparesis and focal EEG changes. The first MR image at that time was normal.

Images (Fig. 7.8)

A. and B.
A month later the child returned to the emergency department with a history of a fall with fractures of the right tibia and fibula. Repeat MR imaging showed multiple areas of subacute infarction on DW (A) and FLAIR (B) images (*arrows*)

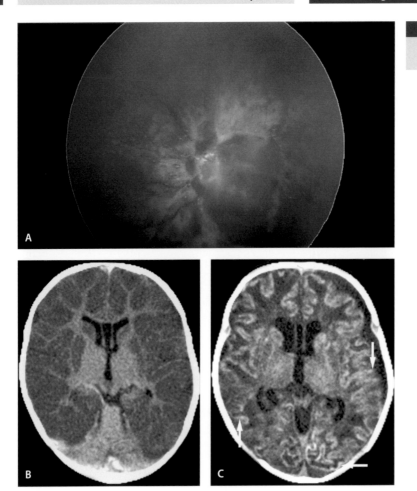

Figure 7.9
Atrophy

Atrophy

Clinical Presentation

A 2-month-old female presenting with seizures and apnea.

Images (Fig. 7.9)

A. Ophthalmologic examination reveals multiple retinal hemorrhages
B. Initial CT scan demonstrates extensive cortical swelling and hypodensity with relative sparing of the basal ganglia and cerebellum, the so-called "reversal sign" or "white cerebellum sign"
C. CT scan obtained 10 days later shows marked generalized cerebral atrophy and linear increased density along the gyri (*arrows*) corresponding to sequelae of laminar necrosis

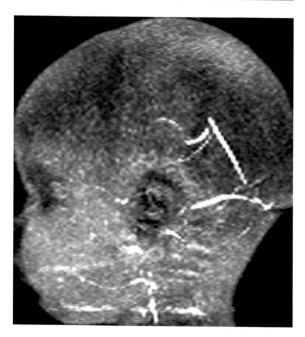

Figure 7.10
Venous sinus thrombosis

Venous Sinus Thrombosis

Clinical Presentation

A 5 month old male found unresponsive. Clinically child abuse is suspected.

Image (Fig. 7.10)

A. MR venogram demonstrates absence of the superior sagittal sinus consistent with sinus thrombosis.

Thalamic Infarcts in a Shaken Infant Syndrome

Clinical Presentation

A 5-month-old female found pulseless with copious bleeding from the nose and seizing. There is clinical suspicion of shaken infant syndrome.

Images (Fig. 7.11)

A. CT scan is unremarkable
B. T1-weighted image fails to demonstrate pathology
C. T2-weighted image is normal
D. On GRE image there is no blood in the parenchyma
E. On DW image there is high signal intensity in both thalami. There are faint areas of diffusion disturbance also involving parts of the basal ganglia as well as the hippocampi
F. On ADC map the thalami and some basal ganglia areas are hypointense
G. Exponential image shows significant hyperintensity of the thalami and parts of the basal ganglia. These areas are consistent with restricted diffusion and cytotoxic edema as seen in HIE

Discussion

It is estimated that in excess of 2000 children in the United States die each year as a result of child abuse. Nonaccidental head injury (NAHI) is largely restricted to children under 3 years of age, with the majority occurring during the first year of life. Inflicted head injury is the most common cause of traumatic death in infancy. With inflicted head injury an accurate history is rarely provided at presentation. The information most commonly reported is usually of a minor nature and the history may be vague or may vary with time. Physical examination although useful may provide little insight regarding underlying brain injury. Consequently, the diagnosis and detection of NAHI usually comes to rest on radiological imaging. Although no single imaging finding is specific for abuse, no other medical condition fully mimics all the features of NAHI in infants and children. If radiographic indicators of abuse or neglect are missed, the consequences are grave for the child who will invariably be returned to a high-risk environment.

Terminology applied to inflicted head injury in children has varied along with the evolution in the

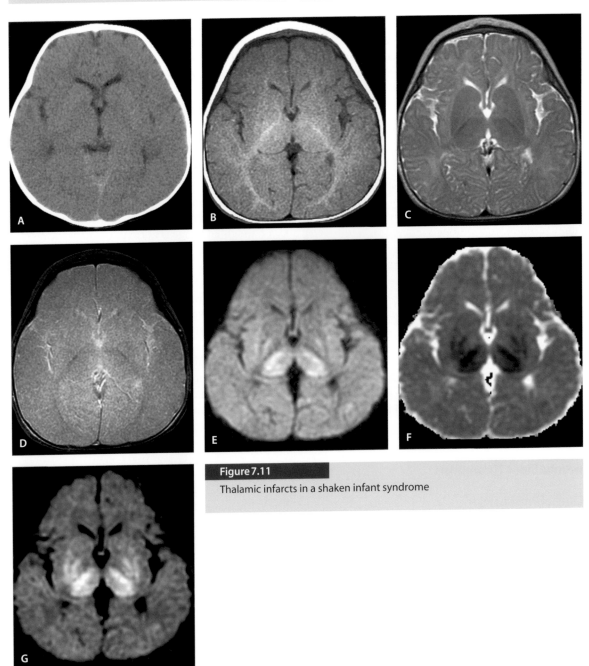

Figure 7.11

Thalamic infarcts in a shaken infant syndrome

understanding of the underlying mechanisms. Regardless of terminology, most inflicted head injuries in children are of the dynamic type. Dynamic injuries may occur in either (a) direct contact trauma (when a stationary head is struck by a moving object, a moving head is struck by a stationary object or when both a moving head and moving object collide) or (b) indirect injury. Contact phenomena result in localized distortion or a fracture of the skull, focal cortical injury, epidural hematoma or subdural hematoma. In contrast to direct trauma, indirect injuries are independent of skull deformation and entail inertial loading which occurs with sudden acceleration or deceleration of the head. Although contact may occur with this mechanism, significant life-threatening injuries may occur without an impact. Head acceleration or deceleration results in a variety of strain deformations of the skull and its contents. Shear strain deformation which produces disruption at tissue interfaces is the most important mechanism in the production of intracranial injury. Furthermore the primary injury occurring with these biomechanical forces may result in other pathophysiological alterations or secondary injury (e.g. edema, swelling, hypoxic ischemia, herniation) and produce additional imaging findings. Other etiological factors may also result in hypoxic-ischemic injury and diffuse cerebral swelling without significant biomechanical force. These include strangulation, suffocation by hand or pillow, and prolonged squeezing of the chest. In these types of injury, external manifestations are minor or nonexistent. Imaging is even more crucial in elucidating severity and mechanisms of injury when the clinical history is not revealing.

Although conventional MR imaging is more sensitive than CT scan in detection of hematomas of various ages and areas of contusions, recent research has proven MR spectroscopy and DW imaging to be informative in the acute phase. MR spectroscopy may distinguish those children who have suffered more significant and long-lasting brain injury by demonstrating lactate or diffusion abnormality. This may help the clinicians more accurately identify those infants who have suffered severe injury, and direct treatment and social services toward these infants.

Suggested Reading

Billmire ME, Myers PA (1985) Serious head injury in infants; accident or abuse? Pediatrics 75:340–342

Buadu L, Ekholm S, Lenane A, Moritani T, Hiwatashi A, Westesson PL (2004) Patterns of head injury in non accidental trauma. Neurographics 3(1):article 2

Caffey J (1974) The whiplash shaken infant syndrome; manual shaking by the extremities with whiplash-induced intracranial and intraocular bleedings, linked with residual permanent brain damage and mental retardation. Pediatrics 54:396–403

Centers for Disease Control (1990) Childhood injuries in the United States. Am J Dis Child 144:627–646

Duhaime AC, Gennarelli TA, Thibault LE, Bruce DA, Margulies SS, Wiser R (1987) The shaken baby syndrome: a clinical, pathological and biomechanical study. J Neurosurg 66:409–415

Kleinman PK (1998) Diagnostic imaging of child abuse, 2nd edn. Mosby, St Louis, pp 286–287

National Clearing House on Child Abuse and Neglect Information (2000) Child fatalities fact sheet. www.calib.com/nc-canch/pubs/factsheet/fatality.html (22 Feb 2000)

Epidural and Subdural Hematoma

Epidural Hematoma (EDH)

Clinical Presentation

A 10-year-old male sustained an injury to the left side of his head after a fall from bike without a helmet. He has known skull fracture on left.

Images (Fig. 7.12)

A. Noncontrast CT scan at presentation demonstrates a shallow extraaxial bleed in left temporal area (*arrow*). Over the right sylvian region, a small amount of subarachnoid blood is present (*arrowhead*)

B. CT scan 9 hours later shows a biconvex EDH in the left temporal area (*arrow*). The central part is low density with a bright periphery. It could be due to active bleeding at the time of the hematoma with swirling blood. The right side lesion is stable

C. On CT scan 24 hours later a hyperdense EDH is seen (*arrow*)

D. T1-weighted image after the third CT scan shows a slightly hyperintense EDH (*arrow*)

E. The EDH is hyperintense on proton density image (*arrow*)

F. T2-weighted image shows hyperintense EDH (*arrow*)

G. Coronal FLAIR image shows heterogeneous but mostly hyperintense EDH (*arrow*)

H. GRE image shows mixed signal hematoma (*arrow*); it varies from iso- to hypointense compared to gray matter

I. b_0 image (SE-EPI) shows also mixed signal intensity in EDH (*arrow*)

J. DW image reveals central low signal with thin peripheral layer of increased signal in EDH (*arrow*). The right temporal findings are stable

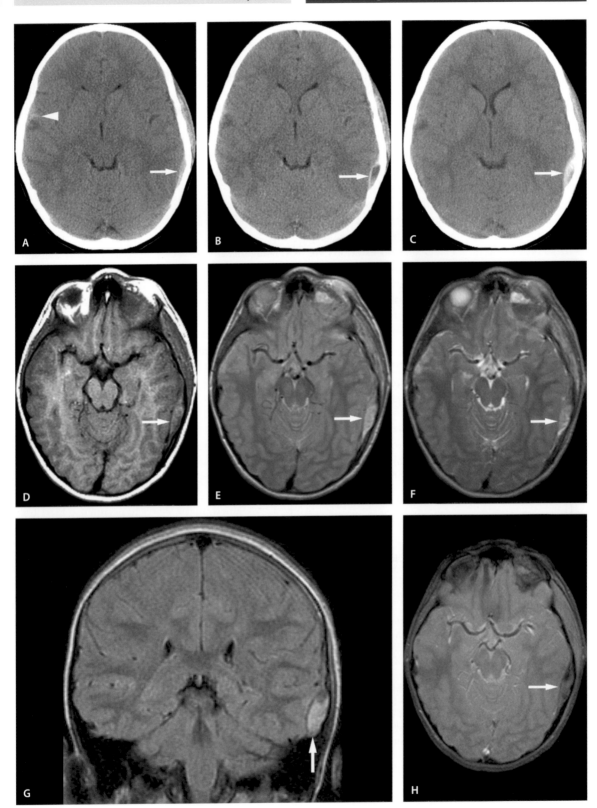

Figure 7.12 A–H

Epidural hematoma

Figure 7.12 I, J

Epidural hematoma

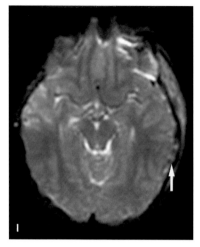
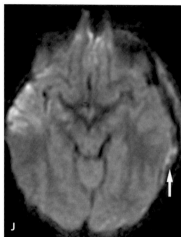

Subdural Hematoma (SDH)

Clinical Presentation

A former 25-week gestational age premature baby, now 9-month-old girl who had 2 weeks extracorporeal membrane oxygenation therapy (ECMO) for chronic lung disease.

Images (Fig. 7.13)

A. Noncontrast CT scan shows mixed density SDH in the right occipital region (*arrow*)
B. Sagittal T1-weighted image 10 days later shows the same SDH to be hyperintense (*arrow*). This is consistent with methemoglobin formation
C. Coronal contrast-enhanced SPGR image shows small right distal ICA with less flow (*arrow*). This is due to the older ECMO treatment technique where right carotid artery was cannulated and sacrificed. The cavernous sinus on right does not fill with contrast as it is thrombosed (*Note:* In the current technique the carotid and jugular vessels are repaired after ECMO treatment)
D. T2-weighted image shows small flow void in the right cavernous carotid artery (*arrow*) that represents collateral flow from left since the right carotid artery has been ligated
E. T2-weighted image shows hyperintense SDH with hemosiderin stain in the medial border of the hematoma (*arrow*). Note good flow void in the sagittal sinus. Low volume of white matter is present as a consequence of prematurity. The corpus callosum is thin. Myelination is seen in the posterior limb of the internal capsule

Discussion

EDH is an uncommon complication of head trauma in children. The potential space between the inner table of the skull and the dura is the location of this hematoma. Classically, a skull fracture that crosses a branch of the middle meningeal artery results in arterial bleeding that dissects the dura from the inner table. However, venous bleeding is also often the reason for an EDH. The characteristic appearance of the hematoma is lens shaped and it respects the sutures. EDH can also be present without a skull fracture. Venous bleeding leading to an EDH is more common in children than in adults. Direct trauma to the venous sinuses or emissary veins may be the reason for the venous bleeding. Most EDHs will be examined with CT imaging and evacuated immediately. It is rare to diagnose an EDH with MR imaging in the hyperacute phase (<24 hours of bleeding). In the hyperacute phase the signal changes are due to oxyhemoglobin that is iso- to slightly hypointense to the gray matter on T1-weighted images and hyperintense on T2-weighted sequences. It is more common to diagnose EDHs in the acute or early subacute phase (24–48 hours after the incident). In that time the hematoma is isointense on T1-weighted image and markedly hypointense on T2-weighted image due to deoxyhemoglobin.

Signal pattern of epidural and subdural hematoma are identical, but they may be very different from those of parenchymal or intraventricular hemorrhage of the same duration. Acute subdural hematomas (SDH) are also mostly diagnosed by CT scan. Also acute SDH may be arterial or venous in nature. Injury to cortical arteries can result in accumulation of blood in the subdural space that will cause a

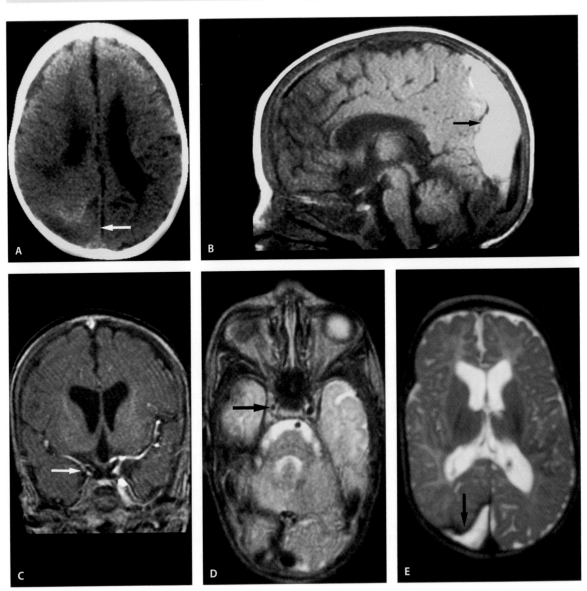

Figure 7.13

Subdural hematoma

mass effect. The bleeding is caused by disruption of the bridging veins coursing the subdural space between the cortex and the dural sinuses. Shallow SDH are sometimes difficult to detect by CT scanning; however, the greater sensitivity of MR imaging for soft-tissue contrast, multiplanar projections and absence of beam hardening bone artifacts, increase the capability of MR imaging to detect even small SDH,

especially if they are subacute. Evolution of SDH follows that of EDH and is discussed above. Oxidation of deoxyhemoglobin to intracellular methemoglobin during the subacute phase causes brightening of the signal first on T1-weighted and later on T2-weighted images as red cell lysis occurs. Chronic SDHs have signal characteristics close to that of CSF, except that they are slightly higher signal due to their protein content. On T2-weighted images the signal of SDH closely resembles that of CSF. Unlike parenchymal hemorrhages there are no hemosiderin-laden macrophages to cause the decrease in the T2 signal.

Subdural hygromas are similar in shape to SDH. They result from a tear in the arachnoid membrane with leaking of CSF into the subdural space. These extraaxial fluid collections closely follow the CSF signal in all sequences. Differentiation of chronic SDH from hygroma is not always possible on CT scan, but MRI imaging is able to make the distinction.

Suggested Reading

Blankenberg FG, Loh N-N, Bracci P, et al (2000) Sonography, CT, and MR imaging: a prospective comparison of neonates with suspected intracranial ischemia and hemorrhage. AJNR Am J Neuroradiol 21:213–218

Bulas DI, Taylor GA, O'Donnell RM, Short BL, Fitz CR, Vezina G (1996) Intracranial abnormalities in infants treated with extracorporeal membrane oxygenation: update on sonographic and CT findings. AJNR Am J Neuroradiol 17: 287–294

Fobben ES, Grossman RI, Atlas SW, Hackney DB, Goldberg HI, Zimmerman RA, Bilaniuk LT. (1989) MR characteristics of subdural hematomas and hygromas at 1.5 T. AJR Am J Roentgenol 3:589–595

Lin DM, Filippi CG, Steever AB, Zimmerman RD (2001) Detection of intracranial hemorrhage: comparison between gradient-echo and b_0 (SE-SPI) images obtained from diffusion-weighted echo-planar sequences. AJNR Am J Neuroradiol 22:1275–1281

Contusion

Clinical Presentation

An 8-year-old male was admitted following a motor vehicle accident. Several days after admission he underwent MR scan to fully evaluate the extent of his injuries.

Images (Fig. 7.14)

A. T2-weighted image reveals left frontal lobe contusion. A shallow subdural hemorrhage is present on left (*arrow*). Hyperintensity is seen in the midbrain (*arrowhead*). This is more likely contusion than DAI, since it involves the dorsolateral brain surface. Soft tissue swelling and contusion is seen on the left

B. Proton density image shows the same left frontal contusion and several smaller contusions in the parenchyma and basal ganglia. Blood is seen in the left lateral ventricle. A shallow subdural hematoma is seen on the left as high signal intensity

C. Proton density image above section shown in B. Again multiple parenchymal hemorrhagic contusions and DAI are seen. Blood layers are seen in the dependent portions of the lateral ventricles (*arrows*)

D. T1-weighted image shows methemoglobin in the left frontal contusion. The extraaxial hematoma is best seen in this sequence. Multiple smaller hemorrhagic contusions are seen. Blood in the occipital horn is present (*arrow*)

Discussion

Acute craniocerebral trauma may reveal several types of lesions: contusion, intracerebral and extracerebral hematomas, general and focal cerebral swelling, and shearing injury (diffuse axonal injury, DAI) of the cerebral white matter. The contusions are caused by direct contact between the skull and brain parenchyma, the floor of the anterior cranial fossa and most often in the temporal and frontal lobes. Contusions also occur at sites where brain parenchyma impacts dural reflexion, in such locations as the splenium of the corpus callosum and dorsolateral brainstem. The contusion may be hemorrhagic or nonhemorrhagic. Hemorrhagic contusions are the most frequent lesion and may result in focal neurological deficits. Contusions are much less likely to be associated with severe initial impairment of consciousness. When cerebral contusions are large or extensive, they may act as mass lesions.

MR imaging is more sensitive in detection of brain contusion that CT imaging. The appearance of the contusions on MR image is variable depending upon the constituents of the contusions. On MR imaging, hemorrhagic contusions appeared as high signal on T1-weighted images and as either low or high signal on T2-weighted images, depending upon the age of hemorrhage. The nonhemorrhagic contusion of the brain is manifest as focal swelling and increased water content of the brain, giving low density on CT images and prolongation on both T1- and T2-weighted images.

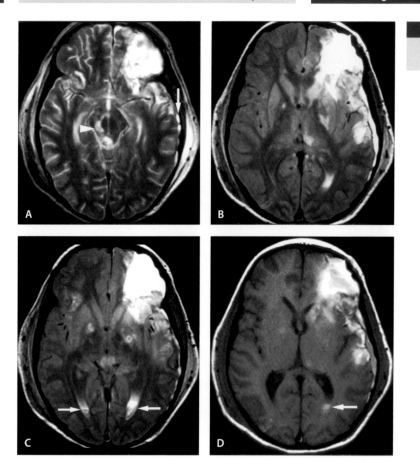

Figure 7.14
Contusion

Suggested Reading

Hesselink JR, Dowd CF, Healy ME, Hajek P, Baker LL, Luerssen TG (1988) MR imaging of brain contusions: a comparative study with CT. AJR Am J Roentgenol 150:1133–1142

Zimmerman RA, Bilaniuk LT, Gennarelli T, Bruce D, Dolinskas C, Uzzell B (1978) Cranial computed tomography in diagnosis and management of acute head trauma. AJR Am J Roentgenol 131:27–34

Diffuse Axonal Injury (DAI)

DAI in Corpus Callosum and Parenchyma

Clinical Presentation

A 10-year-old female with history of car accident.

Images (Fig. 7.15)

A. T2-weighted image shows high signal involving the body and splenium of the corpus callosum (*arrow*)

B. Coronal FLAIR image shows also high signal in the corpus callosum (*arrow*)

C. DAI appears hyperintense on b_0 image (SE-EPI) (*arrow*)

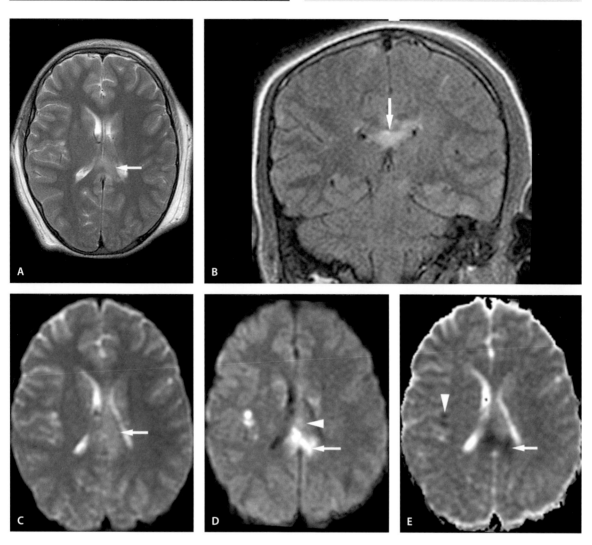

D. DW image demonstrates DAI as high signal (*arrow*) in the splenium. The body of the corpus callosum is less bright (*arrowhead*). A small right gray/white matter junction DAI is also present. It is best seen on DW image

E. The high signal DAI on DW image is hypointense on ADC map (*arrow*) representing cytotoxic edema. The high signal involving the body of the corpus callosum represents T2-shine-through phenomenon. The small gray/white junction DAI is also hypointense on ADC map (*arrowhead*)

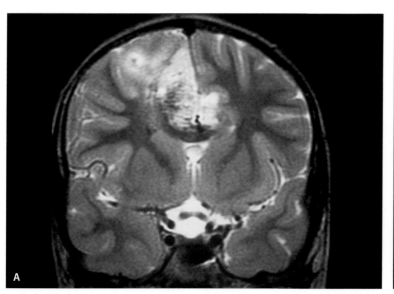
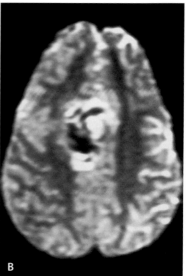

Figure 7.16

Hemorrhagic Contusion with diffuse axonal injury

Hemorrhagic Contusion with DAI

Clinical Presentation

A 9-year-old male was involved with a car accident.

Images (Fig. 7.16)

A. Coronal T2-weighted image shows hemorrhagic contusion in the frontal lobe. Additionally the corpus callosum shows a vague hyperintensity representing DAI

B. b_0 image (SE-EPI) confirms the presence of the hypointense hemorrhage and hyperintense edema at and above the corpus callosum

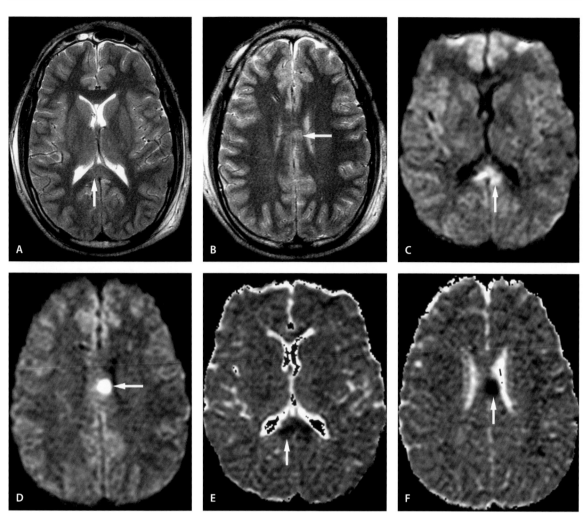

Figure 7.17

Multiple areas of diffuse axonal injury in corpus callosum

Multiple Areas of DAI in Corpus Callosum

Clinical Presentation

A 17-year-old male with history of car accident.

Images (Fig. 7.17)

A. T2-weighted image shows hyperintense lesion in the splenium of the corpus callosum (*arrow*)
B. Another hyperintensity is seen in the body of the corpus callosum on T2-weighted image (*arrow*)
C. and D.
   DW images show these lesions as hyperintense (*arrows*)
E. and F. ADC maps show decreased signal on the DW hyperintensity (*arrows*) representing cytotoxic edema

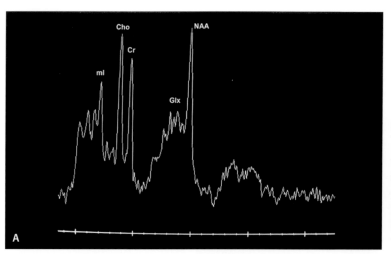
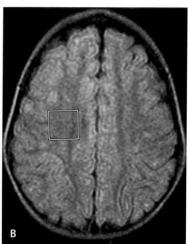

Figure 7.18

Diffuse axonal injury with excitotoxic mechanism

DAI with Excitotoxic Mechanism

Clinical Presentation

A 12-year-old female involved in a car accident. She was referred for MR spectroscopy because of persistent mental status change. The conventional MR study was normal.

Images (Fig. 7.18)

A. Single voxel MR spectroscopy with TE=35 ms. MR spectrum demonstrates prominent glutamate/glutamine peak (*Glx*)
B. Localizer for MR spectroscopy demonstrating the voxel placement. There is no obvious parenchymal injury

Discussion

Diffuse axonal injury is a major form of traumatic brain injury and is caused by shearing stress primarily in the white matter. Diffuse axonal injury results from rotational acceleration and deceleration forces producing diffuse shear-strain deformations of brain tissue, usually at the gray/white matter junction, in the corpus callosum, and at the dorsolateral aspect of the upper brain stem. Diffuse axonal injury is usually related to general poor clinical status.

MR imaging helps in detection of pattern of injury in diffuse axonal injury. The predominant location of these injuries is the white matter of the superior frontal gyrus, at the gray/white matter interface of the frontal and temporal lobes, and in the corpus callosum. Most of these lesions are small (1–5 mm), multiple, bilateral and hemorrhagic. T2-weighted gradient echo MR imaging is an excellent modality for detection of small foci of hemorrhage seen in diffuse axonal injury. Diffusion-weighted imaging shows areas of increased signal with decreased ADC value.

Blunt trauma is a mechanism that elevates the extracellular glutamate levels. This triggers the excitotoxic cascade by allowing excessive accumulation of glutamate in the synaptic space. This can produce disastrous results in the neurons leading to neuronal death. One recent therapeutic approach is to use glutamate receptor blockers to minimize neuronal death.

Suggested Reading

Liu AY, Maldjian JA, Bagley LJ, Sinson GP, Grossman RI (1999) Traumatic brain injury: diffusion-weighted MR imaging findings. AJNR Am J Neuroradiol 20:1636–1641

Mark LP, Prost RW, Ulmer JL, et al (2001) Pictorial review of glutamate excitotoxicity: fundamental concepts for neuroimaging. AJNR Am J Neuroradiol 22:1813–1824

Scheid R, Preul C, Gruber O, Wiggins C, von Cramon DY (2003) Diffuse axonal injury associated with chronic traumatic brain injury: evidence from T2-weighted gradient-echo imaging at 3T. AJNR Am J Neuroradiol 24:1049–1056

Tong KA, Ashwal S, Holshouser BA, et al (2003) Hemorrhagic shearing lesions in children and adolescents with post-traumatic diffuse axonal injury: improved detection and initial results. Radiology 227:332–339

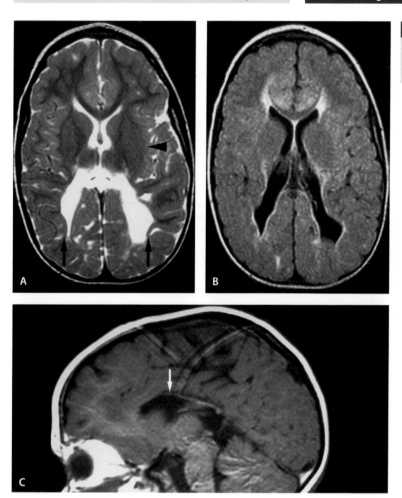

Figure 7.19

Periventricular leukomalacia with white matter aplasia

Periventricular Leukomalacia (PVL), Preterm Hypoxic Ischemic Encephalopathy (HIE)

Periventricular Leukomalacia with White Matter Aplasia

Clinical Presentation

A 3-year-old female, former 33-week gestational age premature baby has developmental delay and spastic diplegia. She presents because of frequent falls.

Images (Fig. 7.19)

A. T2-weighted image shows gray matter extending to the ventricles (*arrows*) from severe white matter loss, mainly in the posterior aspect of the brain. Undulation of the ventricular walls is seen. Demyelination of the external capsule is seen (*arrowhead*)

B. FLAIR image shows periventricular and external capsule demyelination. Again undulation of the ventricular walls is present. Thin genu of corpus callosum is seen

C. Sagittal T1-weighted image shows hypoplasia of the corpus callosum (*arrow*) and cingulate gyrus

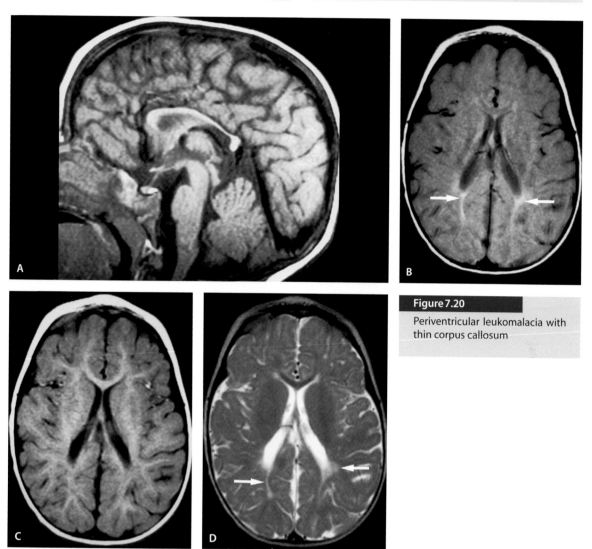

Figure 7.20

Periventricular leukomalacia with thin corpus callosum

Periventricular Leukomalacia with Thin Corpus Callosum

Clinical Presentation

A 12-month-old girl with developmental delay, mixed tone and past history of 33 weeks prematurity with respiratory distress syndrome.

Images (Fig. 7.20)

A. Sagittal T1-weighted image shows thin corpus callosum
B. Proton density image reveals characteristic enlargement of the ventricles with irregular borders and periatrial hyperintensity representing white matter gliosis (*arrows*)
C. T1-weighted image shows deep sulci abutting the irregular ventricles
D. T2-weighted image shows characteristic periatrial gliosis (*arrows*) with deep sulci and white matter volume loss

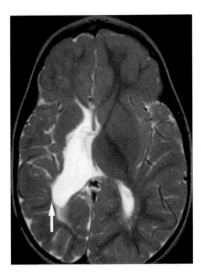

Figure 7.21

Unilateral periventricular leukomalacia

Unilateral Periventricular Leukomalacia

Clinical Presentation

A 2-year-old ex-premature male with left hemiparesis and developmental delay.

Images (Fig. 7.21)

A. Gray matter indents the ventricle wall (*arrow*) due to severe white matter loss on right. Corpus callosum is thin. The right hemisphere is smaller than the left. Typical undulation of ventricular wall is present

Periventricular Leukomalacia with Dystrophic Parenchymal Calcification

Clinical Presentation

A 7-month-old female with developmental delay and a remote history of cardiac arrest and renal failure.

Images (Fig. 7.22)

A. Sagittal T1-weighted image shows thin corpus callosum
B. Proton density image reveals white matter volume loss with low signal calcification (*arrows*) in the frontal region
C. The parenchymal calcification is well seen on SPGR image (*arrows*)

Discussion

Periventricular leukomalacia (PVL) (synonym: preterm hypoxic-ischemic encephalopathy, HIE) in a preterm infant (32–36 weeks) results from extensive necrosis of white matter adjacent to the lateral ventricles in the brain. Before 32 weeks gestational age (28–32 weeks), germinal matrix, intraventricular and intraparenchymal hemorrhages are more common. PVL is seen in 70% of preterm infants with HIE. The determining factor for different patterns of ischemia at the CNS is the time of the anoxic insult. Before 32 weeks gestational age, cavitary PVL and hemorrhages prevail. PVL is rarely seen in term neonates. In term infants the pattern of damage is different. The HIE in term infants is seen in parasagittal, cortical and subcortical regions. In preterm infants the deep periventricular white matter is thought to be at the highest risk of ischemic insult before maturation of centrifugal arteries. Significant risk factors in addition to prematurity include premature rupture of membranes, chorioamnionitis and hyperbilirubinemia. Clinical manifestations include spastic diplegia, quadriparesis, visual disorders, seizures, and cognitive disorders.

Although, ultrasound (US) imaging is used in the acute phase which detects hyperechoic periventricular areas, MR imaging is superior in detection of white matter loss and delayed myelination. The most common findings observed are: abnormally increased periventricular white matter intensity on T2-weighted image, commonly seen in the trigone re-

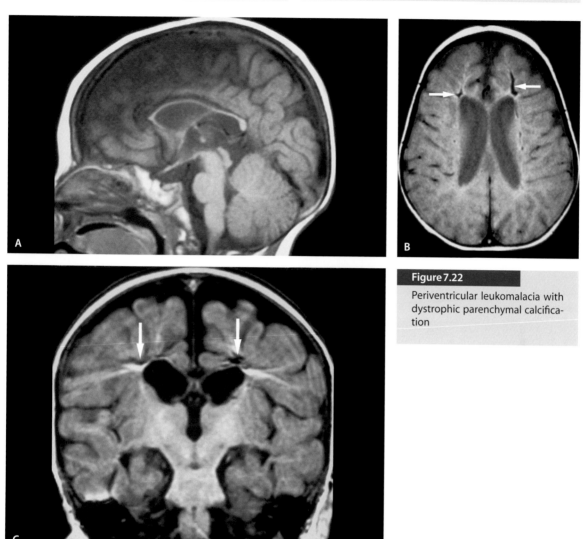

Figure 7.22

Periventricular leukomalacia with dystrophic parenchymal calcification

gions of lateral ventricles, marked loss of periventricular white matter predominantly in periatrial regions, and compensatory focal ventricular enlargement adjacent to regions of abnormal signal intensity. Typically the late findings consist of undulation of ventricular surface, periventricular cysts, callosal thinning, evidence of prior hemorrhage and gliosis. DW images may show signal hyperintensity associated with decreased ADC values. DW imaging may have a higher correlation with later evidence of PVL than conventional MR imaging when performed in the acute phase. Imaging recommendations in suspected cases include early US screening and then MR imaging with DW imaging and MR spectroscopy.

Suggested Reading

Barkovich AJ, Westmark K, Partidge C, Sola A, Ferriero DM (1995) Perinatal asphyxia: MR findings in the first 10 days. AJNR Am J Neuroradiol 16:427–438

Bozzao A, Di Paolo AD, Mazzoleni, et al (2003) Diffusion-weighted MR imaging in the early diagnosis of periventricular leukomalacia. Eur Radiol 13:1571–1576

Wilson DA, Steiner RE (1986) Periventricular leukomalacia: evaluation with MR imaging. Radiology 160:507–511

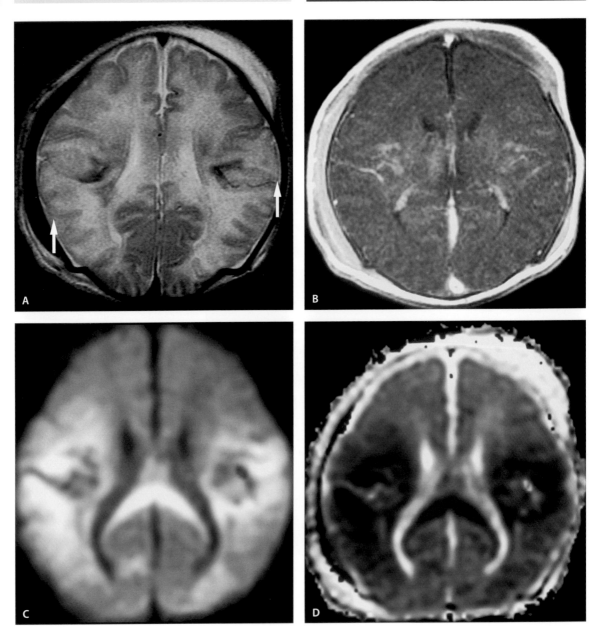

Figure 7.23

Hypoxic ischemic encephalopathy with infarcts

Hypoxic Ischemic Encephalopathy (HIE)

Hypoxic Ischemic Encephalopathy with Infarcts

Clinical Presentation

A 6-day-old full term neonate with traumatic birth and low Apgar scores. Patient is spastic.

Images (Fig. 7.23)

A. T2-weighted image reveals hyperintense and in-distinct cortical gray matter ribbon in both MCA territories (*arrows*)
B. Contrast-enhanced T1-weighted image reveals vague enhancement in both MCA territories
C. DW image shows significant hyperintensity main-ly in both MCA territories and in the splenium of the corpus callosum
D. The hyperintense lesions on DW image are hy-pointense on ADC map consistent with restricted diffusion and cytotoxic edema often seen in is-chemic damage

Hypoxic Ischemic Encephalopathy with Brain Edema

Clinical Presentation

A 9-day-old female infant with hypoglycemia and seizures.

Images (Fig. 7.24)

A. Noncontrast CT scan shows diffuse brain edema, more in the occipital area
B. T1-weighted image shows cortical hyperintensi-ties representing laminar necrosis
C. T2-weighted image shows intense bilateral poste-rior parietal hyperintensity with loss of cortical ribbon (*arrows*)
D. FLAIR image confirms the laminar necrosis (*arrows*)

Hypoxic Ischemic Encephalopathy Post-Surgery

Clinical Presentation

A previously healthy 4-year-old female who experi-enced two seizures leading to anoxia after a minor elective surgery.

Images (Fig. 7.25)

A. Contrast enhanced T1-weighted image shows mild hypointensities in the bilateral frontal and occipi-tal lobes (*arrows*) in watershed distribution
B. DW image shows hyperintense lesions in the bilat-eral frontal and occipital lobes (*arrows*)

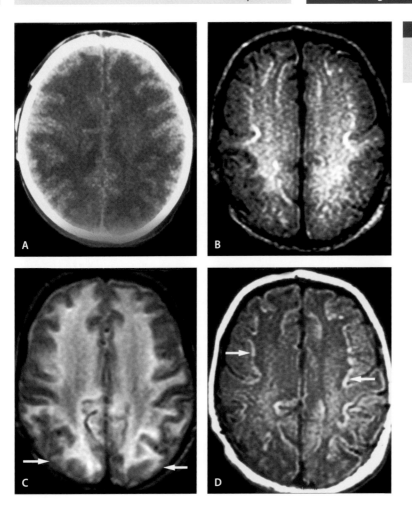

Figure 7.24
Hypoxic ischemic encephalopathy with brain edema

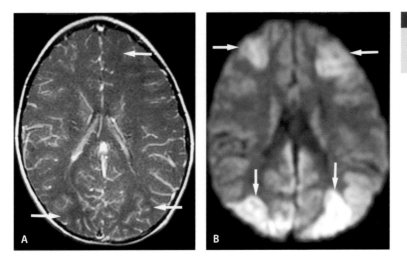

Figure 7.25
Hypoxic ischemic encephalopathy post-surgery

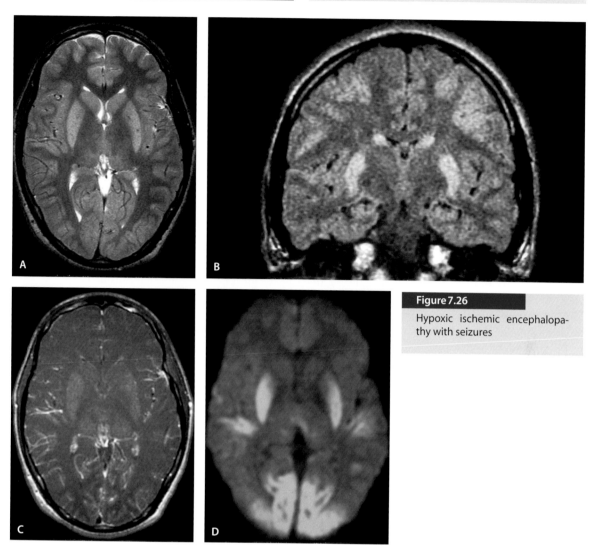

Hypoxic Ischemic Encephalopathy with Seizures

Clinical Presentation

A 15-year-old male with seizure followed by cardiac arrest and decreased mental status.

Images (Fig. 7.26)

A. T2-weighted image reveals significant hyperintensity in both the putamina and the head of the caudate nuclei. The cortical ribbon and gray/white matter junction are indistinct in both occipital lobes

B. Coronal FLAIR confirms the putaminal and caudate hyperintensities. It also reveals focal subcortical white matter hyperintensities

C. Contrast-enhanced T1-weighted image (with magnetization transfer) shows patchy occipital enhancement

D. DW image shows significant hyperintensity involving the putamina, medial thalami, both occipital cortices and superior temporal gyri. Wedge-shaped hyperintensity is seen in insular cortices with relative sparing of the frontal lobes

Discussion

HIE in term infants is an acquired condition in which signs of fetal distress are present prior to delivery, the infant has low Apgar scores, requires resuscitation at birth and has neurological symptoms during the first 24 hours of life. The early recognition, prompt medical intervention, and accurate prognostic prediction of perinatal brain damage are particularly important to decrease morbidity and mortality in affected infants. MR imaging has a large impact on the evaluation of the asphyxiated neonate.

In mild hypoperfusion injury there is redistribution of cerebral blood flow to vital structures in the basal ganglia, brainstem and cerebellum. The white matter is damaged with sparing of the vital gray matter structures. In more profound hypoperfusion, the cerebral blood flow has no time to shift and areas of highest metabolic needs such as the basal ganglia will be damaged. The deep gray matter has been thought to be vulnerable to selective neuronal necrosis in acute total asphyxia. Often the damage is mixed.

Injury in the perinatal period in term infants shows short T1 and T2 in the ventral lateral thalami, posterolateral lentiform nuclei, posterior mesencephalon, and hippocampi, and asphyxia later in infancy shows prolonged T2 in the corpus striatum and most of the cerebral cortex with perirolandic sparing. In term infants diffuse hemispheric parenchymal changes have been associated with severe prolonged partial asphyxia when there is repetitive stress with intermittent recovery. Focal hemispheric changes in the form of infarction may be seen.

Neonatal hypoglycemia is caused by imbalance between supply and utilization of glucose. It can lead to HIE and metabolic strokes. Risk factors include prematurity, mother's diabetes, maternal use of steroids, toxemia, infant sepsis and hypoxia. The classic imaging appearance is that of T2 or FLAIR hyperintensity on the occipito-parietal area posteriorly or DW imaging hyperintensity with hypointense ADC map in the same area. MR spectroscopy is helpful in early ischemia. Glutamine/glutamate peaks are increased in ischemia. Lactate is a normal finding in a developing brain (<37 weeks) as is a low NAA peak.

HIE is not limited to the perinatal period. In older children HIE can follow cardiac arrest, seizures, suffocation, drowning and other condition where hypoxia is present. In all cases of HIE standard MR images may be normal up to 72 hours. However, DW imaging with ADC map is very sensitive in early imaging of ischemia, but the findings pseudonormalize within a week. MR spectroscopy is helpful in early stages of ischemia demonstrating increased glutamine/glutamate peaks.

In preterm infants the ischemic damage is different. Before 32 weeks of gestational age MR imaging can show parenchymal and intraventricular hemorrhage. At 32–36 weeks of gestational age periventricular white matter damage (PVL) and deep gray matter involvement is commonly seen. Subependymal hemorrhage is one of the common sequelae in premature infants which may be depicted as periventricular hemosiderin deposits on initial MR images. Parenchymal encephaloclastic cysts adjacent to hemosiderin deposits may be seen in follow-up MR images. Diffusion tensor imaging may show significant reduction of fractional anisotropy in the posterior limb of the internal capsule.

Suggested Reading

Aida N, Nishimura G, Hachiya Y, Matsui K, Takeuchi M, Itani Y (1998) MR imaging of perinatal brain damage: comparison of clinical outcome with initial and follow-up MR findings. AJNR Am J Neuroradiol 19:1909–1921

Arzoumanian Y, Mirmiran M, Barnes PD, et al (2003) Diffusion tensor brain imaging findings at term-equivalent age may predict neurologic abnormalities in low birth weight preterm infants. AJNR Am J Neuroradiol 24:1646–1653

Barkovich AJ (1992) MR and CT evaluation of profound neonatal and infantile asphyxia. AJNR Am J Neuroradiol 13:959–972

Barkovich AJ, Westmark K, Partridge C, Sola A, Ferriero DM (1995) Perinatal asphyxia: MR findings in the first 10 days. AJNR Am J Neuroradiol 16:427–438

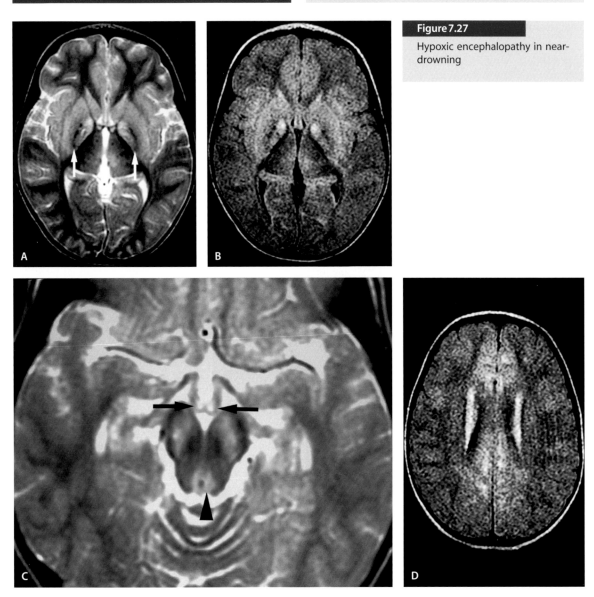

Figure 7.27

Hypoxic encephalopathy in near-drowning

Hypoxic Encephalopathy in Near-Drowning

Clinical Presentation

A 3-year-old boy, near-drowning victim found in swimming pool. The study was obtained 4 days after the accident.

Images (Fig. 7.27)

A. T2-weighted image shows partially hemorrhagic, partially necrotic lesions in the globus pallidi (*arrows*), caudate nuclei and posterior putamen
B. FLAIR image confirms the necrotic findings in globus pallidi
C. T2-weighted image through the midbrain reveals hyperintensity involving the corticospinal tracts, compact substantia nigra and periaqueductal gray matter (*arrowhead*). Mamillary bodies also demonstrate abnormal hyperintensity (*arrows*)
D. FLAIR image shows hyperintensity in the caudate body

Discussion

Drowning is defined as death by asphyxia due to submersion in a liquid medium. The term "near-drowning" is applied to patients with cardiac arrest and asphyxia after submersion in water, who are resuscitated and survive beyond 24 hours. Of those who survive prolonged submersion, the majority have severe neurological impairment, but as many as 30% may remain neurologically intact. During a drowning episode, neurological damage may be caused by a variety of factors, including cerebral hypoxia, carbon dioxide narcosis, laryngospasm, pulmonary reflexes, or vagally mediated cardiac arrest.

MR imaging findings include focal (particularly occipital) and generalized edema, basal ganglia changes, cortical abnormalities, and brain stem infarcts. The earliest basal ganglia changes are of diffuse T1 hyperintensities, which may be seen as early as 1 day after the hypoxic event. Later, the areas of hyperintensity become more focal and show a characteristic distribution involving the posterior lentiform nuclei and ventrolateral thalamus. The indistinct basal ganglia margins on T2-weighted images are a common finding and are an early sensitive indicator of an anoxic-ischemic event. In the first 24 hours, the presence of edema or T2 changes in the basal ganglia is both sensitive and specific for poor outcome. In severe cases, the basal ganglia margins may progress to invisible basal ganglia. In infants, laminar necrosis occurs more commonly and high intensity subcortical lines are more frequent in older children.

DW imaging with ADC map often depicts acute or subacute ischemic brain lesions when CT and MR images are normal or near normal. The prognosis of HIE depends on the severity and extension of the lesions. Since cytotoxic edema is usually irreversible, DW is helpful in estimating a patient's prognosis and management, especially if it is combined with MR spectroscopy. MR imaging and MR spectroscopy are complementary studies and they measure different aspects of hypoxia. Gray matter MR spectroscopy in cases with poor outcome shows a markedly decreased NAA peak and elevation of glutamine/glutamate and lactate.

Suggested Reading

Dubowitz DJ, Bluml S, Arcinue E, Dietrich RB (1998) MR of hypoxic encephalopathy in children after near-drowning: correlation with quantitative proton MR spectroscopy and clinical outcome. AJNR Am J Neuroradiol 19:1617–1627

Kreis R, Arcinue E, Ernst T, Shonk TK, Flores R, Ross BD (1996) Hypoxic encephalopathy after near-drowning studied by quantitative 1H-magnetic resonance spectroscopy. J Clin Invest 97:1142–1154

Multicystic Encephalomalacia

Clinical Presentation

A 3-month old male with history of right hemispheric stroke. At the age of 3 years he presents in the emergency room with seizures.

Images (Fig. 7.28)

A. T1-weighted image shows a thin corpus callosum
B. DW image shows hypointensity in right hemisphere cystic lesions
C. Axial FLAIR image reveals small right hemisphere and multiple CSF containing spaces with dilated lateral ventricle
D. Coronal FLAIR image confirms the encephalomalacia and ex vacuo atrophy displacing the midline to right
E. T2-weighted image shows diffuse hyperintense cysts throughout the right hemisphere that is smaller
F. T1-weighted image shows hypointensity in the right cerebral hemisphere. This is consistent with an area of encephalomalacia and gliosis due to a prior insult such as infarct or infection. Minimal hyperintensity is noted in the area of encephalomalacia consistent with mineralization
G. T1-FLAIR image shows multiple CSF containing cysts. The thin cortex is better appreciated in this sequence
H. CT at the age of 3 years shows multicystic encephalomalacia with small right hemicranium

Figure 7.28 ▶

Multicystic encephalomalacia

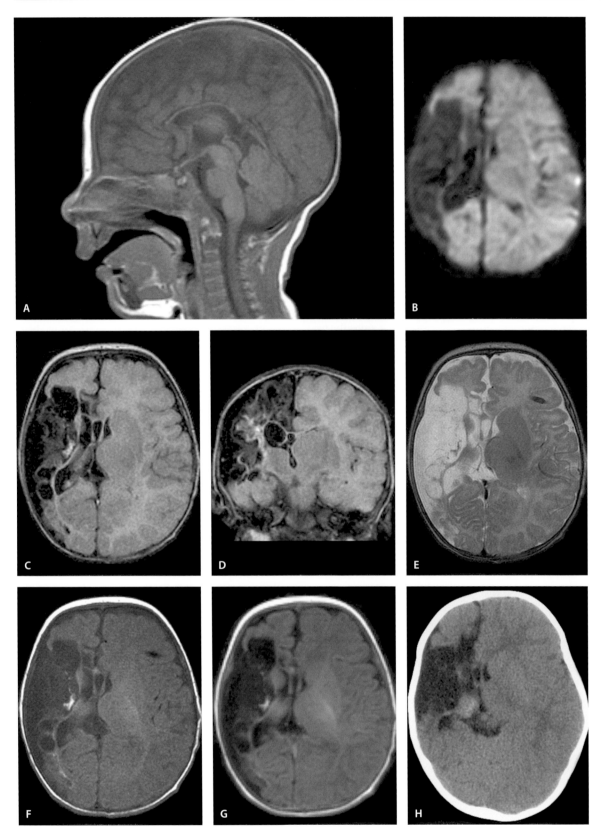

Discussion

The developing brain is susceptible to injury from infectious, ischemic and inflammatory insults. Multicystic encephalomalacia results from insult to the brain late in gestation, during birth or after birth. Encephalomalacia, in contradistinction to porencephaly, is characterized by astrocytic proliferation and glial septations within the damaged brain. The location of the cysts varies with the nature of the lesion. In the early 1980s, diagnosing periventricular (PVL) and multicystic leukomalacia in neonates using cranial sonography was possible for the first time. The more wide use of MR imaging in the late 1980s allowed more detailed brain imaging even in small preterm babies often vulnerable to brain injury from many causes. MR imaging being more accurate shows more numerous or more extensive cysts compared to US studies. MR images are also able to show cysts not present on sonograms. CT scans show initially hypointensity leading later to cyst formation. Calcification may be present. On early MR images ill-defined T1 and T2 prolongation is present leading later to multiple cystic lesions with strands of glial septae. MR spectroscopy shows low metabolites.

Suggested Reading

Inder TE, Anderson NJ, Spencer C, Wells S, Volpe JJ (2003) White matter injury in the premature infant: a comparison between serial cranial sonographic and MR findings at term. AJNR Am J Neuroradiol 5:805–809

Resch B, Vollaard E, Maurer U, Haas J, Rosegger H, Muller W (2000) Risk factors and determinants of neurodevelopmental outcome in cystic periventricular leucomalacia. Eur J Pediatr 9:663–670

Status Epilepticus and Postictal Stage

Status Epilepticus with Partially Reversible Tissue Changes

Clinical Presentation

A 19-year-old male who has epilepsy, had an episode of status epilepticus. Patient was transferred from an outside hospital due to prolonged status epilepticus. He is still having impaired cognitive function after 5 days of ictus and hypoxic injury is suspected clinically.

Images (Fig. 7.29)

A. There is diffuse increased signal intensity in the right temporal parietal cortex and right hippocampus (*arrows*). The cortex is swollen
B. On coronal FLAIR image the hippocampus is hyperintense and swollen (*arrow*). Cortical swelling is also demonstrated
C. On DW image the same areas are hyperintense
D. ADC values are decreased in these areas, confirming restricted diffusion
E. and F.
   In the follow-up study 12 days later the large diffusion abnormality involving the right temporal and parietal cortices has largely resolved
G. and H.
   There is persistent gyral swelling and T2 prolongation involving the right temporal cortex seen on axial T2-weighted (G) and coronal FLAIR (H) images

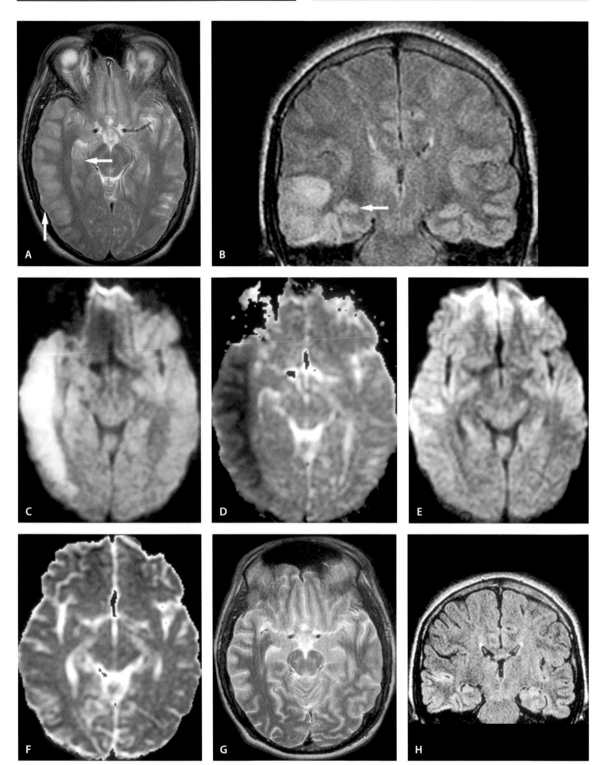

Figure 7.29 A–H

Status epilepticus with partially reversible tissue changes

Status Epilepticus
with Permanent Tissue Damage

Clinical Presentation

A 2-year-old female with Rasmussen's encephalitis and developmental delay presents with focal seizures involving the right face and hand. The girl subsequently underwent hemispherectomy.

Images (Fig. 7.30)

A. On T2-weighted image there is diffuse thalamic and cortical hyperintensity on the left side
B. Coronal FLAIR image shows better the abnormal increased signal within the swollen gyri
C. DW image shows a gyriform area of high signal involving the thalamus and entire cortical area on the left side
D. ADC values are decreased in hyperintense lesion on DW image (C), confirming restricted diffusion as seen in cytotoxic edema
E. Contrast-enhanced image demonstrates slight hyperemia on the left
F. MR angiography (noncontrast study, 3D TOF) shows increased flow-related enhancement on the left MCA, especially at the peripheral branches (*arrowheads*). The left MCA is also dilated (*arrow*) consistent with hyperperfusion
G. Single voxel proton MR spectroscopy on the left side 9 days later shows questionable lactate peak. There is increased choline with relatively low NAA compared to the uninvolved right side. Short echo MR spectroscopy showed increased glutamine/glutamate peaks (not shown)
H. Localizer for the MR spectroscopy demonstrating the analyzed voxel
I. DW image 9 days later shows a gyriform area of high signal involving mainly the occipital cortex on the left side. The frontoparietal cortex is near normal
J. The corresponding ADC map shows still hypointensity in the occipital area (*arrow*). The frontoparietal hypointensity on the initial study (D) is near normal

K. T2-weighted image 5 months later shows interval increase in the ventricular size especially on the left temporal and parietal lobes with no associated sulcal effacement. This is consistent with tissue loss. There is a persistent hyperintensity of the left hemisphere on T2-weighted images
L. On contrast-enhanced image, there is persistent enhancement of the gray matter of the left cerebral hemisphere especially in the occipital region
M. DW image shows no abnormal signal
N. ADC map shows parenchymal hyperintensity

Discussion

MR imaging is widely used to evaluate patients with seizures. In the early development of MR imaging the studies were obtained to detect anatomical, developmental and structural brain abnormalities and evaluate patients for seizure surgery. MR imaging is especially useful in the diagnosis of mesial temporal sclerosis. Also parahippocampal structures are well visualized in MR imaging. On the standard MR image, signal alterations related to ictal or postictal situation can be misdiagnosed as cerebritis, infarctions, MELAS, herpes encephalitis, neoplastic lesions or even demyelinating diseases. DW imaging is helpful in evaluating patients with epilepsy, as it will discriminate between cytotoxic edema and vasogenic edema in ictal and postictal brain. Standard MR imaging can demonstrate transient increase in T2 signal and cortical swelling in addition to hippocampus, corpus callosum, thalamic and cerebellar signal alterations. During ictus there is increased metabolic activity and consumption of oxygen and glucose in the seizure focus. This hypermetabolic state results in metabolic ischemia, hypercarbia and lactic acidosis, which impair vascular autoregulation in the affected areas leading to vasogenic edema and disruption of the blood-brain barrier.

If the patient suffers from a continuous seizure lasting longer than 30 minutes or two or more consecutive seizures together lasing longer than 30 minutes without full recovery, the situation is called status epilepticus. This is a serious condition. Several investigators have found reversible lesions in MR images after status epilepticus. Research has shown that there is increase in the release of glutamate from the presynaptic terminal of neuronal axons. Cytotoxic edema in status epilepticus and acute ischemia presents with restricted diffusion. A cascade of events in status epilepticus result in cytotoxic edema that can

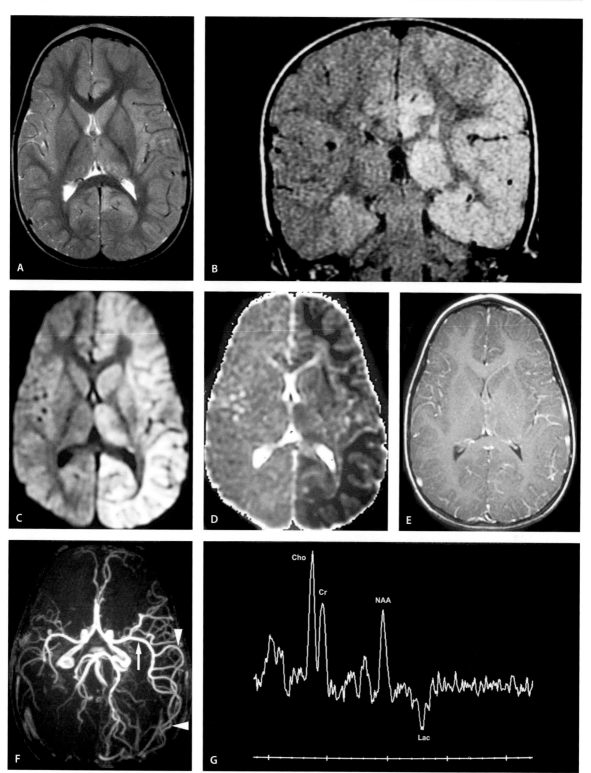

Figure 7.30 A–G

Status epilepticus with permanent tissue damage (H–N see next page)

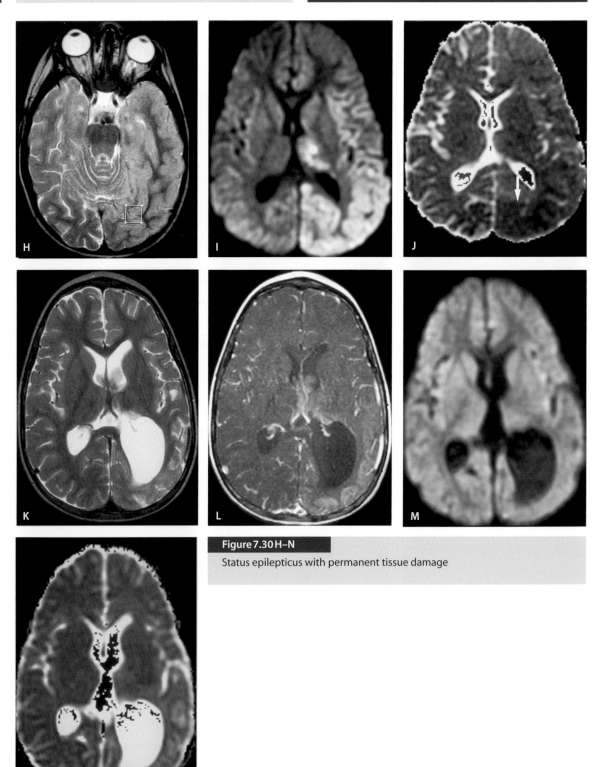

Figure 7.30 H–N

Status epilepticus with permanent tissue damage

be at least partially reversible. This is in contrast to considerable ischemia where changes are usually irreversible. In the ischemic process there is significant compromise of the blood supply to the brain; however, in status epilepticus there is an increase in cerebral metabolism with an increase in the blood flow seen in MR angiography and MR perfusion studies. This will maintain the energy supply of the neurons provided that there is sufficient oxygen supply. Although some lesions are reversible, most lesions in status epilepticus are permanent with neuronal necrosis, gliosis and delayed neuronal death with subsequent atrophy.

DW imaging and ADC maps are more sensitive than conventional MR imaging to visualize gray and white matter involvement and discriminate between cytotoxic and vasogenic edema following status epilepticus. DW image reveals an acute postictal depression of ADC (low signal), interictal normalization and then chronic elevation (high signal) in the seizure focus. Distinction between vasogenic and cytotoxic edema is important since cytotoxic edema following a seizure indicates more extensive brain damage that is often irreversible leading to tissue loss and atrophy.

Suggested Reading

Bronen RA (2000) The status of status: seizures are bad for your brain's health. AJNR Am J Neuroradiol 21:1782–1783

Flacke S, Wullner U, Keller E, Hamzei F, Urbach H (2000) Reversible changes in echo planar perfusion- and diffusion-weighted MRI in status epilepticus. Neuroradiology 42:92–95

Kim JA, Chung JI, Yoon PH, et al (2001) Transient MR signal changes in patients with generalized tonicoclonic seizure or status epilepticus: periictal diffusion-weighted imaging. AJNR Am J Neuroradiol 22:1149–1160

Cortical Laminar Necrosis

Clinical Presentation

A 6-month-old male who suffered status epilepticus, brain edema followed with subsequent diffuse volume loss and laminar necrosis.

Images (Fig. 7.31)

A. Sagittal T1-weighted image reveals characteristic laminar hyperintense lesions of the cerebral cortex (*arrows*)
B. Significant volume loss is seen on T2-weighted image, especially in the fontal lobes
C. Coronal T2-weighted image shows significant cortical atrophy, thinning of the corpus callosum and extensive white matter changes that are often progressive

Discussion

Cortical laminar necrosis is a histopathological entity, related to conditions of cerebral energy depletion, especially hypoxia-ischemia and hypoglycemia, either in the perinatal period or later in life. Neurons are more vulnerable to energy depletion than glial cells and vascular elements, and among the layers of gray matter, the third layer is more vulnerable than superficial layers. White matter abnormalities tend to be more frequent in premature children, and cortical laminar abnormalities tend to be more common in term neonates and older children.

Cerebral edema is seen in the acute stage. Early cortical changes usually show low signal intensity on T1-weighted MR images which could be due to acute ischemic changes. Unenhanced T1-weighted images reveal characteristic laminar hyperintense lesions of the cerebral cortex in the late subacute stage. Usually, cortical high-intensity lesions on both T1-weighted and FLAIR images appear 2 weeks after the ictus, indicating short T1 and long T2 lesions. On proton density images, cortical laminar necrosis may be seen as high intensity due to increased mobile protons in the reactive tissue. In the chronic stage, cortical atrophy and delayed but progressive white matter changes are present.

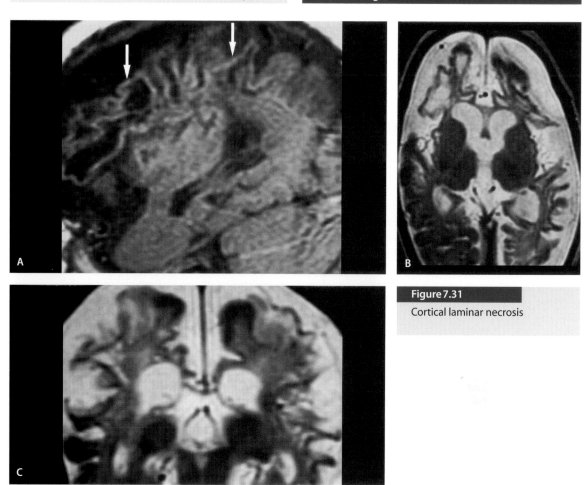

Figure 7.31
Cortical laminar necrosis

In severe HIE, subtle changes may be difficult to see with conventional MR imaging. DW images are helpful for evaluating and dating diffuse cerebral anoxia, and therefore aid in the determination of prognosis and management of these patients. During the acute period, DW images may show abnormalities in the basal ganglia, cerebellum, and cortex. During the early subacute period, gray matter abnormalities dominate in the DW images. During the late subacute period, DW images may show mostly white matter abnormalities. During the chronic stage, the results of DW imaging are normal, but conventional MR imaging shows laminar necrosis, atrophy and volume loss.

Suggested Reading

Komiyama M, Nishikawa M, Yasui T (1997) Cortical laminar necrosis in brain infarcts: chronological changes on MRI. Neuroradiology 39:474–479

Valanne L, Paetau A, Suomalainen A, Ketonen L, Pihko H (1996) Laminar necrosis in MELAS syndrome: MR and neuropathological observations. Neuropediatrics 27:154–160

Van der Knaap MS, Smit LS, Nauta JJ, Lafeber HN, Valk J (1993) Cortical laminar abnormalities – occurrence and clinical significance. Neuropediatrics 24:143–148

Figure 7.32

Cyclosporin-induced encephalopathy

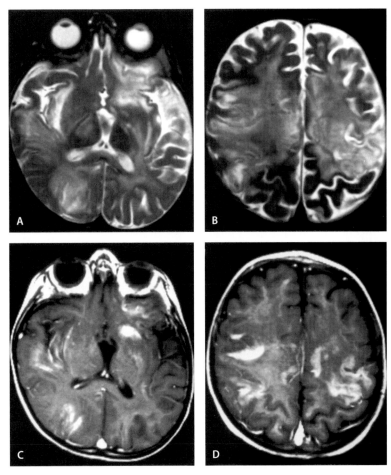

Cyclosporin-Induced Encephalopathy

Clinical Presentation

A 1-year-old male with altered mental status and muscle weakness following cyclosporin treatment.

Images (Fig. 7.32)

A. T2-weighted image shows extensive white matter hyperintensity with some gray matter involvement and insular cortex involvement. No mass effect is present

B. T2-weighted image through the centrum semiovale shows near complete involvement of the white matter with some cortical gray matter involvement on the left

C and D. T1-weighted image with contrast enhancement shows diffuse white matter enhancement

Discussion

The incidence of cyclosporin-induced neurotoxicity has been reported to be 10–25%. Endothelial injury is thought to be the main causative factor. The clinical features may include headache, tremor, hallucinations, and altered level of consciousness, seizures, cerebellar ataxia, transient aphasia, muscle weakness and visual disturbance. Cyclosporin-induced toxicity is often reversible.

Both cortical gray and white matter involvement has been described. CT images show hypodense areas in the subcortical white matter or gray matter. Focal subcortical areas of hemorrhage may be seen in advanced cases. T2-weighted images typically show areas of high signal intensity in the subcortical white matter mainly in the occipital-parietal regions. Rarely, other locations such as the frontal lobes, corpus callosum, brain stem, pons and cerebellum may also be involved. The cortical gray matter can also be involved. Cortical laminar necrosis has been described to develop following cyclosporin treatment and polychemotherapy. Contrast enhancement may be seen due to disruption of the blood-brain barrier. The imaging features of cyclosporin-induced cytotoxicity closely mimic those of hypertensive encephalopathy and can be seen in many conditions such as eclampsia, renal disease, use of immunosuppressants, following chemotherapy, and increased blood pressure.

Suggested Reading

Jansen O, Krieger D, Krieger S, Sartor K (1996) Cortical hyperintensity on proton density-weighted images: an MR sign of cyclosporine-related encephalopathy. AJNR Am J Neuroradiol 17:337–344

Yamamoto A, Hayakawa K, Houjyou M (2002) CT and MRI findings of cyclosporine-related encephalopathy and hypertensive encephalopathy. Pediatr Radiol 32:340–343

Pontine and Extrapontine Myelinolysis in the Setting of Rapid Correction of Hyponatremia

Clinical Presentation

A 4-month-old male with Chiari II malformation received intravenous hypertonic saline which was followed by severe global brain edema requiring shunting of the ventricles. This follow-up study was obtained 2 months later.

Images (Fig. 7.33)

A. T1-weighted image through the pons shows a large low-intensity cavity replacing the fourth ventricle with patchy mixed signal involving the cerebellar hemispheres, but sparing the pons

B. T1-weighted image through midbrain shows replacement of all white matter with abnormal low signal and outlined by high signal

C. T2-weighted image through the midbrain at the same level as B reveals no normal-appearing brain

D. T1-weighted image through the basal ganglia reveals significant brain damage with atrophy and multiple cystic lesions throughout the white matter with a small amount of normal-appearing cortex between the cystic areas. These findings are compatible with cystic encephalomalacia

E. T2-weighted image (at the same level as D) shows marked tissue loss, more prominently in the left with cystic encephalomalacia and a small left occipital extraaxial fluid collection. Blood products are seen in both occipital horns (*arrows*)

Discussion

Severe hyponatremia with hypoosmolality carries a high morbidity and mortality with severe neurological complications. Rapid correction of severe hyponatremia can lead to demyelinating lesions and may be the cause of central pontine myelinolysis (CPM) or extra pontine myelinolysis (EPM), which may occur with or without accompanying CPM. The entity has been known since its first description in 1959; however, before the time of MR imaging, early diagnosis was difficult. It was first known with alcoholism, but malnutrition and transplantation encephalopathy with rapid serum sodium changes have also been implicated for a 10% to 13% incidence of CPM. Pathologically, it is characterized by myelin loss with relative neuronal sparing. The central pons is the most common site of involvement (90%) but it can also be seen affecting extrapontine locations such as the basal ganglia, thalami, and cerebral cortex/subcortex. Histological studies have shown oligodendroglial cells to be most susceptible to CPM-caused osmotic stress, and myelinolysis parallels the distribution of these cells in the central pons, and the above-mentioned extrapontine locations. Histologically there is preservation of neurons and axons, differentiating this from pontine infarct.

CPM/EPM is an osmolar disturbance resulting in demyelination that is initially difficult to detect with CT and routine MR imaging. Since the underlying process is osmotic disturbance of water and electrolytes, it is understandable that DW imaging shows positive before the routine MR imaging sequences. DW images show restricted diffusion before the other sequences show changes. MR imaging changes are secondary to increased water content, with enhancement patterns varying. T2-weighted and FLAIR images are more sensitive than CT imaging in detection of changes of demyelinating lesions of pontine and extrapontine locations. Characteristically, there is no mass effect. The classic appearance is hyperintense triangular central pontine abnormality sparing the ventrolateral pons and corticospinal tracts. Follow up MR imaging should be performed as these changes may be completely reversible. Differential diagnosis

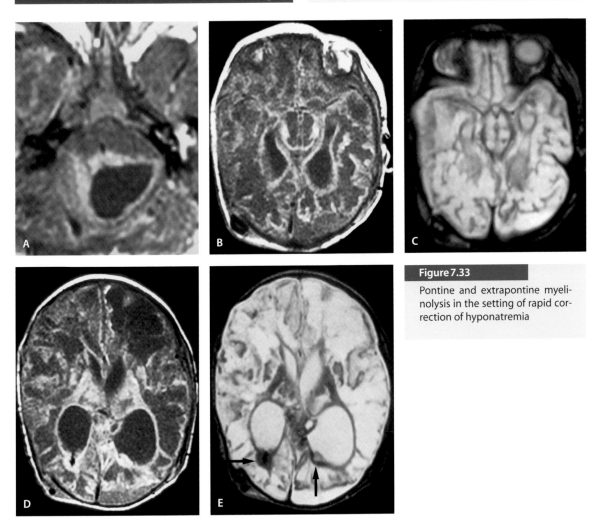

Figure 7.33

Pontine and extrapontine myelinolysis in the setting of rapid correction of hyponatremia

includes pontine glioma, ischemic changes, and multiple sclerosis. Absence of a mass effect helps in differentiating myelinolysis from glioma. The central location is not typically seen in infarcts. Multiple sclerosis usually exhibits additional characteristics along the margins of the lateral ventricles.

Suggested Reading

Kumar SR, Mone AP, Gray LC, Troost BT (2000) Central pontine myelinolysis: delayed changes on neuroimaging. J Neuroimaging 10:169–172

Morlan L, Rodriguez E, Gonzalez J, Jimene-Ortiz C, Escartin P, Liano H (1990) Central pontine myelinolysis following correction of hyponatremia: MRI diagnosis. Eur Neurol 30:149–152

Ruzek KA, Campeau NG, Miller GM (2004) Early diagnosis of central pontine myelinolysis with diffusion-weighted imaging. AJNR Am J Neuroradiol 25:210–213

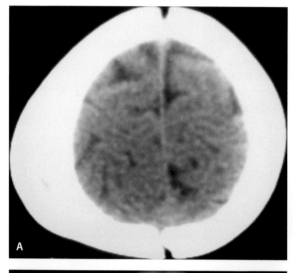

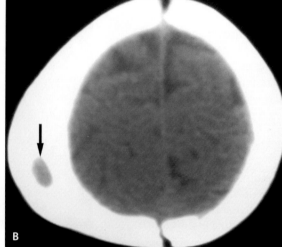

Figure 7.34

Cephalhematoma, CT scan

Cephalhematoma

CT Scan of Cephalhematoma

Clinical Presentation

A 3-month-old boy who had a cephalhematoma at birth which has diminished in size. Over the past month he has had an enlarging lesion in this area.

Images (Fig. 7.34)

A. CT scan with brain window shows calvarial thickening on right. The brain is normal
B. Intermediate window shows lytic-appearing center of the cephalhematoma (*arrow*). No underlying brain hematoma is seen
C. Bone window reveals a prominent lesion involving the posterior right parietal bone corresponding to the lesion noted on the recent skull series. The lesion has a lytic-appearing center with bony proliferation along its outer margin. The inner table remains intact. This is characteristic of the healing cephalhematoma that represents subperiosteal hemorrhage with a thin calcified peripheral rim of bone

MR Imaging of Cephalhematoma

Clinical Presentation

A 3-month-old male with a calcified lesion of the left calvarium on plain films. The examination is requested due to clinical suspicion of cephalhematoma.

Images (Fig. 7.35)

A. Sagittal T1-weighted image demonstrates a lentiform lesion immediately deep to the scalp overlying the left parietal lobe (*arrow*). It is isointense to the brain

B. On T2-weighted image the hematoma is clearly extraaxial (*arrow*) with normal-appearing underlying brain. The signal is iso- to slightly hypointense to the gray matter

C. On GRE image the blood is low signal (*arrow*)

D. This 3-month-old cephalhematoma is iso- to hypointense on T1 FLAIR image

E. On FLAIR image the lesion is low signal

F. Coronal contrast-enhanced SPGR image demonstrates this lesion to be extracranial and adjacent to the outer table of the left parietal bone in a manner consistent with a cephalhematoma. The center of the hematoma is isointense to the brain without enhancement. The periphery enhances with contrast

G. The hematoma is hypointense on DW image

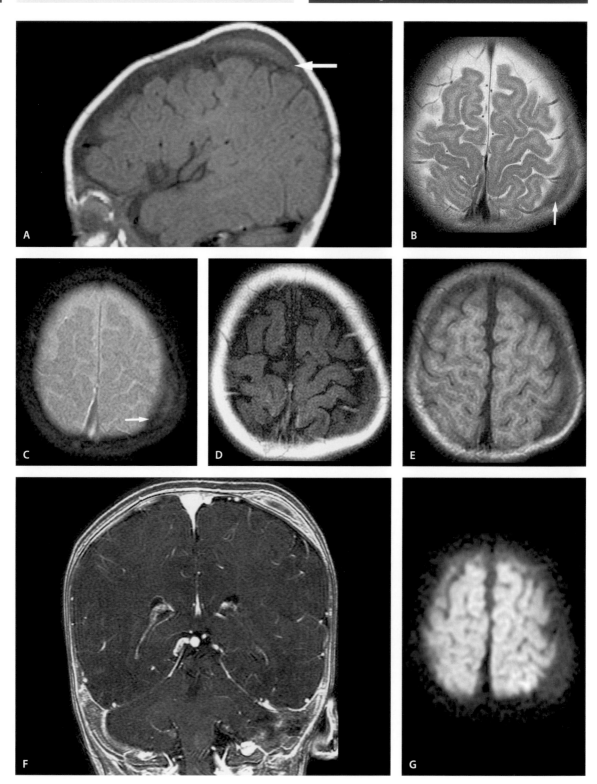

Figure 7.35

Cephalhematoma, MR imaging

Cephalhematoma and Hypoxic-Ischemic Insult

Clinical Presentation

A 2-day-old baby girl who has a history of seizures and has hematoma on the head. She has cardiac anomalies and HIE is suspected.

Images (Fig. 7.36)

A. Sagittal T1-weighted image shows hematoma isointense to the cortex
B. T2-weighted image shows ill-defined cortical ribbon in the left occipital area (*arrow*)
C. The hematoma is hypointense on T2-weighted image
D. DW image reveals an area of focal hyperintensity in the left occipital lobe (*arrow*)
E. DW image also shows multiple areas of focal hyperintensities in the left cerebral hemisphere (*arrows*)
F. The hematoma is hypointense on DW image (*arrow*)
G. The hyperintensity on DW image is hypointense on ADC map consistent with HIE and cytotoxic edema
H. ADC map through the cephalhematoma shows mixed signal

Follow-up MR imaging was performed 4 days later:
I. Sagittal T1-weighted image 4 days later. The hematoma is hyperintense consistent with methemoglobin formation
J. T2-weighted image shows high signal in the occipital white matter (*arrow*)
K. The hematoma is less hypointense on T2-weighted image
L. T1-FLAIR image shows hypointensity in the left occipital lobe
M. Coronal T2-weighted image shows hypointense hematoma
N. Coronal gradient echo shows darker core and isointense periphery of the hematoma
O. On T1-weighted image there is gyriform hyperintensity consistent with cortical necrosis
P. The previously seen hyperintensity has pseudonormalized on DW image
Q. The left occipital hypointensity is not hyperintense on ADC
R. The correct calculation of ADC in the T2-dark hematoma is difficult

Discussion

Cephalhematoma represents subperiosteal hemorrhage. It is usually related to birth trauma or instrumentation during the delivery. The periosteum of the involved bone, usually parietal or occipital bone, is elevated by the underlying hematoma. Therefore, the hematoma is strictly limited by the margins of the bone and does not cross suture lines. In its earliest stages (first 2 weeks), the hematoma is of soft tissue density due to its blood content. As healing progresses, there is formation of a shell of bone by the elevated periosteum and the calcification becomes visible on CT scan and plain radiograph of the skull. It initially appears as a thin calcified rim covering the hematoma. The layer of calcification subsequently thickens as it matures. Following complete resorption of the hematoma, the calcified rim is incorporated into the outer table of the skull. This may persist for months or years as a palpable (and radiographically visible) thickening of the outer table of the skull. Subtle skull fractures underlying the cephalhematoma may coexist but are usually not clinically significant. The findings may persist for years, even into adulthood. A lytic-appearing lesion at the site of old cephalhematoma may also persist, and this entity should be kept in mind when evaluating lytic or cyst-like skull lesions.

MR imaging can also identify subperiosteal cephalhematomas. Plain radiographs, bone scans, and enhanced CT scans are limited in their ability to determine if a cephalhematoma is infected unless associated osteomyelitis exists. Until now aspiration has been the diagnostic procedure of choice for cephalhematomas suspected of being infected. MR imaging may be helpful, especially if a DW sequence is used. The relationship of the hematoma and the temporal muscle may be a key MR imaging finding for the diagnosis of cephalhematoma.

Suggested Reading

Aoki N (1983) Epidural hematoma communicating with cephalhematoma in a neonate. Neurosurgery 13:55–57

Fujiwara K, Saito K, Ebina T (2002) Bilateral cephalhematomas in juvenile – case report. Neurol Med Chir (Tokyo) 42: 547–549

LeBlanc CM, Allen UD, Ventureyra E (1995) Cephalhematomas revisited. When should a diagnostic tap be performed? Clin Pediatr 2:86–89

Reeves A, Edwards-Brown M (2000) Intraosseous hematoma in a newborn with factor VIII deficiency AJNR Am J Neuroradiol 21:308–309

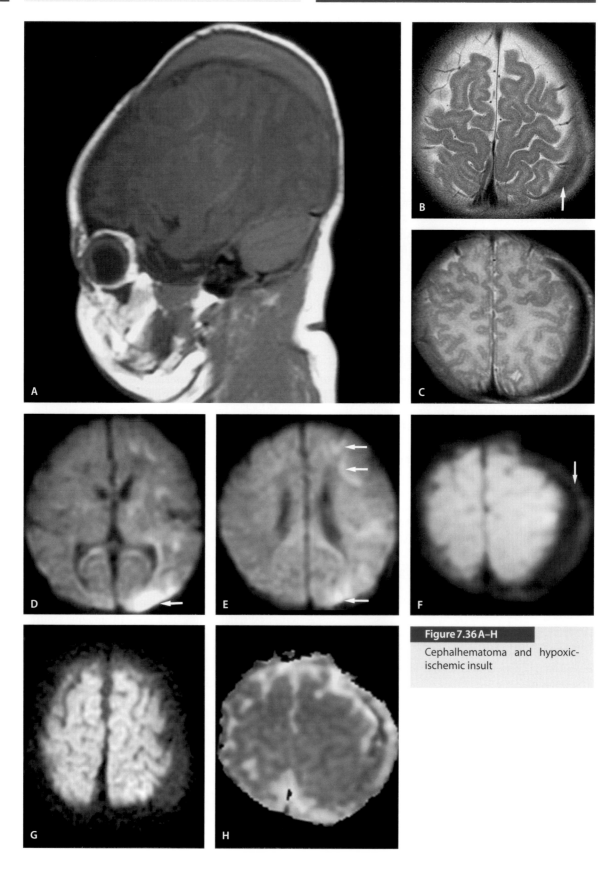

Figure 7.36 A–H

Cephalhematoma and hypoxic-ischemic insult

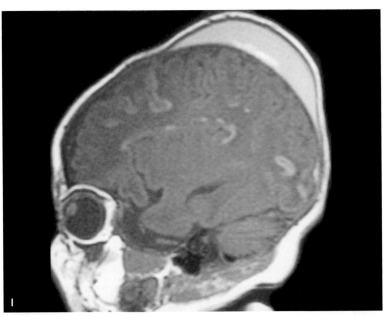

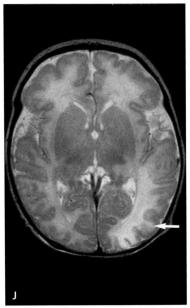

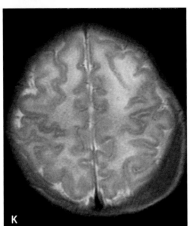

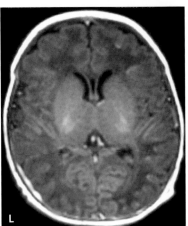

Figure 7.36 I–M

Cephalhematoma and hypoxic-ischemic insult

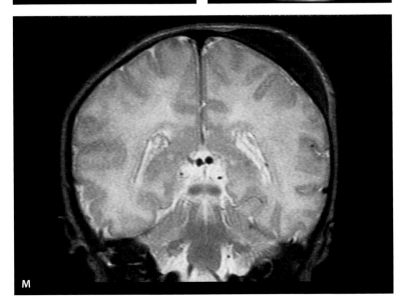

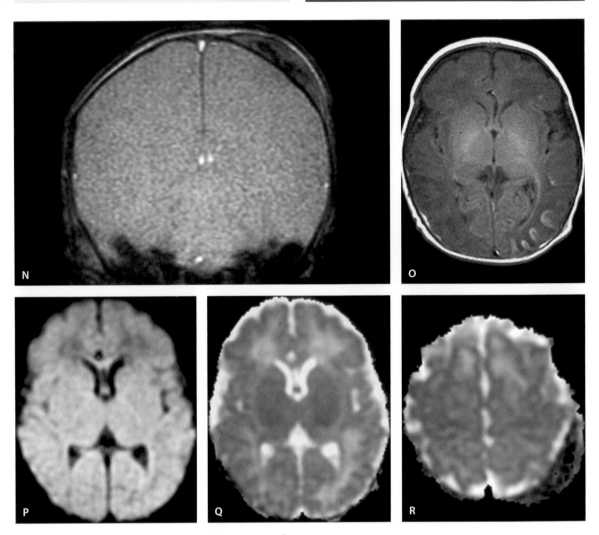

Figure 7.36 N–R

Cephalhematoma and hypoxic-ischemic insult

Vascular Disorders

Introduction

A large variety of lesions affect the pediatric intracranial vascular system. They range from congenital arterial and venous developmental anomalies to vascular malformations and acquired conditions. Many generalized childhood diseases also affect the CNS vasculature. Many of these manifestations are often overshadowed by the disease process itself and therefore remain unrecognized. Cerebrovascular diseases account for significant morbidity and mortality in children. Early and accurate recognition is vital for the best outcome.

Vascular malformations is a large group diseases subdivided to true arteriovenous malformations (AVM), cavernous malformations, capillary telangiectasias, dural arteriovenous fistulas (AVF) and developmental venous anomalies (DVA). DVA are considered as a normal variant of venous drainage and are seldom symptomatic. The two first categories account for most spontaneous (nontraumatic) hemorrhages of childhood. Aneurysmal bleed in childhood is extremely rare. Dural AVF are uncommon in the pediatric population. Association of cavernous malformations and DVA has been reported; the coexistence is higher in the posterior fossa.

Stroke in children is one of the commonest causes of hemiplegia. The incidence of pediatric stroke is 2.6 yearly cases per 100,000 population in Caucasian children and slightly higher among African-American children. Stroke in children may be classified into two categories: perinatal stroke and childhood stroke. Pediatric strokes can be also arterial or venous, in the same way as adult strokes. Perinatal strokes are caused by inherited clotting disorders or coagulation abnormalities. Congenital or acquired cardiac disorders and sickle cell disease are common causes of stroke. However, other diseases such as autoimmune disorders, post-varicella angiopathy, inborn errors of metabolism and mitochondrial encephalopathy with lactic acidemia may also be a few of the etiological factors. Autoimmune disorders may lead to ischemic infarcts through vasculitis or by inducing a hypercoagulable state. Traumatic dissection of major vessels is uncommon, but has to be considered as an etiological factor also in childhood stroke. Antecedent varicella infection should be considered as an etiological factor in childhood basal ganglia infarct.

The clinical presentation of an infarct may vary depending upon the location involved. The ischemic stroke is more common than hemorrhagic stroke in children. Mortality from stroke in US children has decreased dramatically over the last 20 years. Black children are at greater risk of death from all stroke types than are white children. Although controlling the known stroke risk factors has improved the mortality and morbidity, it is unlikely that this alone accounts for declining stroke mortality; ethnic differences in children and still-unrecognized stroke risk factors may play important roles.

Radiographic diagnosis of acute arterial ischemic stroke is challenging. CT scan may be normal in 50–60% of hyperacute infarct (<12h). However, hyperdense artery with obscuration of lentiform nuclei may be seen in 25–50% of cases. In acute infarct (12 to 24h), there may be loss of gray-white matter interfaces and sulcal effacement. A wedge-shaped low-density area that involves both gray and white matter with a mass effect is usually seen after 1–3 days. Hemorrhagic transformation may occur. Within a period of 4–7 days of infarct, postcontrast-enhanced CT shows gyral enhancement. Transient calcification may occur after 1–8 weeks with encephalomalacia changes and volume loss.

MR imaging is more sensitive than CT in identifying acute infarct. The earliest findings are absence of normal flow void and slow flow with intravascular arterial enhancement following intravenous contrast injection. Acute infarct is seen as anatomic alterations on T1-weighted images. T2-weighted MR images show hyperintense signal with meningeal enhancement on T1-weighted gadolinium-enhanced images. MR venography is a rapid and noninvasive method to evaluate the patency of major dural sinuses. It is not well-suited to visualizing smaller cortical veins with slow flow. Even though conventional catheter angiography still is the gold standard for evaluation of brain and neck vessels, MR arteriogram and CT angiogram provide fast, sensitive and noninvasive alternatives for vascular examinations. DW image can detect signal intensity changes within minutes of arterial occlusion. DW image and cerebral blood volume (CBV) best predict final infarct volume. DW-CBV mismatch predict lesion growth into the CBV abnormality, thus outlining the full extent and severity of the ischemic lesion.

Suggested Reading

Abe T, Singer RJ, Marks MP, Norbash AM, Crowley RS, Steinberg GK (1998) Coexistence of occult vascular malformations and developmental venous anomalies in the central nervous system: MR evaluation. AJNR Am J Neuroradiol 19:51–57

Carvalho KS, Garg BP (2002) Arterial strokes in children. Neurol Clin 20:1079–1100

Fullerton HJ, Chetkovich DM, Wu YW, Smith WS, Johnston SC (2002) Deaths from stroke in US children, 1979 to 1998. Neurology 59:34–39

Roach ES (2000) Etiology of stroke in children. Semin Pediatr Neurol 7:244–260

Schaefer PW, Hunter GJ, He J, Hamberg LM, Sorensen AG, Schwamm LH, Koroshetz WJ, Gonzalez RG (2002) Predicting cerebral ischemic infarct volume with diffusion and perfusion MR imaging. AJNR Am J Neuroradiol 23:1785–1794

Truwit CL (1992) Venous angioma of the brain: history, significance, and Images. AJR Am J Roentgenol 159:1299–1307

Childhood Cerebrovascular Diseases with Infarct

Dissection

Brain Infarct Due to Traumatic Dissection of Internal Carotid Artery

Clinical Presentation

A 6-year-old with headache and right hemiparesis following a minor blunt trauma to the upper neck.

Images (Fig. 8.1)

A. Axial T2-weighted image reveals hyperintense lesion (*arrow*) in the left frontal lobe, head of caudate nucleus, lentiform nucleus and anterior limb of the internal capsule. This is consistent with subacute infarct

B. Coronal MIP image of MR arteriogram shows better narrowing of the left distal internal carotid artery (*arrow*) with poor flow-related enhancement in the left middle cerebral artery and the anterior cerebral artery (*arrows*).

C. MR angiography (3D TOF) demonstrates poor visualization of the left distal internal carotid artery, middle cerebral artery and in its frontal and anterior temporal branches (*arrowheads*)

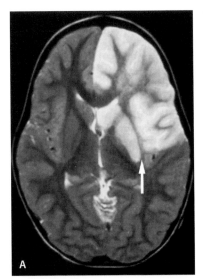

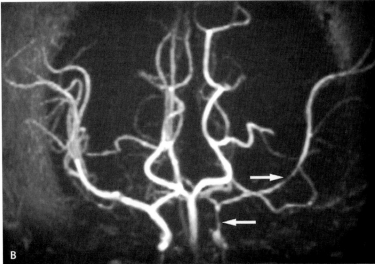

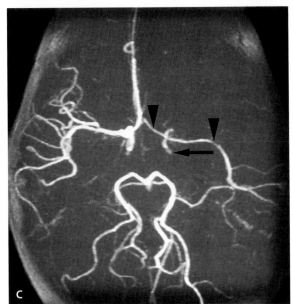

Figure 8.1

Brain infarct due to traumatic dissection of internal carotid artery

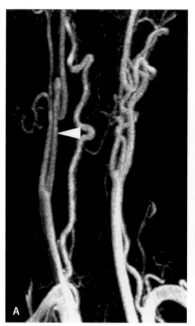
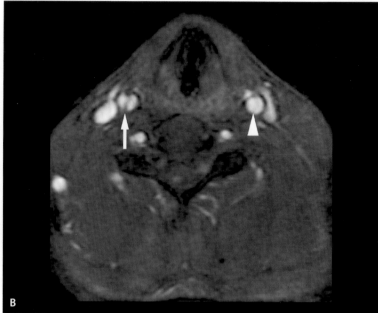

Figure 8.2

Bilateral common carotid dissection in patient with Marfan syndrome

Bilateral Common Carotid Dissection in Patient with Marfan Syndrome

Clinical Presentation

A young adult male with history of stroke and aortic dissection repair with carotid dissections years previously. Patient presents with new symptoms of dissection.

Images (Fig. 8.2)

A. Contrast enhanced MR arteriogram of the neck reveals smaller right common carotid artery. Decreased size of the right internal carotid artery (*arrowhead*) is seen in comparison with the left

B. Axial gradient echo image below the carotid bifurcation shows the two lumens with a flap in between (*arrow*). A dissection is also present in the left common carotid artery with a flap in between the two lumens (*arrowhead*).

Discussion

Traumatic dissection may follow only minimal physical trauma (such as sports activity), but also blunt trauma to the neck or falling onto a blunt object carried in the mouth are common etiologies. Involvement of the internal carotid artery may be either extracranial or intracranial from the dura at the skull base to the carotid terminus. Patients with Marfan syndrome have often dissections of major vessels. Pain is more common in the extracranial dissection. Propagation of thrombosis or distal embolization can lead to hemiplegia

Posterior circulation vascular occlusive disease in children is a rare event. Traumatic injury to the cervical vertebral artery is the most commonly reported cause of injury. The most vulnerable location for intimal injury of the cervical vertebral artery is the point at which the artery exits from the C2 transverse foramen before piercing the atlantooccipital membrane. Cervical spine anomalies and/or instability are thought to increase the risk of vertebral artery injury at this site after trauma. Vasoreactivity caused by migraine, and emboli may also be associated with posterior circulation stroke.

Suggested Reading

Husson B, Lasjaunias P (2004) Radiological approach to disorders of arterial brain vessels associated with childhood arterial stroke – a comparison between MR arteriogram and contrast angiography. Pediatr Radiol 34:10–15

Lanthier S, Carmant L, David M, Larbrisseau A, de Veber G (2000) Stroke in children: the coexistence of multiple risk factors predicts poor outcome. Neurology 54:371–378

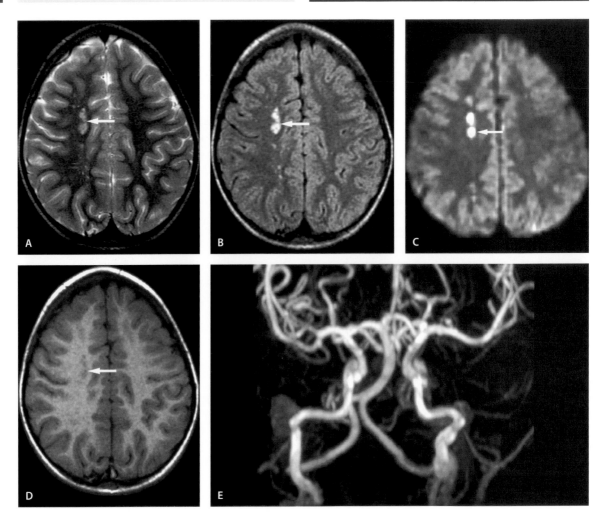

Figure 8.3
Sickle cell hemoglobinopathy with infarct: single area involvement

Sickle Cell Hemoglobinopathy with Infarct

Single Area Involvement

Clinical Presentation

A 4-year-old child with known sickle cell disease (SCD) presents with new onset of headaches.

Images (Fig. 8.3)

A. T2-weighted image shows multifocal areas of high signal within the centrum semiovale (*arrow*). This is consistent with small vessel injury frequently seen in this location in children with SCD
B. FLAIR image shows hyperintensity in the same area (*arrow*)
C. DW image shows the hyperintense areas to have restricted diffusion consistent with small subacute infarcts (*arrow*)
D. The lesions are of decreased signal on T1-weighted image (*arrow*)
E. MR arteriogram (3D TOF) reveals normal flow in major vessels of the circle of Willis

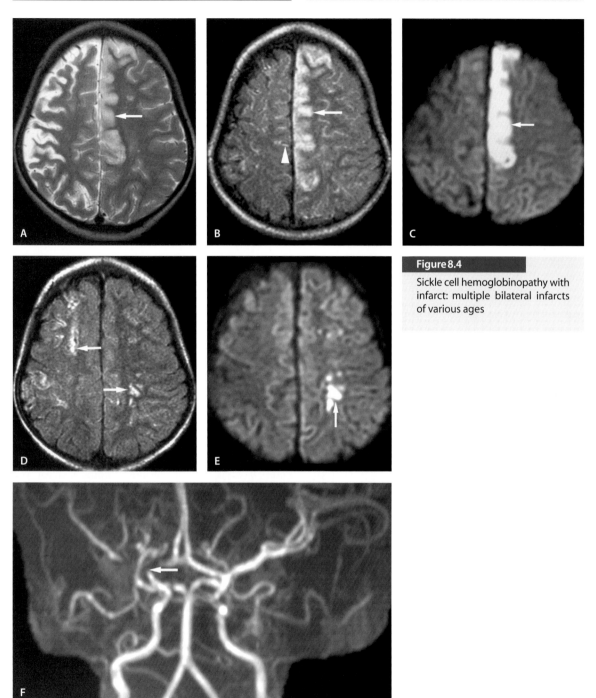

Figure 8.4

Sickle cell hemoglobinopathy with infarct: multiple bilateral infarcts of various ages

Multiple Bilateral Infarcts of Various Ages

Clinical Presentation

A 3-year-old male with SCD presents with acute on-set of right-sided weakness.

Images (Fig. 8.4)

A. T2-weighted image through the upper centrum semiovale shows an abnormal high signal with swelling in cortical gyri in the distribution of the left anterior cerebral artery (*arrow*). Note the cortical atrophy in the right

B. FLAIR image of the same area shows high signal lesions (*arrow*). Note also the thin linear areas of high signal in right side gyri (*arrowhead*)

C. DW image through the upper centrum semiovale reveals restricted diffusion in the same area (*arrow*). This is consistent with subacute infarction

D. FLAIR image through a lower area reveals multiple areas of abnormal high signal (*arrows*)

E. DW image through the lower centrum semiovale reveals restricted area also in the left semiovale

F. Coronal MR arteriogram (3D TOF) shows patent vessels on the left. The right M1 segment of the right middle cerebral artery is absent (*arrow*) with collateral circulation to supply the M2 segment and more distal branches.

Sickle Cell Disease and with Low Hematocrit and CNS Infarct

Clinical Presentation

A 19-month-old male with known SCD presents with left-sided neurological deficits, very low hematocrit and respiratory distress.

Images (Fig. 8.5)

A. T2-weighted image shows increased signal in the medial temporal lobe lateral to internal capsule (*arrows*)

B. T2-weighted image shows areas of vague increased signal adjacent the left lateral ventricle (*arrow*)

C. T1-weighted image is normal

D. DW image shows restricted diffusion in the left medial temporal lobe and lateral to the trigone (*arrows*). These are consistent with acute and subacute infarcts

E. DW image through the ventricle shows an area of restricted diffusion (*arrow*)

F. FLAIR image reveals hyperintensity (*arrow*) that partially shows hyperintensity in the DW image, but is partially visible on T2-weighted image and thus subacute infarct in nature

G. Contrast enhanced T1-weighted image shows multiple areas of abnormal enhancement bilaterally (*arrows*)

H. Multiple areas of abnormal enhancement are also seen in both centrum semiovale areas

I. MR arteriogram reveals normal circle of Willis with some irregular appearing vessels in both peripheral branches of posterior cerebral arteries (*arrows*)

Discussion

Sickle cell anemia (SCA) is a disease caused by production of abnormal hemoglobin, which binds with other abnormal hemoglobin molecules within the red cells to cause rigid deformation of the cell. This impairs the red cells' ability to pass through small vascular channels causing infarctions. The sickled cells can also cause turbulent flow with abrasive action to the vessel wall with endothelial damage. Approximately 25% of all patients with SCA suffer a neurological complication over their lifetime; 11% of these complications will occur by age 20 years. Rarely stroke has been reported in children with sickle cell trait. Stroke, atrophy, and cognitive impairment are major consequences of SCA. Other less-common neurological complications are intraparenchymal and subarachnoid hemorrhage, aneurysm and moyamoya disease. Hemorrhagic events have been reported more in older children whereas ischemic infarcts are more common in younger children.

Reduced blood flow (from any cause) may result in the development of a fine collateral network of vascular channels. This process is called moyamoya. Silent infarctions are twice as common as clinical infarction and may occur in up to 22% of children by 12 years of age. Infarction in SCA is usually ischemic. Ischemia is believed to result from sickled cells in the cerebral vessels, with resultant adherence of red blood cells, intimal damage, intimal hyperplasia, and endoluminal narrowing. Infarcts in SCA tend to occur in the white matter and at the peripheral supply zones of the anterior cerebral and middle cerebral arteries.

Suggested Reading

Dobson SR, Holden KR, Nietert PJ, et al (2002) Moyamoya syndrome in childhood sickle cell disease: a predictive factor for recurrent cerebrovascular events. Blood 99:3144–3150

Earley CJ, Kittner SJ, Feeser BR, et al (1998) Stroke in children and sickle-cell disease: Baltimore-Washington Cooperative Young Stroke Study. Neurology 51:169–176

Riggs JE, Ketonen LM, Wang DD, Valanne LK (1995) Cerebral infarction in a child with sickle cell trait. J Child Neurol 10:253–254

Figure 8.5 ▶

Sickle cell disease and with low hematocrit and CNS infarct

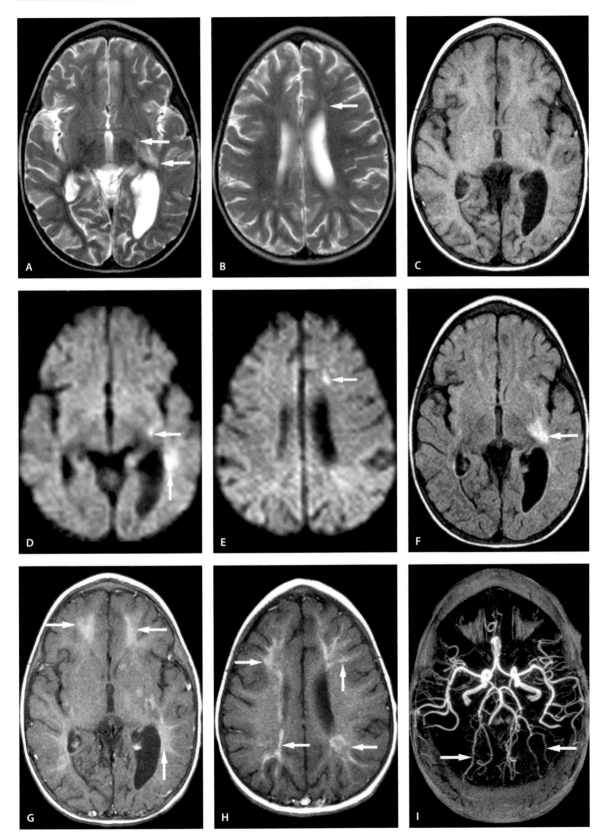

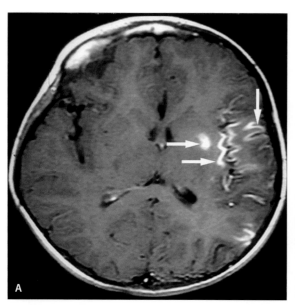
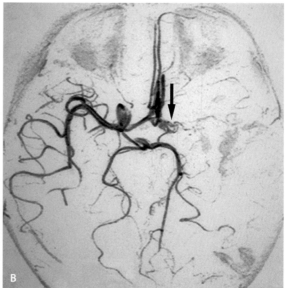

Figure 8.6

Herpes simplex virus vasculopathy and infarction

Herpes Virus Infections of the CNS and Vascular Thrombosis

Herpes Simplex Virus Vasculopathy and Infarction

Clinical Presentation

A 2-year-old male with a 2-week history of herpes simplex virus encephalitis (HSVE), confusion and new onset of right hemiparesis.

Images (Fig. 8.6)

A. Contrast-enhanced T1-weighted image reveals enhancement in left temporal infarction region. Some areas were hemorrhagic and bright in the precontrast image
B. A collapsed image from the MR arteriogram (3D TOF, video reversal) shows lack of flow related enhancement in the left middle cerebral artery.

Discussion

HSVE is caused by type I virus on older children whereas neonatal HSVE is caused by type 2 virus. The family of herpesviruses consists of a large group of double-stranded DNA viruses that includes HSV type 1, HSV type 2, cytomegalovirus (CMV), Epstein-Barr virus, varicella zoster virus, HSV 6, and HSV 7. It is spread by salivary or respiratory contact. It is the most common sporadic encephalitis in North America and other industrialized countries. Infection may result from primary infection or reactivation of latent infection in the trigeminal ganglion. The mesial temporal lobes, insular cortex, cingulated gyrus and inferior frontal lobes are typical areas of involvement. Edema and hemorrhagic lesions are seen in the affected areas. Recently new imaging findings have been reported in a group of infants and young children. In this age group, the cortex and adjacent white matter of the cerebral hemispheres were involved, without classic medial temporal lobe involvement. Thus this group differs from the previously reported pattern in neonates and older children and adults.

CT is often normal in the early phase of the disease. MR imaging plays an important role in the time-

Figure 8.7

Varicella vasculopathy
and infarction

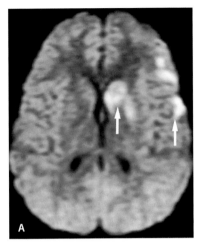
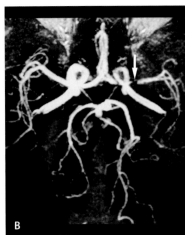

ly diagnosis of postnatal CNS infections and their complications. In some patients the imaging findings are sufficiently specific to suggest a cause. The sequelae of CNS infection, including hydrocephalus, abscess, subdural collections, ischemia/infarction, demyelination, and vascular thrombosis, can be accurately imaged and serially followed with MRI. Diffusion imaging is more sensitive than conventional MRI alone in detection of changes due to infections and ischemic lesions, especially mapping the anatomic distribution of the lesions. Ischemic lesions/infarctions are a known complication of HSVE. HSV type 1 and CMV alter the phenotype of the endothelium in vitro from anticoagulant to procoagulant, thereby promoting the adherence of neutrophils and platelets to the endothelium. The thrombotic process includes multifactorial enhanced procoagulant effects with associated loss of anticoagulants. Thus virus infection in vivo promotes vascular injury and thrombosis, which may contribute to ischemic lesions often seen in association with viral infections.

Suggested Reading

Leonard JR, Moran CJ, Cross DT III, Wippold FJ II, Schlesinger Y, Storch GA (2000) MR imaging of herpes simplex type I encephalitis in infants and young children: a separate pattern of findings. AJR Am J Roentgenol 174:1651–1655

Teixeira J, Zimmerman RA, Haselgrove JC, Bilaniuk LT, Hunter JV (2001) Diffusion imaging in pediatric central nervous system infections. Neuroradiology 43:1031–1039

Tien RD, Felsberg GJ, Osumi AK (1993) Herpesvirus infections of the CNS: MR findings. AJR Am J Roentgenol 161:167–176

Vercellotti GM (1998) Effects of viral activation of the vessel wall on inflammation and thrombosis. Blood Coagul Fibrinolysis [Suppl] 2:S3–S6

Varicella Vasculopathy and Infarction

Clinical Presentation

A 13-year-old male presents with confusion several weeks after varicella infection.

Images (Fig. 8.7)

A. DW image reveals restricted diffusion in both deep and cortical areas (*arrows*). These are consistent with areas of acute infarcts
B. MR arteriogram (3D TOF) shows normal vessels on right. There is poor flow-related enhancement in the M1 (*arrow*) and M2 segments of the left middle cerebral artery. There is lack of flow-related enhancement in the peripheral vessels on left. Additionally there is irregularity in the visualized peripheral vessels.

Discussion

Varicella-zoster virus (VZV) belongs to the family of herpes viruses. It may produce a wide variety of neurological diseases in children, including diffuse meningoencephalitis, vasculopathy, Reye's syndrome, acute cerebellar ataxia, transverse myelitis, polyradiculopathy, and optic neuritis. In young children with acute ischemic stroke, there is a threefold increase in preceding varicella infection compared with published population rates. Varicella-associated ischemic stroke accounts for nearly one-third of childhood ischemic strokes. Varicella-associated stroke has characteristic features, including a twofold increase in recurrent ischemic strokes and transient ischemic attacks. Thus varicella infection is an important risk factor for childhood stroke. The recurrence of varicella virus in the trigeminal and cervical distribution may be associated with a vasculopathy affecting both large and small vessel arteries, typically producing stroke or stroke-like symptoms weeks to months after eruption of the vesicles. Pathologically, there is infiltration of the intima and adventitia with giant and mononuclear cells thereby leading to complications. The infarcts have the tendency to be deep in the hemispheres in the pediatric population. MR imaging is the most sensitive neuroimaging tool in these children (see also the previous Discussion on Herpes simplex virus vasculopathy and infarction).

Suggested Reading

Askalan R, Laughlin S, Mayank SA, et al (2001) Chickenpox and stroke in childhood: a study of frequency and causation editorial comment: pediatric stroke. Stroke 32:1257–1262

Bodensteiner JB, Hille MR, Riggs JE (1992) Clinical features of vascular thrombosis following varicella. Am J Dis Child 146:100–102

Caruso JM, Tung GA, Brown WD (2001) Central nervous system and renal vasculitis associated with primary varicella infection in a child. Pediatrics 107:E9

Schwid S, Ketonen L, Betts R, Richfield E, Kieburtz K (1992) Cerebrovascular complications after primary varicella-zoster infection. Lancet 340:669

CNS Vasculitis and Infarct

CNS Vasculitis with Basal Ganglia Infarct

Clinical Presentation

A 6-year-old female with a 7-hour history of headaches and progressive loss of function of the left side of the body. Patient has also a 2-week history of sinusitis and fatigue without fever.

Images (Fig. 8.8)

A. Noncontrast CT scan demonstrates vague right basal ganglia and insular cortex edema (*arrow*)
B. T2-weighted image later on the same day demonstrates significant edema involving the right insular region and head of the caudate nucleus. Only mild involvement of the internal capsule and lentiform nucleus is seen
C. Axial 3-D TOF MR arteriogram demonstrates poor flow-related enhancement in the right middle cerebral artery (*arrow*). Patient had also a neck vessel MR arteriogram with normal appearing vessels
D and E. Conventional carotid arteriograms demonstrate irregular and beading appearance of the right middle cerebral artery (*arrows*)
F. T2-weighted follow-up study 10 days later demonstrates a well-defined infarction in the right basal ganglia

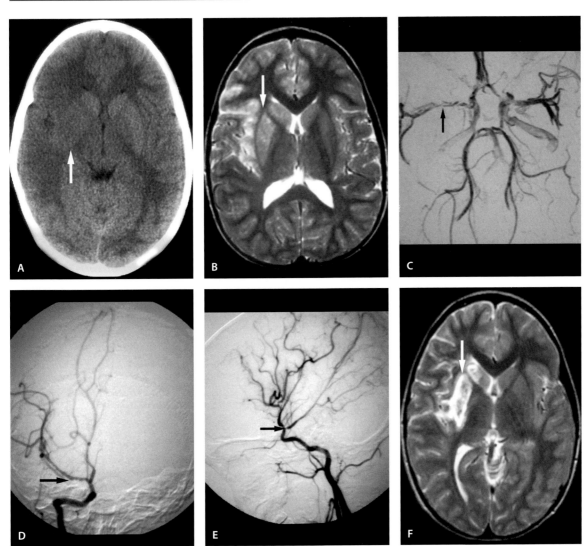

Figure 8.8

CNS vasculitis with basal ganglia infarct

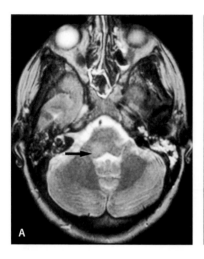
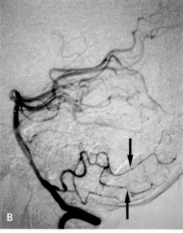

Figure 8.9

CNS vasculitis and posterior circulation infarct in patient with primary Sjögren's syndrome

CNS Vasculitis and Posterior Circulation Infarct in Patient with Primary Sjögren's Syndrome (PSS)

Clinical Presentation

A young adult female with PSS presents with acute onset of multiple cranial nerve palsies (CN 5, 6, 7) on right and headache. She has also left body numbness.

Images (Fig. 8.9)

A. T2-weighted image shows area of hyperintensity in the pons (*arrow*). The medulla had a similar lesion (not shown). Neither lesion showed abnormal enhancement or mass effect
B. Conventional catheter angiography shows beaded appearance in some of the vessels in the posterior circulation (*arrows*)

Discussion

Posterior circulation vascular occlusive disease in children and young adults is rare. When a young person presents with abrupt onset of neurological signs and symptoms indicative of posterior circulation ischemia a history of traumatic injury to the neck and head should be elicited. Radiographs of the cervical spine should be taken to exclude associated anomalies. MR imaging is the modality of choice for assessment of posterior circulation infarcts. MR arteriogram being a noninvasive modality should be performed for assessment of vertebral and basilar artery patency.

CNS involvement in PSS is controversial with regard to frequency, significance, and etiology. Cerebral dysfunction depends on the number and location of lesions. CNS involvement may be acute, remittent or progressive. Cognitive dysfunction and psychiatric manifestations seem to be frequent in PSS. In CNS involvement, there is no correlation between clinical findings and results of CSF study or MRI which can be normal or disclose nonspecific abnormalities. Neuropathological studies suggest that MRI abnormalities are associated with mononuclear inflammatory ischemic vasculopathy resulting in small or major infarcts. Angiographically confirmed vasculitic changes are seen in 20% of cases with PSS and CNS symptoms. Autopsy and biopsy results have documented active CNS involvement in PSS patients with normal MRI and cerebral angiograms. Although pediatric PSS is rare, it is important to consider Sjögren's syndrome in a child or young adult with unexplained facial weakness and in the differential diagnosis of pediatric and young adult stroke.

Suggested Reading

Ganesan V, Chong WK, Cox TC, Chawda SJ, Prengler M, Kirkham FJ (2002) Posterior circulation stroke in childhood: risk factors and recurrence. Neurology 59:1552–1556

Gottfried JA, Finkel TH, Hunter JV, Carpentieri DF, Finkel RS (2001) Central nervous system Sjogren's syndrome in a child: case report and review of the literature. J Child Neurol 6:683–685

James CA, Glasier CM, Angtyuaco EE (1995) Altered vertebrobasilar flow in children: angiographic, MR, and MR angiographic findings. AJNR Am J Neuroradiol 16:1689–1695

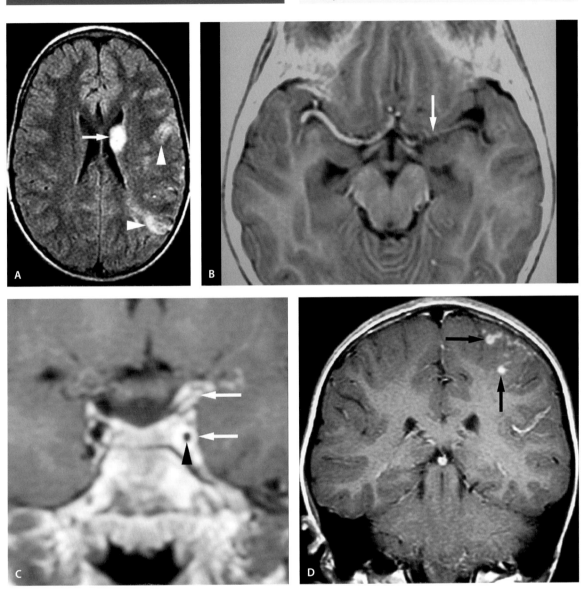

Figure 8.10

Wiskott-Aldrich syndrome, vasculitis and infarct

Wiskott-Aldrich Syndrome (WAS), Vasculitis and Infarct

Clinical Presentation

An 8-year-old male with WAS presents with recent loss of right side motor skills and speech.

Images (Fig. 8.10)

A. FLAIR image shows T2 hyperintensity in the left corona radiata (*arrow*). Two additional areas of hyperintensity are seen in the middle cerebral artery distribution (*arrowheads*)

B. T2-weighted (reversed) image shows decreased flow (decreased flow void) in the left M1 segment of the middle cerebral artery

C. Coronal contrast-enhanced T1-weighted image of the cavernous carotid arteries reveals significant narrowing (decreased flow void) of the distal left internal carotid artery (*arrowhead*) with vessel wall enhancement (*arrows*)

D. Contrast-enhanced image shows areas of enhancement (*arrows*) in the left middle cerebral artery distribution

Discussion

WAS is an uncommon X-linked immunodeficiency disorder characterized by eczema, thrombocytopenia, and immunodeficiency. Autoimmune inflammatory complications in WAS are common – up to 71% has been reported. Vasculitides and autoimmune hemolytic anemias are the most common manifestations. However, vasculitic complications of the brain are rare, in fewer that 10% of cases. WAS includes dysfunction of nearly all effector arms of the immune system, as well as thrombocytopenia with platelet dysfunction. As a consequence of these abnormalities, these children have bleeding, recurrent and severe infections with common and opportunistic organisms, autoimmune disease, and lymphoreticular malignancies. Long-surviving patients may have progressive multifocal leukoencephalopathy.

Suggested Reading

Conley ME, Saragoussi D, Notarangelo L, Etzioni A, Casanova JL; PAGID; ESID (2003) An international study examining therapeutic options used in treatment of Wiskott-Aldrich syndrome. Clin Immunol 109:272–277

Matsushima T, Nakamura K, Oka T, et al (1997) Unusual MRI and pathological findings of progressive multifocal leukoencephalopathy complicating adult Wiskott-Aldrich syndrome. Neurology 48:279–282

Schurman SH, Candotti F (2003) Autoimmunity in Wiskott-Aldrich syndrome. Curr Opin Rheumatol 15:446–453

Sullivan KE (1999) Recent advances in our understanding of Wiskott-Aldrich syndrome. Curr Opin Hematol 6:8–14

Arteriovenous Malformations (AVMs)

Clinical Presentation

An autistic child with developmental delay and seizures and known AVM since the age of 4 years when he was examined for seizures.

Images (Fig. 8.11)

A. T2-weighted image shows an extensive AVM involving the right occipital lobe (*arrow*). The pretreatment images were obtained in 2001, immediately before treatment

B. DW image shows decreased signal and prominent vessels in the right occipital lobe (*arrow*)

C. Contrast-enhanced T1-weighted image shows enhancement of the AVM nidus

D., E. and F.
Axial (D), coronal (E) and sagittal (F) MR venography (phase contrast technique) shows prominent venous drainage from the AVM into the straight sinus (*arrow*), vena Galen (*arrow*) and torcular region (*arrow*)

G. 3D TOF shows flow-related enhancement in the large arteries (*arrow*) from the posterior cerebral artery to the region of the AVM. A large vein is seen posteriorly (*black arrowhead*). Note the large posterior communicating artery on right (*white arrowhead*)

H. T2-weighted image 26 months after the second stereotactic radiosurgery shows minimal hyperintensity, mainly involving the white matter and to lesser extent the medial gray matter (*arrow*)

I. On posttreatment FLAIR image there is abnormal signal in the AVM area (*arrow*)

J. DW image shows minimal asymmetry on the white matter tracts without significant signal abnormality (*arrow*)

K. Axial contrast-enhanced T1-weighted image shows small area of residual enhancement (*arrow*) in the occipital lobe

L. In the MR arteriogram (3D TOF) following radiosurgery the AVM is no longer seen. Incidentally, there is absent A1 of the right anterior cerebral artery

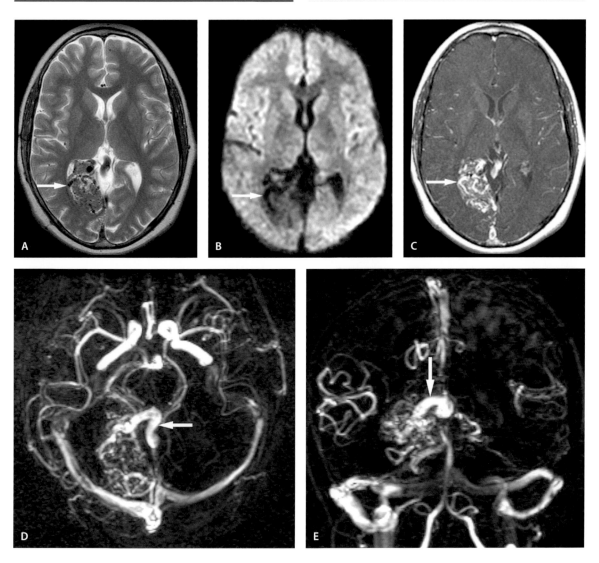

Figure 8.11 A–E

Arteriovenous malformation (F–L see next page)

Discussion

AVMs are composed of arteries that communicate directly with veins rather than feeding into progressively smaller blood vessels. Because of this abnormality the veins contain blood under abnormally high pressure. This leads to enlargement of the thin-walled veins to deal with the increased pressure and flow. These thin walled veins can rupture.

Intracranial AVMs are subdivided into two types, brain parenchymal (pial) malformations and dural malformations. A third type, mixed pial-dural AVMs occur when a parenchymal malformation gets its blood supply from dural sources. AVMs are congenital lesions presenting commonly between 20 and 40 years of age. The majority of the AVMs are solitary; however, multiple AVMs are seen in Rendu-Osler-Weber and Wyburn-Mason syndromes. Of all pial AVMs, 85% are found in the cerebral hemispheres,

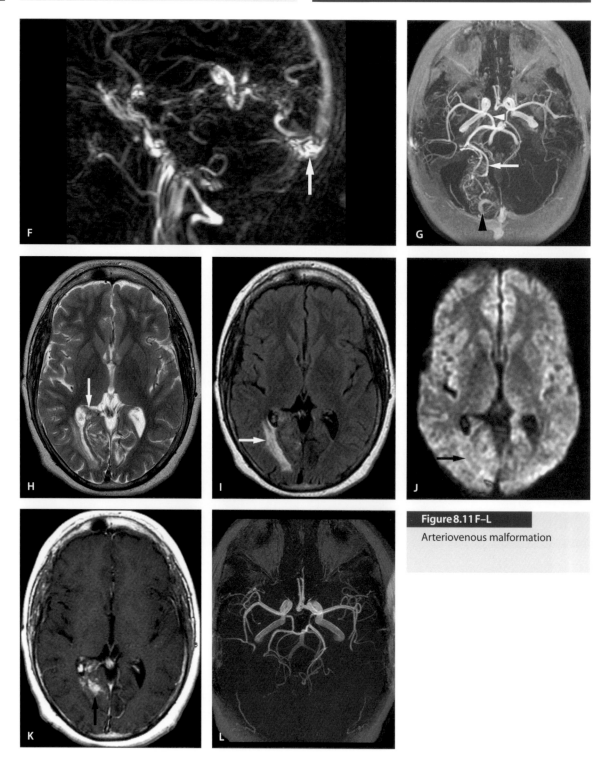

Figure 8.11 F–L

Arteriovenous malformation

and 15% occur in the posterior fossa. There is a 2–4% risk of rupture of an AVM per year.

On CT, AVM is seen as serpiginous isodense or slightly hyperdense vessels that enhance strongly following contrast administration. A prominent draining vein may be seen. CT is particularly useful in showing acute hemorrhage, and calcification may be seen in 25–30% of cases.

MR in the subacute stage or later allows a better anatomic analysis of the lesion and provides more thorough information about prior hemorrhage, pseudoaneurysms and the condition of the surrounding brain tissue. On conventional sequences, AVMs are seen as flow-voids due to high-velocity signal loss. MR arteriogram may show nidus with an early draining vein. MRI cannot exclude the presence of micro-AVMs, even if the localization is known beforehand. Cerebral digital subtraction angiography (DSA) is still considered the gold standard to establish the diagnosis and is used in the work-up of endovascular treatment. MRI, MR arteriogram and CT angiogram play an important role in follow-up examination.

Suggested Reading

Kupersmith MJ, Vargas ME, Yashar A, Madrid M, Nelson K, Seton A, Berenstein A (1996) Occipital arteriovenous malformations: visual disturbances and presentation. Neurology 46:953–957

Soderman M, Andersson T, Karlsson B, Wallace MC, Edner G (2003) Management of patients with brain arteriovenous malformations. Eur J Radiol 46:195–205

Tranchida JV, Mehall CJ, Slovis TL, Lis-Planells M (1997) Imaging of arteriovenous malformation following stereotactic radio surgery. Pediatrics 27:299–304

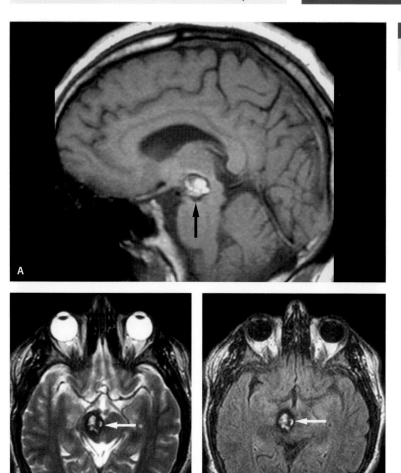

Figure 8.12

Cavernous malformation

Cavernous Malformation

Solitary Intrinsic Parenchymal Lesion

Clinical Presentation

An asymptomatic young adult male who had first CT scan for a minor head trauma (assault). CT showed mixed density lesion in the right cerebral peduncle.

Images (Fig. 8.12)

A. Sagittal T1-weighted image shows a rounded lesion (*arrow*) with intrinsic high signal and peripheral low signal. No mass effect is present

B. T2-weighted image shows typical "popcorn"-like bright lesion surrounded with a low signal intensity hemosiderin rim with variable thickness (*arrow*)

C. FLAIR image shows the "popcorn"-like lesion (*arrow*).

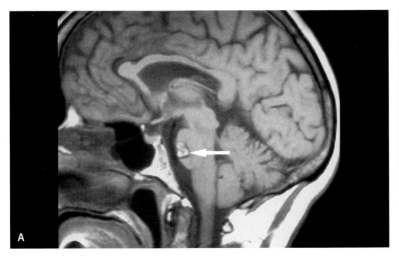 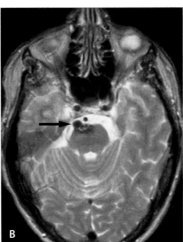

Figure 8.13

Solitary exophytic cavernous malformation

Solitary Exophytic Cavernous Malformation

Clinical Presentation

Adult male presented with dizziness.

Images (Fig. 8.13)

A. Sagittal T1-weighted image shows a high-signal lesion surrounded by a low-signal rim (*arrow*)

B. T2-weighted image shows the typical "popcorn"-like lesion with exophytic growth into the prepontine cistern (*arrow*)

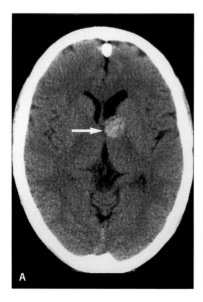
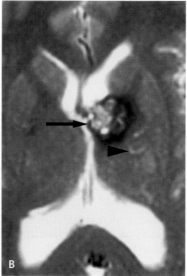
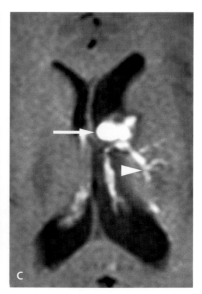

Figure 8.14

Solitary cavernous malformation with developmental venous anomaly

Solitary Cavernous Malformation with Developmental Venous Anomaly

Clinical Presentation

Adult male presented with headache.

Images (Fig. 8.14)

A. Noncontrast CT scan shows calcified lesion in the left basal ganglia (*arrow*). No surrounding edema is seen

B. T2-weighted image shows typical mixed signal lesion with hemosiderin stain of variable thickness (*arrow*). Associated developmental venous malformation is vaguely seen (*arrowhead*). There is mass effect upon the foramen of Monro, causing enlargement of the left lateral ventricle

C. Contrast-enhanced T1-weighted image shows enhancement in the cavernous malformation (*arrow*). Classic "Medusa head" appearance of large venous malformation is seen (*arrowhead*) draining the left basal ganglia

Multiple Cavernous Malformations

Clinical Presentation

Young adult female with a several-year history of dizziness.

Images (Fig. 8.15)

A. T2-weighted image through cerebellum reveals multiple cavernous malformations throughout the white matter. May lesions have the typical popcorn appearance. Note, however, that there are also multiple small hypointense lesions without central areas of high signal intensity representing hemosiderin depositions (*arrows*)

B. Coronal T2-weighted image through posterior fossa shows multiple foci of cavernous malformations (*arrows*). The appearances of the lesions are typical mixed signal intensity lesions with high signal center and peripheral low signal hemosiderin

C. T2-weighted image through brainstem shows a large pontine lesion (*arrow*). Multiple small hypointense lesions are also seen in the white matter

D. T2-weighted image through the basal ganglia reveals multiple cavernous malformations distributed through the white matter and basal ganglia

E. Sagittal noncontrast T1-weighted image demonstrates the large pontine lesion (*arrow*) with scattered smaller parenchymal lesions.

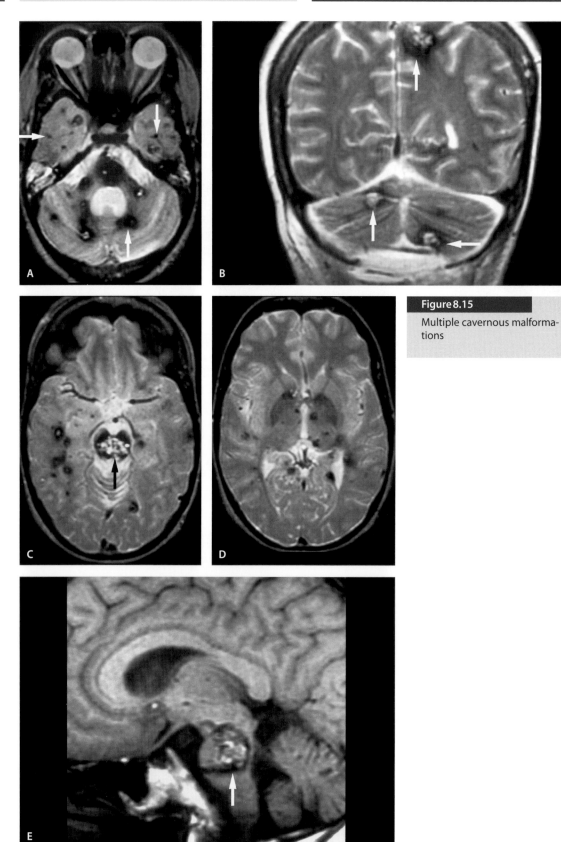

Figure 8.15

Multiple cavernous malformations

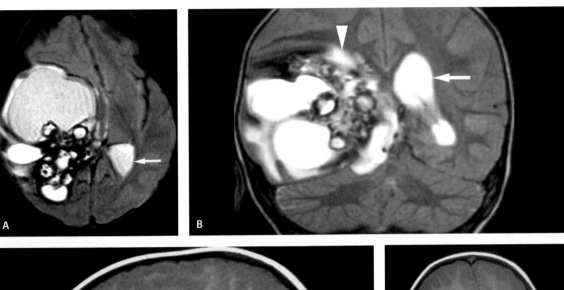

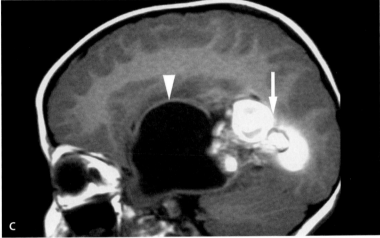
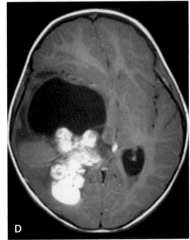

Figure 8.16

Cavernous malformation simulating neoplasm with major bleed

Cavernous Malformation Simulating Neoplasm with Major Bleed

Clinical Presentation

A 2-year-old male with acute onset of hemiparesis and mental status change. At surgery a large cavernous malformation was found that had bled.

Images (Fig. 8.16)

A. Proton density image demonstrates a mixed signal intense lesion in the right hemisphere with significant midline shift. The lesion is composed of multiple small round hyperintensities with a peripheral low signal intensity rim. The left temporal horn is significantly dilated (*arrow*)

B. Coronal T2-weighted image demonstrates enlargement of the left lateral ventricle (*arrow*). The right temporal lobe mass lesion has some surrounding edema (*arrowhead*). The lesion is composed of multiple small cystic areas with a thin peripheral low signal intensity rim. There is also mass effect upon the cerebellum

C. Sagittal T1-weighted image demonstrates the lesion to be mainly hemorrhagic (*arrow*). The temporal horn is trapped and dilated (*arrowhead*)

D. Contrast-enhanced T1-weighted image through the same area as image A. Although the lesion is mainly hemorrhagic, minimal enhancing areas are also present

Discussion

Cavernous malformations (synonyms: cavernous angiomas, cavernoma) are angiographically occult vascular malformations that typically appear as discrete multilobulated berry-like lesion(s) consisting of widely open spaces with little intervening tissue and evidence of recent or old hemorrhage. Cavernous malformations can be found in any part of the brain, but 80% are found in a supratentorial location. Deep cerebral white matter, corticomedullary junction, and basal ganglia are common supratentorial locations, whereas pons and cerebellar hemispheres are common infratentorial locations. Multiple lesions can be seen in 50–80% of cases, particularly in familial cases, which are more frequent among people of Hispanic origin. The typical age of presentation is between 20 and 40 years. MR imaging with contrast has shown that cavernous malformations frequently appear to arise at the distal end radicles of venous anomalies. This association is seen in 30–50% of cases. Patients usually present with seizures, focal neurological deficits or headaches.

On CT, cavernous malformations are usually isodense to moderately hyperdense on noncontrast-enhanced scans. Calcification is seen in about 30% of cases. On MR imaging, cavernous malformation is seen as a complex reticulated popcorn-like mixed intensity mass representing hemorrhage in different stages of evolution. A low-signal hemosiderin rim that commonly surrounds the lesion is a characteristic feature of cavernous malformation. Variable contrast enhancement occurs in post-gadolinium images. Gradient echo sequences should always be performed when a solitary intracranial hemorrhagic lesion is identified for detection of multiple lesions. If cavernous malformation is suspected, high field-strength MR units (1.5 T and over) should be used to optimize lesion detection. The lesions may remain undetected with low field-strength MR units. It is also important to perform a gadolinium-enhanced study to look for DVA. The presence of DVA may affect the

surgical plan, as it drains normal brain parenchyma and their ligation may lead to venous infarction.

Suggested Reading

Dillon WP (1997) Cryptic vascular malformations: controversies in terminology, diagnosis, pathophysiology, and treatment. AJNR Am J Neuroradiol 18:1839–1846

Novak V, Chowdhary A, Abduljali A, Novak P, Chakeres D (2003) Venous cavernoma at 8 Tesla MRI. Magn Reson Imaging 21:1087–1089

Villani RM, Arienta C, Caroli M (1989) Cavernous angiomas of the central nervous system. J Neurosurg Sci 33:229–252

Developmental Venous Anomaly

Clinical Presentation

Young adult with headaches.

Images (Fig. 8.17)

A. T2-weighted image shows poorly defined area of increased signal intensity in the right periventricular area (*arrow*)

B. Contrast-enhanced T1-weighted image reveals a typical venous malformation in the right frontal lobe. Central vein (arrow) drains towards the medullary veins

C. Sagittal contrast enhanced T1-weighted image shows multiple enhancing venous radicles coalescing to a central vein (*arrow*), which then drains to the medullary veins

Discussion

DVA (synonyms: venous angioma, venous malformation) are composed of radially arranged, dilated anomalous veins that form a common trunk that passes through brain parenchyma and usually empties into a cortical vein or dural sinus. Many abnormal medullary veins coalesce into one large trunk giving the angiographic appearance of "caput Medusa" (head of Medusa – goddess with "hair" of snakes). Venous angiomas are often located in deep cerebral or cerebellar white matter, near the ventricular margin. The most common location is adjacent to the frontal horn of the lateral ventricle followed by the cerebellum. These lesions rarely bleed unless as-

Figure 8.17

Developmental venous anomaly

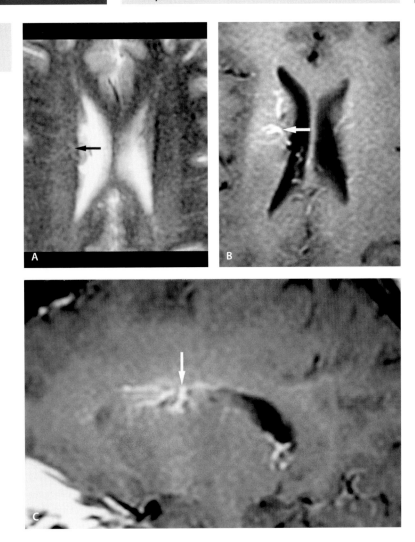

sociated with cavernous malformation which may be seen in 30–40% of cases of solitary venous angioma.

Contrast-enhanced CT shows tuft of vessels near the ventricular surface with a dilated draining vein. Contrast-enhanced MR imaging along with MR arteriogram is the imaging modality of choice. Vessels are seen as tubular and stellate strongly enhancing structures with variable signal. Associated hemorrhagic or gliotic changes may be seen in 10–15% of cases. A venous malformation is important to normal venous drainage of the brain. Its presence may affect the surgical plan, as ligation of the veins may lead to venous infarction.

Suggested Reading

Truwit CL (1992) Venous angioma of the brain: history, significance, and images. AJR Am J Roentgenol 159:1299–1307

Konan AV, Raymond J, Bourgouin P, Lesage J, Milot G, Roy D (1999) Cerebellar infarct caused by spontaneous thrombosis of a developmental venous anomaly of the posterior fossa. AJNR Am J Neuroradiol 20:256–258

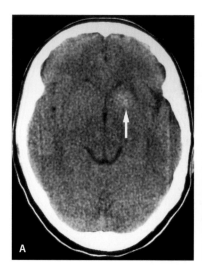 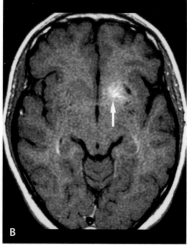

Figure 8.18

Capillary telangiectasia

Capillary Telangiectasia

Clinical Presentation

A 15-year-old female with history of seizures and movement disorder. A selective carotid arteriogram was performed and it shows a vague capillary blush in the region of the left basal ganglia. The lesion drains via several small veins into a single larger vein, which then drains into the basal vein of Rosenthal. These findings suggest that this lesion is perhaps a transitional malformation and not a pure capillary telangiectasia.

Images (Fig. 8.18)

A. Noncontrast CT scan shows slight hyperattenuation in the left basal ganglia with punctate calcification (*arrow*). No mass effect is present
B. Contrast-enhanced T1-weighted image shows diffuse enhancement in the left basal ganglia lesion (*arrow*). The lesion has been stable over several years.

Discussion

Capillary telangiectasias are small areas of abnormally dilated capillaries with otherwise normal brain tissue. Capillary telangiectasias are different from venous malformations mainly in their compact nature and the size of the anomalous vessels. They have been described throughout the brain; however, the pons is the most classical location. Capillary telangiectasias represent 16–20% of all brain vascular malformations; however autopsy series have provided estimates that the prevalence of capillary telangiectasias is around 0.4%, although they may not be visible on imaging studies. Capillary telangiectasias are usually solitary, but they may also be found in association with other brain vascular malformations such as cavernous and venous angiomas. They can occur at any age without specific sex/race predilection. Most of them are asymptomatic but have been associated with minor symptoms such as vertigo, headache and dizziness.

Contrast-enhanced CT may show subtle areas of enhancement. Rarely, tiny specks of calcification may be seen on noncontrast-enhanced CT. Contrast-enhanced MR images characteristically show brush-/lace-like enhancement without any mass effect. T2-weighted images may not show any significant signal alteration. Gradient echo sequences are useful in cases of capillary telangiectasia associated with hemorrhage. The differential diagnosis for an enhancing pontine lesion includes infection, demyelinating lesion, neoplasm, or rarely central pontine myelinolysis. Absence of mass effect or significant T2 prolongation is an important finding to differentiate capillary telangiectasia from other conditions.

Suggested Reading

Barr RM, Dillon WP, Wilson CB (1996) Slow-flow vascular malformations of the pons: capillary telangiectasia? AJNR Am J Neuroradiol 17:71–78

Castillo M, Morrison T, Shaw JA, Bouldin TW (2001) MR imaging and histologic features of capillary telangiectasia of the basal ganglia. AJNR Am J Neuroradiol 22:1553–1555

Lee RR, Becher MW, Benson ML, Rigamonti D (1997) Brain capillary telangiectasia: MR imaging appearance and clinicohistopathologic findings. Radiology 205:797–805

Sinovenous Thrombosis

Transverse Sinus Thrombosis Extending Into Superior Sagittal, Sigmoid and Jugular Sinus

Clinical Presentation

A 12-year-old female with acute lymphatic leukemia suffered from posterior reversible leukoencephalopathy syndrome (PRES) four months previously. Now she presents with a several-week episode of headaches and vomiting.

Images (Fig. 8.19)

A. Noncontrast CT scan shows an increased density along the expected course of the right transverse sinus (*arrow*) that is dominant in this patient

B. Contrast-enhanced T1-weighted image shows enhancement of dural collaterals in the wall of the thrombosed sinus resulting in the "empty delta" sign (*arrow*), but no enhancement is seen in the sinus itself

C. FLAIR image demonstrates abnormal hyperintensity in the right transverse sinus (*arrow*)

D. DW image reveals high signal in the transverse and sigmoid sinuses (*arrows*)

E. Sagittal projection of 2D (time-of-flight) MR venography demonstrates absence of flow-related enhancement in the superior sagittal sinus (*arrowheads*). Smaller vascular channels are seen and they most likely represent dilated dural collaterals and/or partially recanalized superior sagittal sinus

F. Coronal projection of the MR venography shows absent flow in the right transverse and jugular sinus (*arrow*). According to CT scan (prominent sigmoid sinus groove in the bone), the right transverse sinus is the dominant one

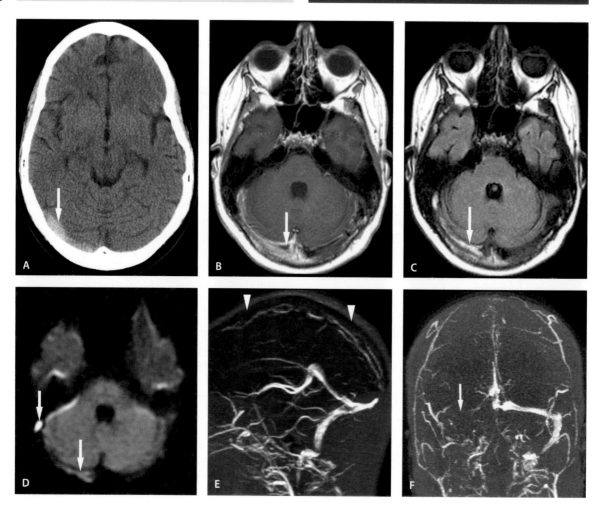

Transverse sinus thrombosis extending into superior sagittal, sigmoid and jugular sinus

Evolution of Transverse Sinus Thrombosis

Clinical Presentation

Young adult female presents with pain over the right occipital region. She has opacification in the right mastoid air cells, best seen on T2-weighted image.

Images (Fig. 8.20)

A. T1-weighted image demonstrates minimally hyperintensity in the right transverse sinus (*arrow*) consistent with slow flow in the sinus or early venous sinus thrombosis

B. T2-weighted image shows hypointensity in the transverse sinus (*arrow*)

C. Contrast-enhanced T1-weighted image demonstrates lack of expected enhancement in the right transverse sinus. The sinus signal is dark. There is enhancement of dural collaterals in the wall of the thrombosed sinus (*arrow*) resulting in the "empty delta" sign

D. T1-weighted image 4 days later shows abnormal increased signal intensity in the transverse sinus (*arrow*) consistent with venous sinus thrombosis

E. Sagittal T1-weighted image confirms the sinus thrombosis (*arrows*)

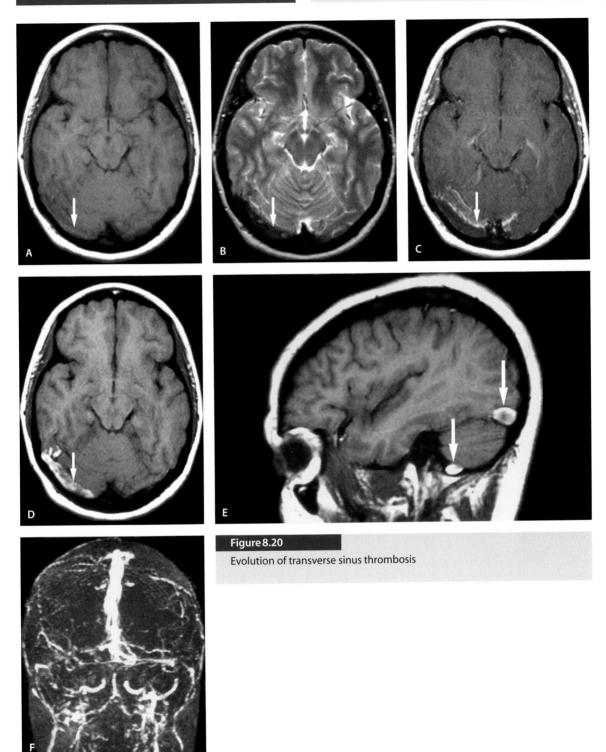

Figure 8.20

Evolution of transverse sinus thrombosis

F. Coronal projection of MR venography (2D TOF) shows lack of flow-related enhancement in the transverse sinus, with flow enhancement in smaller dural collateral vessels. The left transverse sinus is hypoplastic

Discussion

Veno-occlusive disease of the brain most commonly affects the superior sagittal sinus, followed by transverse, sigmoid, and straight sinuses. Trauma, tumors, infection, dehydration, hypercoagulable states such as pregnancy, and oral contraceptives are the most common causes. Nephrotic syndrome is an uncommon cause of sinus thrombosis.

Noncontrast-enhanced CT may demonstrate increased attenuation in the thrombosed veins known as the "cord sign". Contrast-enhanced CT may show the "empty delta" sign, which occurs when the thrombus fails to enhance within the dural sinus and is outlined by enhanced collateral channels in the falx and dura. On MR imaging, hyperacute thrombus is seen as low signal on both T1- and T2-weighted images. MR venography may show loss of vascular flow signal or a frayed appearance of the venous sinus. Indirect signs of thrombus include the presence of collateral channels.

Suggested Reading

Yuh WT, Simonson TM, Wang AM, et al (1994) Venous sinus occlusive disease: MR findings. AJNR Am J Neuroradiol 15:309–316

Sturge-Weber (SWS) Syndrome and Lack of Flow Through the Superior Sagittal Sinus Simulating Chronic Superior Sagittal Sinus Thrombosis

Clinical Presentation

An 18-year-old male with SWS had MRI because of increased frequency of seizures. Conventional catheter angiography confirmed the finding that there is no flow through the superior sagittal sinus. It also confirmed hat the large vascular channels represent collateral veins.

Images (Fig. 8.21)

A. T2-weighted image demonstrates enlarged medullary veins (*arrow*)
B. Coronal T2-weighted image shows multiple flow voids in the central region consistent with enlarged medullary veins and enlarged deep venous drainage (*arrows*)
C. Sagittal T1-weighted image demonstrates transparenchymal flow voids consistent with draining veins (*arrows*)
D. Contrast-enhanced T1-weighted image demonstrates linear enhancement in the transcortical and transparenchymal (*arrows*) veins draining into the deep system
E. Sagittal MR venography (2D phase-contrast) demonstrates lack of a flow-related enhancement in the superior sagittal sinus (*arrowheads*). Prominent central collateral venous channels are present (*arrow*).

Discussion

SWS (synonym: encephalotrigeminal angiomatosis) is a rare neurocutaneous disorder that involves the skin, CNS, leptomeningeal vasculature and retina. The gene locus has not yet been mapped. The classic presentation is a facial port-wine nevus involving the first division of trigeminal nerve branches on the ipsilateral side of the leptomeningeal angioma. Choroidal involvement leading to buphthalmos is present in one-third of patients. The patients usually have seizures. The seizure activity will usually increase over time and often becomes refractory to medication. Patients usually present with developmental delay. The leptomeningeal malformation consists of abnormal venous structures and lack of development of cortical veins leading to impaired venous drainage that leads to cortical atrophy and calcium depositions in the junction of the gray and white matter. They usually involve the cortical layers of two through four. The meningeal angioma is usually in the pia mater. Angiomas may also involve the choroids plexus that is enlarged and demonstrates significant enhancement. Scleral enhancement is also common. Due to the calcification the cortical enhancement is difficult to visualize with CT; however, it is well visualized on MRI.

Suggested Reading

Comi AM (2003) Pathophysiology of Sturge-Weber syndrome. J Child Neurol 8:509–516

Griffiths PD, Coley SC, Romanowski CA, Hodgson T, Wilkinson ID (2003) Contrast-enhanced fluid-attenuated inversion recovery imaging for leptomeningeal disease in children. AJNR Am J Neuroradiol 4:719–723

Lin DD, Barker PB, Kraut MA, Comi A (2003) Early characteristics of Sturge-Weber syndrome shown by perfusion MR imaging and proton MR spectroscopic imaging. AJNR Am J Neuroradiol 9:1912–1915

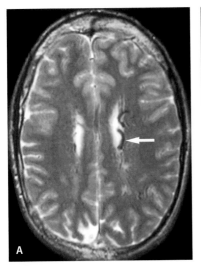
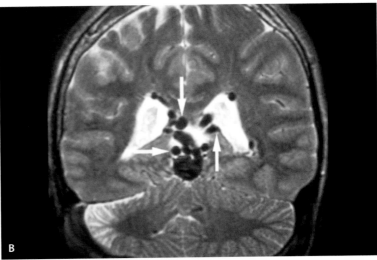
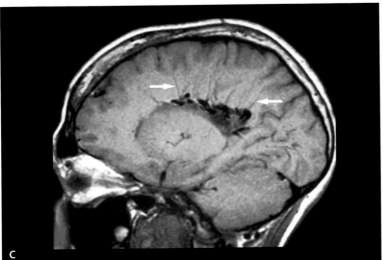
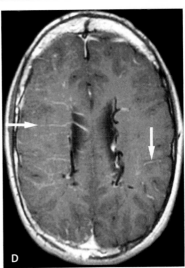
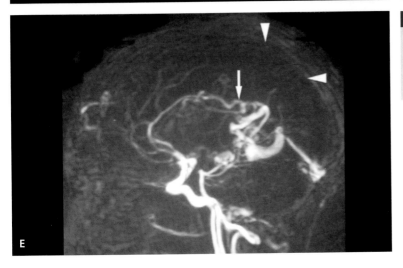

Figure 8.21

Sturge-Weber syndrome and lack of flow through the superior sagittal sinus simulating chronic superior sagittal sinus thrombosis

Iatrogenic Sinus Thrombosis in an Infant Treated with Extracorporeal Membrane Oxygenation (ECMO)

Clinical Presentation

A 2-week-old near full-term baby underwent venoarterial ECMO therapy, where ligation of both internal carotid artery and jugular vein are part of the procedure. MRI shows normal brain parenchyma without diffusion abnormality or parenchymal bleed. The patient's clinical condition was good.

Images (Fig. 8.22)

A. Axial noncontrast CT shows a hyperdense right transverse sinus (*arrow*). Contrast-enhanced CT (not shown) demonstrated the empty delta sign. The study was performed 2 days before the MRI scan
B. Axial FLAIR image reveals high signal intensity in both transverse sinuses (*arrows*)
C. Axial T1-weighted image shows abnormal increased signal in both transverse sinuses (*arrows*) consistent with venous sinus thrombosis and/or slow flow
D. The DW image shows no evidence of venous infarcts
E. Coronal MR venography (phase-contrast) shows lack of flow in the thrombosed dominant right transverse sinus. There is flow in the left transverse sinus (*arrow*)
F. Axial MR venography (phase-contrast) shows flow in the partially thrombosed left transverse sinus (*arrow*).

Discussion

ECMO treatment is a commonly used therapy for neonates in respiratory failure. In venoarterial ECMO both internal carotid artery and jugular vein are ligated when ECMO catheters are placed. The ECMO procedure results in significant alteration in cerebral blood flow, which increases the risk of intracranial infarction or hemorrhage. Internal jugular vein ligation can lead to increased sagittal sinus pressure leading to additional subarachnoid space enlargement by decreasing CSF absorption at the arachnoidean villi. Approximately one-third of treated patients have intracranial hemorrhage located mainly in the brain parenchyma or in the cerebellum. Extraaxial hemorrhages are rare. These patients have increased rate of infarcts of the same side as the carotid ligation and hemorrhages on the side opposite the carotid ligation. The ligation of the jugular vein results in abnormal venous drainage and stasis within the deep medullary veins. Jugular vein ligation and thrombosis leads also to transverse sinus thrombosis.

Suggested Reading

Bulas DI, Taylor GA, O'Donnell RM, Short BL, Fitz CR, Vezina G (1996) Intracranial abnormalities in infants treated with extracorporeal membrane oxygenation: update on sonographic and CT findings. AJNR Am J Neuroradiol 17: 287–294

Provenzale JM, Joseph GJ, Barrborial DP (1998) Dural sinus thrombosis: findings on CT and MR imaging and diagnostic pitfalls. AJR Am J Roentgenol 170:777–783

Yuh WT, Simonson TM, Wang AM, et al (1994) Venous sinus occlusive disease: MR findings. Am J Neuroradiol 15:309–316

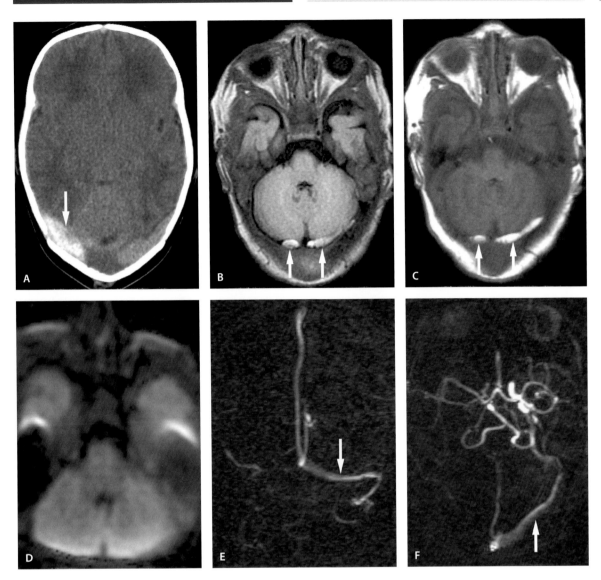

Figure 8.22

Iatrogenic sinus thrombosis in an infant treated with extracorporeal membrane oxygenation

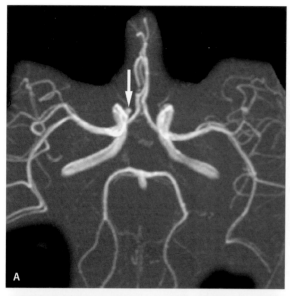

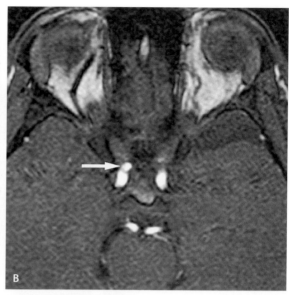

Figure 8.23

Berry aneurysm

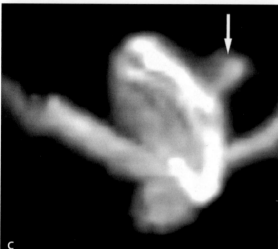

Intracranial Aneurysm

Berry Aneurysm

Clinical Presentation

A 16-year-old male presents with tingling of left side of the body, extremities and headaches. Symptoms were considered to be consistent with complex migraine and the aneurysm is an incidental finding.

Images (Fig. 8.23)

A. MR arteriogram (3D TOF) shows a round outpouching involving the junction of right internal carotid artery and right ophthalmic artery (*arrow*). It measures approximately 4 mm in diameter. The diagnosis was confirmed with conventional catheter angiography

B. Source image demonstrates the aneurysm more clearly (*arrow*)

C. Magnified image of MR arteriogram demonstrating the aneurysm (*arrow*)

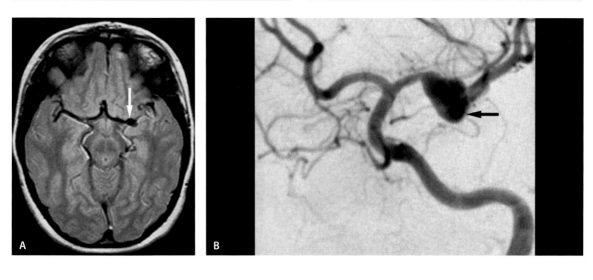

Figure 8.24
Fusiform aneurysm

Fusiform Aneurysm

Clinical Presentation

A 9-year-old female with headaches.

Images (Fig. 8.24)

A. Proton density image shows a fusiform dilatation of the left middle cerebral artery (*arrow*)
B. Cerebral angiography confirmed the presence of fusiform ectasia of the left middle cerebral artery

Berry Aneurysm with Significant Vasospasm

Clinical Presentation

A 22-month-old comatose male presents with sub-arachnoid bleed on CT scan.

Images (Fig. 8.25)

A. T1-weighted image shows high intensity blood in the suprasellar cistern and in the left frontal lobe (*arrows*)
B. T2-weighted image shows a round decreased signal intensity area corresponding to the distal internal carotid artery (*arrow*). Hyperintense blood is seen in the subarachnoid space along both middle cerebral arteries (*arrowheads*) and in the left frontal lobe parenchyma
C. DW image shows hyperintensity in the left frontal lobe and along the left middle cerebral artery. A round decreased signal is seen at the assumed tip in the left internal carotid artery (*arrow*)
D. ADC map shows hypointense lesion in the left frontal lobe adjacent the Sylvian fissure and anteriorly (*arrow*). These areas are consistent with restricted diffusion secondary to vasospasm
E. Echoplanar T2-weighted (b_0) image from the DW image shows also round decreased signal at the distal internal carotid artery (*arrow*) where surgery confirmed the presence of an aneurysm that was successfully clipped
F. An axial collapsed image from a MR angiogram demonstrates poor flow in the left internal carotid artery (*arrow*) and left middle cerebral artery (*arrowheads*)
G. Coronal MIP of the MR angiogram reveals significant vasospasm and tapering appearance of the left internal carotid artery (*arrow*), later confirmed on two conventional catheter angiograms
H. Axial postcontrast T1-weighted image suggests a curvilinear enhancement (*arrow*), suggestive of aneurysm wall enhancement. An 8-mm aneurysm was later clipped in this location

Discussion

Intracranial aneurysms are rare in childhood, occurring at a frequency of approximately 0.5–4.6% with a slight male preponderance. Less than 1% of all aneurysms are found in children below 15 years of age, a low prevalence contributing to common delays in diagnosis. Although childhood aneurysms are found in the same locations as in adults, posterior circulation aneurysms are more common in children. Approximately 3–45% are giant aneurysms with an average size of 17 mm. Approximately 75–80% of childhood cerebral aneurysms are congenital, 15–20% are traumatic, and 5–10% are mycotic. Traumatic aneurysms develop from shearing injuries in the cavernous carotid artery, in pericallosal artery adjacent to the falx, or distally in superficial vessels damaged by penetrating injuries. Mycotic aneurysms are usually secondary to septic emboli originating in the heart, or to the hematogenous spread of infection; they are typically multiple and found in peripheral vessels, often deep in the brain parenchyma. Spontaneous fusiform middle cerebral artery aneurysms are mainly seen in adults. Dissection is proposed as the underlying cause of these lesions. Subarachnoid hemorrhage is the commonest clinical presentation, although cranial nerve symptoms are also common, especially in aneurysms at the cavernous sinus.

CT is the first line investigation in diagnostic workup, especially in patients with acute symptoms. MR arteriogram and CT angiogram being noninvasive are good tools for detailed anatomic evaluation of vessels. However, sometimes, severe spasm may not be able to show the lesion. In those cases delayed contrast-enhanced T1-weighted images are important to outline the aneurysmal wall and confirm the diagnosis. Conventional angiography is still the gold standard in aneurysm work-up.

Suggested Reading

Day AL, Gaposchkin CG, Yu CJ, Rivet DJ, Dacey RG Jr (2003) Spontaneous fusiform middle cerebral artery aneurysms: characteristics and a proposed mechanism of formation. J Neurosurg 99:228–240

Sungarian A, Rogg J, Duncan JA III (2003) Pediatric intracranial aneurysm: a diagnostic dilemma solved with contrast-enhanced MR imaging. AJNR Am J Neuroradiol 24:370–372

Wojtacha M, Bazowski P, Mandera M, Krawczyk I, Rudnik A (2001) Cerebral aneurysms in childhood. Childs Nerv Syst 17:37–41

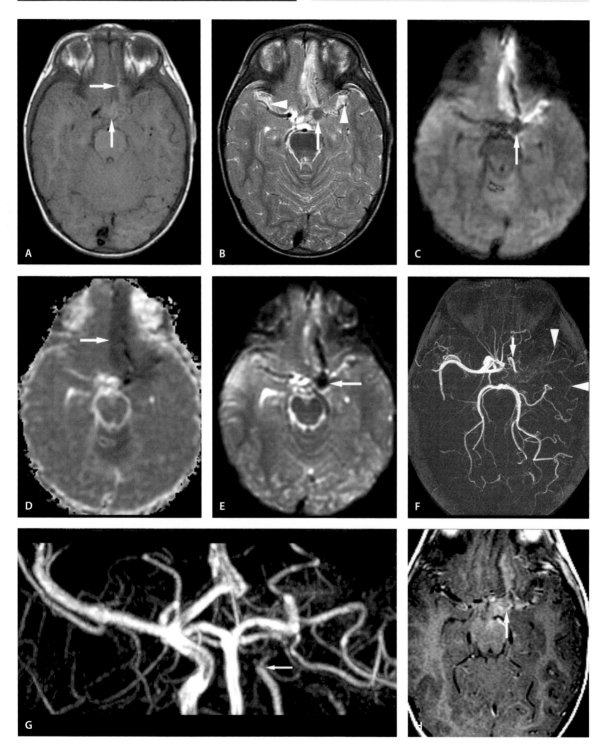

Figure 8.25

Berry aneurysm with significant vasospasm

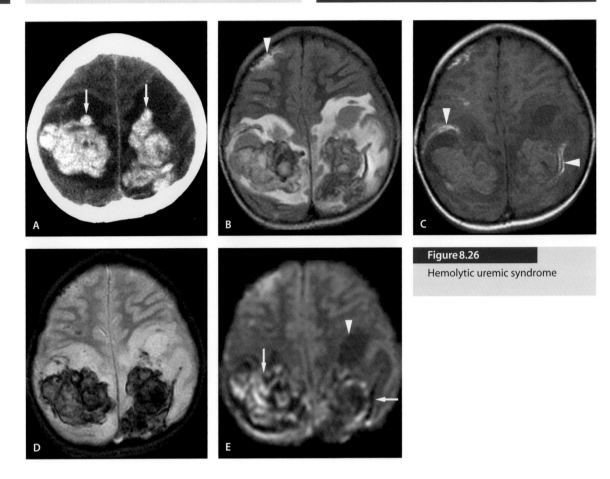

Figure 8.26

Hemolytic uremic syndrome

Hemolytic Uremic Syndrome (HUS)

Clinical Presentation

A 5-year-old girl with pneumococcal sepsis, hypertension and hemolytic uremic syndrome. She presented with acute onset of headaches, nausea and vomiting.

Images (Fig. 8.26)

A. Noncontrast CT scan demonstrates bilateral intraparenchymal hemorrhages (*arrows*) in both centrum semiovale areas with surrounding low density edema
B. FLAIR image reveals the large bilateral parenchymal hemorrhages to have mainly low signal with hyperintense surrounding edema. An additional small right frontal hemorrhagic focus is seen in this image (*arrowhead*)

C. On the T1-weighted image the hematomas are near isointense to the gray matter with peripheral hyperintensity (*arrowheads*) corresponding to methemoglobin formation in early subacute intracerebral hematoma
D. Gradient echo image defines better the parenchymal blood products
E. DW image shows mixed signal in the hematoma (*arrows*) with low signal in the vasogenic edema (*arrowheads*)

Discussion

Hemolytic uremic syndrome (HUS) is caused most commonly by O-157 *E. coli* enteritis, but diarrhea-negative HUS has been associated with other infections such as *Streptococcus pneumoniae* and noninfectious conditions, such as that associated with tacrolimus. Pneumococcus-induced HUS carries an increased risk of mortality and renal morbidity compared with *E. coli*-induced HUS. HUS is a general microangiopathic disorder, which potentially causes fatal CNS complications in infants and children. Neurological manifestations occur in early and acute stages of the disease. Clinical symptomatology includes altered level of consciousness, focal or generalized seizures, cortical blindness, hemiplegia, and hemorrhage.

Radiologically, a heterogeneous spectrum of CNS lesions is seen in HUS, including petechial and parenchymal hemorrhages, hemorrhagic and/or nonhemorrhagic infarctions, spongiosis and gliosis, and cerebral edema. CT may show cortical infarction with hemorrhage, extensive BBB disturbance in the gray-white matter interface, and diffuse cerebral edema. In the acute stage, T1-weighted images show low signal intensity lesions and T2-weighted images demonstrate diffuse high-signal foci in cerebral white matter. Basal ganglia involvement is common. Many of these lesions are partially reversible if treated well in time.

Suggested Reading

Ogura H, Takaoka M, Kishi M, Kimoto M, et al (1998) Reversible MR findings of hemolytic uremic syndrome with mild encephalopathy. AJNR Am J Neuroradiol 19:1144–1145

Signorini E, Lucchi S, Mastrangelo M, Rapuzzi S, Edefonti A, Fossali E (2000) Central nervous system involvement in a child with hemolytic uremic syndrome. Pediatr Nephrol 14:990–992

Taylor CM, Chua C, Howie AJ, Risdon RA (2004) Clinico-pathological findings in diarrhoea-negative haemolytic uraemic syndrome. Pediatr Nephrol 19:419–425

Theobald I, Kuwertz-Broking E, Schiborr M, Heindel W (2001) Central nervous system involvement in hemolytic uremic syndrome (HUS) – a retrospective analysis of cerebral CT and MRI studies. Clin Nephrol 56:S3–S8

Intracerebral Hematoma

Clinical Presentation

A 1-day-old full-term female with hydrocephalus and intracerebral bleed.

Images (Fig. 8.27)

A. Noncontrast CT scan shows dilated lateral and third ventricles. A slightly hyperdense hematoma with peripheral lower density is present in the region of the germinal matrix (*arrow*). A large porencephalic cyst is present on the right

B. T2-weighted image shows ventricular enlargement and right hyperintense germinal matrix hematoma (*arrow*) with central darker signal intensity

C. FLAIR image better shows the extent of the intraventricular bleed. Note that the CSF in the ventricles is not dark. There is blood level in the left occipital horn (*arrowhead*). The periphery of the hematoma is bright with a darker central area

D. Contrast-enhanced T1-FLAIR image demonstrates ependymal enhancement (*arrowheads*). The center of the hematoma is darker and isointense to the brain

E. The ependymal enhancement is best appreciated in the coronal SPGR image. The central dark area of the hematoma corresponds to the CT hyperdensity

F. The hematoma is hyperintense in the DW image. This is usually seen in late subacute hematomas

Discussion

Intracranial hemorrhage among full-term infants is a rare event. A number of etiological factors have been proposed such as vascular malformations (AVM, cavernous angiomas and aneurysms), impairment in coagulation, hypoxic-ischemic injury, septicemia, and birth-related trauma. The symptoms include seizure, impaired consciousness, focal neurological deficits, headache and vomiting. Onset of symptoms may be acute or subacute. The predominant location of spontaneous hemorrhage in the full-term infant is cerebral, followed by intraventricular, subarachnoid, and infratentorial. Subdural hemorrhage is commonly seen in birth-related injuries.

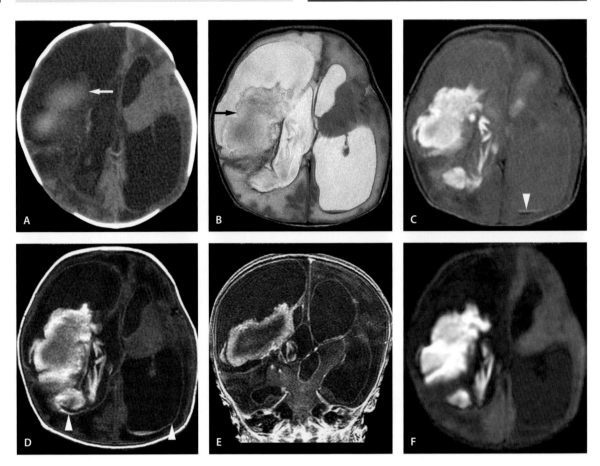

Figure 8.27

Intracerebral hematoma

CT image accurately depicts acute neonatal hemorrhage. On MR imaging, the intensities of hemorrhagic lesions are variable depending upon the age of the hematoma, oxygenation stage of the hemoglobin, status of red cell membranes, hematocrit, proteins and clot formation. The environment also contributes to the signal intensity. On long repetition time and long echo time (long TR/TE, T2-weighted image) images at 1.5 T, the acute hematoma is usually hypointense, whereas in the hyperacute hematoma only a thin hypointense rim is seen. It is mandatory to perform MR arteriogram in cases of large hematoma for suspected underlying vascular malformations.

Suggested Reading

Atlas SW, DuBois P, Singer MB, Lu D (2000) Diffusion measurements in intracranial hematomas: implications for MR imaging of acute stroke. AJNR Am J Neuroradiol 21:1190–1194

Fenichel GM, Webster DL, Wong WK (1984) Intracranial hemorrhage in the term newborn. Arch Neurol 41:30–34

Jhawar BS, Ranger A, Steven D, del Maestro RF (2003) Risk factors for intracranial hemorrhage among full-term infants: a case-control study. Neurosurgery 52:581–590

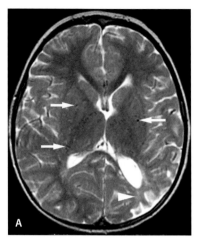 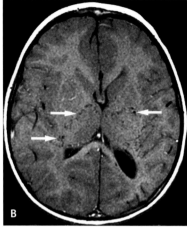 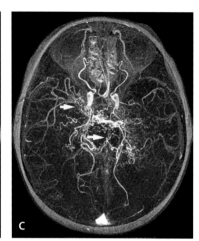

Figure 8.28

Bilateral moyamoya disease

Moyamoya Disease

Bilateral Moyamoya Disease

Clinical Presentation

A 3-year-old with left-side motor seizures and forget-fulness.

Images (Fig. 8.28)

A. T2-weighted image shows multiple flow voids in both basal ganglia consistent with enlarged lenticulostriate vessels (*arrows*). Focal cortical atrophy is seen in the left watershed between the middle cerebral artery and posterior cerebral artery (*arrowhead*). This is consistent with an old infarct

B. T1-weighted image shows better the multiple basal ganglia flow voids consistent with enlarged collateral vessels (*arrows*)

C. A collapsed maximum intensity projection image from MR arteriogram demonstrates narrowing of the supraclinoid carotid arteries bilaterally with poor visualization of the M1 and A1 segments of the middle cerebral artery and anterior cerebral artery. There is prominent collateral circulation in the skull base (*arrows*) at the region of the posterior communicating arteries and thalamoperforating arteries, and along the assumed course of the proximal M1 of middle cerebral artery.

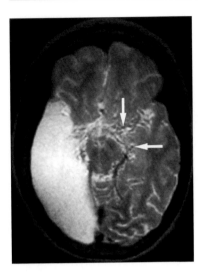

Bilateral Moyamoya Disease with a Major Infarct

Clinical Presentation

An 11-year-old female with left hemiparesis and worsening of seizures. Arteriogram in an outside hospital confirmed the diagnosis of moyamoya.

Images (Fig. 8.29)

A. T2-weighted image shows right hemiatrophy and a large middle cerebral artery infarct. Multiple irregular flow voids are seen at the circle of Willis (*arrows*) consistent with collateral circulation without a well-defined M1 trunk. She has been neurologically stable for the past 6 years

Unilateral Moyamoya (Variant)

Clinical Presentation

Progressive left hemiparesis in a 4-month-old male with NF-1.

Images (Fig. 8.30)

A. MR arteriogram (3D TOF) shows decreased flow-related enhancement in the right internal carotid artery and M1 of the middle cerebral artery and A2. A1 is not visible (*arrowhead*). There are collateral vessels at the skull base in the region of lenticulostriate arteries (*arrows*) corresponding to the angiographically seen vascular blush ("moyamoya")

B. Conventional catheter angiography confirms the MR arteriogram findings. Note the anterior cerebral artery filling through collateral circulation. The fine collateral network in the basal ganglia shows a vascular blush ("moyamoya") (*arrow*)

Sickle cell Disease Leading to Moyamoya Disease

Clinical Presentation

A 13-year-old male with sickle cell disease presents with seizures.

Images (Fig. 8.31)

A. T2-weighted image shows right hemiatrophy, an old cortical infarct and thickened calvaria. There are multiple small "flow voids" in the splenium of the corpus callosum (*arrow*) representing collateral vessels. Collaterals are also seen in the right thalamus and subependymal area (*arrowheads*)

B. A collapsed maximum intensity projection of (3D TOF, video reversed image) MR angiogram demonstrates a nonvisualized right internal carotid artery with prominent collateral vessels in the region of the right thalamoperforating arteries, left posterior communicating arteries and splenium of the corpus callosum. There is poor visualization of A1 segments bilaterally

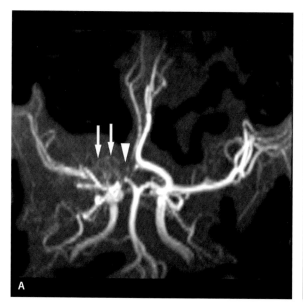

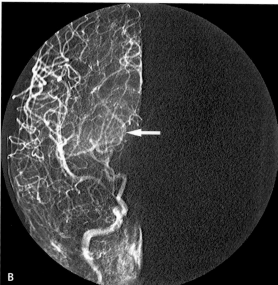

Figure 8.30

Unilateral moyamoya (variant)

Figure 8.31

Sickle cell disease leading to moyamoya disease

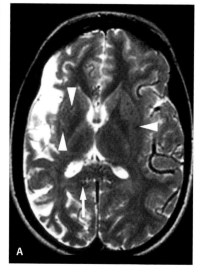

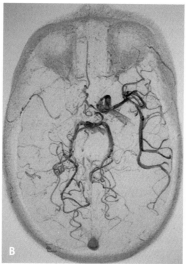

Discussion

Primary moyamoya disease (synonym: progressive
occlusive cerebrovascular disease) is an idiopathic
slowly progressive, bilateral occlusion of the supraclinoid portion of internal carotid arteries. Since the occlusion is slowly progressive, multiple anastomoses
develop between the internal and external carotid arteries. A vascular network is formed at the base of the
brain composed of collaterals from the anterior or
posterior choroidal arteries, the basilar artery and
the meningeal arteries giving the angiographic ap-

pearance of "puff of smoke". They may also arise from the thalamoperforating arteries and lenticulostriate arteries. Moyamoya disease has a bimodal peak. A peak in children is associated with ischemic cortical infarcts whereas a peak in adults is associated with deep white matter infarcts and hemorrhagic strokes. The ischemic strokes are repetitive and affect both the cerebral cortex, often in watershed areas, and deeper structures.

CT imaging demonstrates multiple ischemic infarcts in more than 80% of cases with abnormal enhancement. Cerebral atrophy may be seen in 50–60% of cases. MR imaging is more sensitive than CT imaging, particularly with the use of diffusion and perfusion MR imaging which allow the identification of early ischemic areas for the diagnosis of infarcts. MR arteriogram shows gradual narrowing of the supraclinoid and cavernous portions of the internal carotid artery with numerous enlarged lenticulostriate and thalamoperforating arteries, as well as dural, leptomeningeal, and pial collateral vessels simulating "puff of smoke". The term "moyamoya" (secondary moyamoya) is also used more widely: any process leading to reduced blood flow (such as sickle cell disease, NF-1, and radiation vasculopathy) may result in the development of fine collateral vascular channels, moyamoya.

Suggested Reading

Akgun D, Yilmaz S, Senbil N, Aslan B, Gurer YY (2000) Moyamoya syndrome with protein S deficiency. Eur J Paediatr 4:185–188

Cramer SC, Robertson RL, Dooling EC, Scott RM (1996) Moyamoya and Down syndrome. Clinical and radiological features. Stroke 27:2131–2135

Robertson RL, Burrows PE, Barnes PD, Robson CD, Poussaint TY, Scott RM (1997) Angiographic changes after pial synangiosis in childhood moyamoya disease. AJNR Am J Neuroradiol 18:837–845

Vein of Galen Malformation

Clinical Presentation

A 15-month-old male with cardiomegaly.

Images (Fig. 8.32)

A. T2-weighted image shows a rounded, strikingly hypointense mass in the region of the vein of Galen (*arrow*). There is mild dilatation of the lateral ventricles
B. Proton density-weighted image better appreciates the hypointensity of the lesion
C. Sagittal T1-weighted image through the midline demonstrates the aneurysmal dilatation of the vein of Markowski (*arrow*). This patient has also suprasellar arachnoid cyst
D. Sagittal paramedian image shows the dilated vein leading to the dilated vein of Markowski (*arrow*)
E. MR arteriogram (video reversed image) demonstrates dilated feeding arteries and enlarged persistent embryonic median prosencephalic vein of Markowski (*arrow*). This is not a true vein of Galen. There is a persistent median vein that drains into the sagittal sinus via the falcine vein

Discussion

Vein of Galen malformations (synonym: vein of Galen "aneurysm") are rare congenital vascular malformations characterized by shunting of the arterial flow into an enlarged cerebral vein dorsal to the tectum. Although vein of Galen malformations constitute only 1% of all cerebral vascular malformations, they comprise up to 30% of all pediatric vascular malformations. Vein of Galen malformations develop between the 6th and the 11th week of gestation, after the development of the circle of Willis before the true vein of Galen develops. There is an arteriovenous connection between primitive choroidal vessels and embryonic median prosencephalic vein of Markowski. A persistent median vein drains into the sagittal sinus via the falcine vein. Other venous anomalies such as anomalous dural sinuses and sinus stenosis are commonly present in association with vein of Galen malformations. Most of these malformations present in early childhood, often causing congestive heart failure in the neonate.

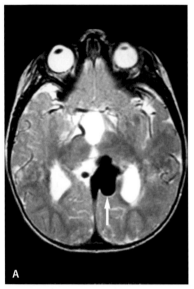

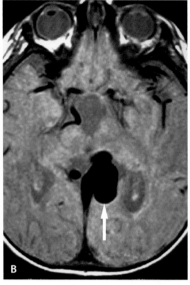

Figure 8.32

Vein of Galen malformation

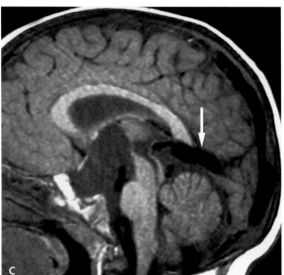

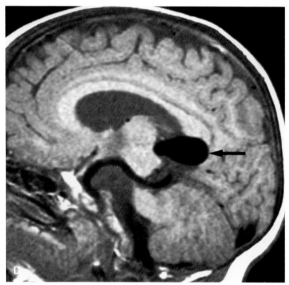

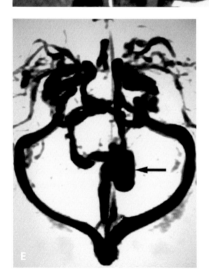

Antenatal ultrasound and color Doppler can make the diagnosis of vein of Galen malformation. MR imaging is the modality of choice since it can show the malformation in three dimensions and depict the exact anatomy of the dilated channels and thrombosis if any. MR arteriogram with 2D-TOF may be a useful additional technique for evaluating fetal vein of Galen malformations. MR imaging also helps in evaluating any associated parenchymal damage and thrombosis to a better extent. MR angiography demonstrates the major vessels of supply, tortuosity of accessible arteries, and venous anatomy.

Embolization of the feeding arteries is the preferred therapeutic modality for a patient with severe cardiac failure. MR imaging is mandatory before endoarterial treatment, to assess brain parenchyma. Angiography is performed only at the time of endovascular treatment, while MR arteriogram and MR imaging have a role in follow-up examination.

Suggested Reading

Bhattacharya JJ, Thammaroj J (2003) Vein of Galen malformations. J Neurol Neurosurg Psychiatry 74 [Suppl 1]:42–44

Jones BV, Ball WS, Tomsick TA, Millard J, Crone KR (2002) Vein of Galen aneurysmal malformation: diagnosis and treatment of 13 children with extended clinical follow-up. AJNR Am J Neuroradiol 23:1717–1724

Raybaud CA, Strother CM, Hald JK (1989) Aneurysms of the vein of Galen: embryonic considerations and anatomical features relating to the pathogenesis of the malformation. Neuroradiology 31:109–128

Konno S, Numaguchi Y, Shrier DA, Qian J, Sinkin RA (1996) Unusual manifestation of a vein of Galen malformation: value of CT angiography. AJNR Am J Neuroradiol 17:1423–1426

Head and Neck

Introduction

This book is primarily a book on MR imaging of the pediatric central nervous system including the spine. However, going through neuroradiology cases, we stumbled on a number of unusual and interesting head and neck cases and decided to include a short chapter on MR imaging of the pediatric head and neck.

The chapter contains congenital malformation, developmental anomalies, and unusual inflammatory neoplastic disease in the pediatric head and neck area. This chapter does not have the ambition of being a complete head and neck chapter, but rather a chapter on miscellaneous conditions that can be well imaged with contemporary techniques. CT is the primary cross-sectional imaging technique for the pediatric head and neck but with newer development and rapid sequences MR imaging will be more and more useful. The lack of radiation is a significant advantage in this group of patients. Degenerative, inflammatory, neoplastic and congenital abnormalities are presented in this chapter

Multinodular Goiter

Clinical Presentation

An 18-year-old presenting with hyperthyroidism.

Images (Fig. 9.1)

A. Coronal T1-weighted image shows marked enlargement of the left and right thyroid glands with narrowing of the trachea
B. Axial T2-weighted image with fat suppression shows a multilobulated enlargement of the entire thyroid gland with narrowing of the trachea
C. Coronal T1-weighted image with contrast shows enlargement of the thyroid gland without abnormal enhancement

Discussion

Goiter is a clinical diagnosis that implies an enlargement of the thyroid gland. Goiter develops because the thyroid gland compensates for inadequate thyroid hormone output. In goiter the thyroid tissue hypertrophies to achieve an euthyroid state. Often the regulation is not optimal and the patient may show either hypothyroidism or hyperthyroidism. Multinodular goiter can also be evaluated with nuclear scintigraphy and ultrasound. CT and MR imaging are useful in evaluating secondary manifestations of goiter such as compression and displacement of trachea, esophagus and adjacent vessels. It is often important to determine the substernal and mediastinal extension which is best seen on CT or MR images.

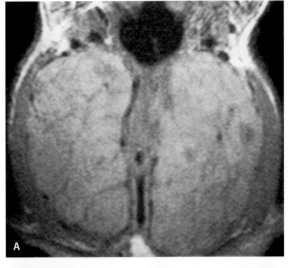

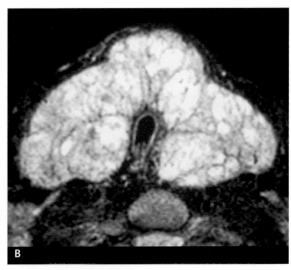

Figure 9.1

Multinodular goiter

Suggested Reading

Dworkin HJ, Meier DA, Kaplan M (1995) Advances in the management of patients with thyroid disease. Semin Nucl Med 25:205–220

Huysmans DA, Hermus AR, Corstens FH, et al (1994) Large, compressive goiters treated with radioiodine. Ann Intern Med 121:757–762

Noma S, Kanaoka M, Minami S, et al (1988) Thyroid masses: MR imaging and pathologic correlation. Radiology 168:759–764

Thyroglossal Duct Cyst

Clinical Presentation

A 3-year-old female presents with a mass at the base of the tongue.

Images (Fig. 9.2)

A. Sagittal T2-weighted image shows a cystic lesion at the base of the tongue. It has high signal intensity on the T2-weighted images and is located in the region of foramen sacrum
B. Axial T2 fat-suppressed image shows a high signal in the lesion at the base of the tongue
C. Contrast-enhanced axial image demonstrates no enhancement in the lesion
D. Coronal contrast-enhanced image confirms the location of the nonenhancing lesion to the base of the tongue

Discussion

The developing thyroid gland is initially connected to the tongue by a narrow tube called the thyroglossal duct. This duct extends from the junction between the anterior two-thirds and the posterior one-third of the tongue down to the hyoid bone and further to the thyroid bed. In a normal situation the thyroglossal duct begins to degenerate and eventually atrophy between the fifth and sixth fetal weeks. The foramen sacrum at the tongue is the normal remnant of this duct. Thyroglossal duct cyst is the most common congenital neck mass and accounts for nearly 90% nonodontogenic congenital cysts.

It is usually located in the midline and can occur anywhere along the path of the thyroglossal duct. On MR imaging the T1-weighted signal intensity can vary from low to high while the T2-weighted images in general are high signal intensity. The variation in signal intensity reflects the variable protein content of the cyst. Treatment is surgical. It is important to remove not only the cyst but the sinus tract as well to avoid recurrence. The general operation for thyroglossal duct cyst is called the Sistrunk procedure. By this procedure the body of the hyoid bone is removed with the thyroglossal duct and its cyst. This procedure has reduced the recurrence rate from nearly 50% to less than 4%.

The symptoms for thyroglossal duct cyst are often related to infections, but others present with dysphagia or a palpable mass.

Suggested Reading

Blandino A, Salvi L, Scribano E, Chirico G, Longo M, Pandolfo I (1990) MR findings in thyroglossal duct cysts: report of two cases. Eur J Radiol 11:207–211

Pound L (1981) Neck masses of congenital origin. Pediatr Clin North Am 28:841–844

Ward G, Hendrick J, Chamber R (1949) Thyroglossal tract abnormalities, cysts, and fistula. Surg Gynecol Obstet 89:727–734

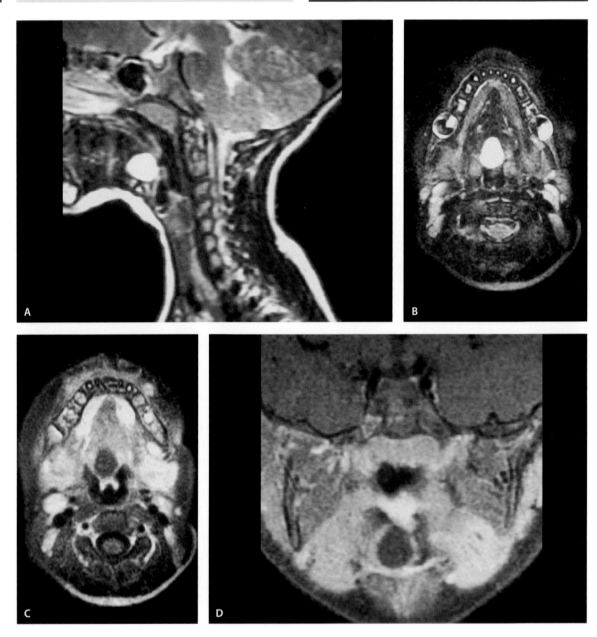

Figure 9.2

Thyroglossal duct cyst

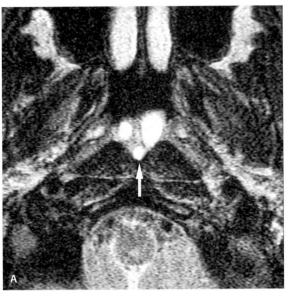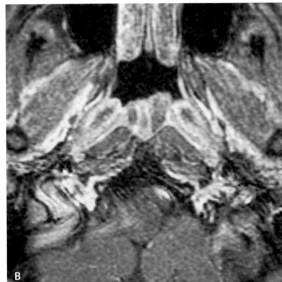

Tornwaldt Cyst

Clinical Presentation

An 18-year-old presenting with the incidental finding of a Tornwaldt cyst.

Images (Fig. 9.3)

A. T2-weighted axial image with fat suppression demonstrates three cysts in the posterior nasopharynx (*arrow*). This is high signal on T2-weighted images
B. Contrast-enhanced image demonstrates no enhancement and low signal in the center of the cyst. FLAIR image demonstrate the high signal on the cyst in the posterior nasopharynx

Discussion

Tornwaldt cyst occurs when the pharyngeal bursa ectoderm retracts with the notochord into the clivus. Thus this is a developmental cyst. It is seen in approximately 3% of healthy adults and most of the time is asymptomatic. Occasionally a patient may complain of occipital pain, purulent nasal drainage, ear fullness or odynophagia. A cyst that gets infected causes symptoms that are consistent with infection. The infection can spread inferiorly towards the mediastinum. They are often bright on T2-weighted images, presumably due to high protein content. There is usually no need for treatment. The cyst is named after Gustav Ludwig Tornwaldt (1843–1910).

Suggested Reading

Miyahara H, Matsunaga T (1994) Tornwaldt's disease. Acta Otolaryngol [Suppl] 517:36–39
Mukherji SK (2003) Pharynx. In: Som PM, Curtin DH (eds) Head and neck imaging, 4th edn. Mosby, St Louis, pp 1507–1509
Yousem DM (1998) Case review: head and neck imaging. Mosby, St Louis

Cystic Hygroma in Neck of Newborn

Clinical Presentation

A 3-week-old male presents with apnea and cyanosis. On palpation there was a soft subtle mass in the left neck. This was vaguely visible on inspection.

Images (Fig. 9.4)

A. Sagittal T2-weighted image shows a 5 cm high signal intensity multiloculated mass (*arrow*) in the anterior neck extending from the mandible to almost the thoracic inlet
B. Coronal contrast-enhanced T1-weighted image shows no enhancement but high proteinaceous content of the mass lesion with a fluid-fluid level (*arrow*)
C. Axial contrast-enhanced T1-weighted image with fat suppression demonstrates again no enhancement but high signal intensity fluid with a fluid-fluid level (*arrow*)
D. Axial T2-weighted image with fat suppression shows a lesion with high signal in the anterior neck displacing the normal structures. There are multiple fluid levels with low signal indicating blood products

Discussion

Cystic hygroma is the most common form of lymphangioma. It consists of dilated cystic lymphatic spaces. The most common location is in the neck. Cystic hygromas are often isolated with the remainder of the lymphatic system being normal. The differential diagnosis of a large neck mass in a newborn includes lymphangioma, teratoma and epidermoid. An isolated cystic hygroma may develop when one of several potential lymphatic venous anastomoses fail to form. An isolated cystic hygroma can also form if an aberrant bud loses its connection to the primordial lymphatic sac from which it arose.

On imaging cystic hygromas are typically multiloculated masses in the neck. The cyst wall is rarely seen unless the lesion has been infected. Typically the T1 is low and T2 signal intensity is high. If hemorrhage has occurred fluid levels are best seen on MR imaging and a fluid level is characteristic of a cystic hygroma.

Lymphangiomas can be subclassified histologically into cystic hygroma or lymphangioma, cavernous lymphangioma, capillary or simple lymphangioma and vasculolymphatic malformation or lymphangiohemangioma. It is often best to consider these four types as a spectrum of manifestations of the same pathological process. Each case often has combinations and they are often separated by the size of the lymphatic spaces. Pathologically they are very similar since all of them are composed of endothelium-lined lymphatic channels that are separated by connected tissue stroma.

Suggested Reading

Anderson NG. Kennedy JC (1992) Prognosis in fetal cystic hygroma. Aust N Z J Obstet Gynaecol 32:36–39

Gallagher PG, Mahoney MJ, Gosche JR (1999) Cystic hygroma in the fetus and newborn. Semin Perinatol 23:341–356

Koeller KK, Alamo L, Adair CF, Smirniotopoulos JG (1999) Congenital cystic masses of the neck: radiologic-pathologic correlation. Radiographics 19:121–146; quiz 152–153

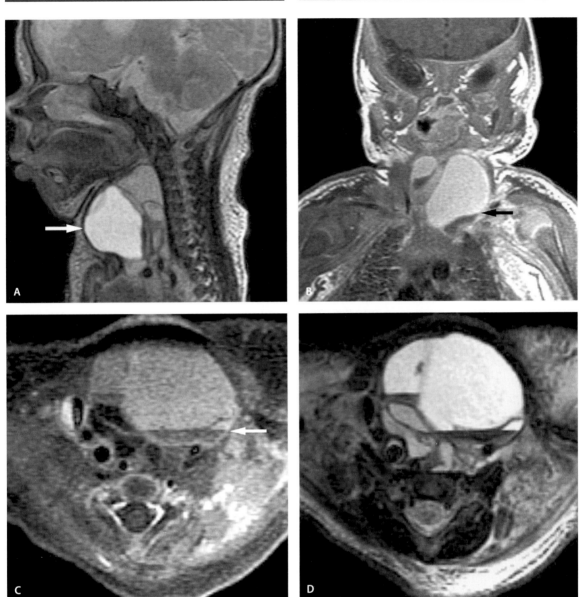

Cystic hygroma in neck of newborn

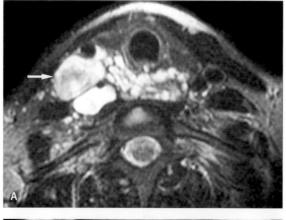

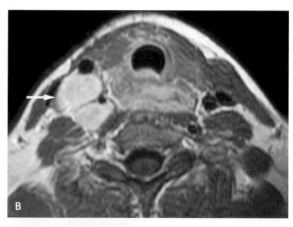

Figure 9.5

Plexiform neurofibromatosis of the neck

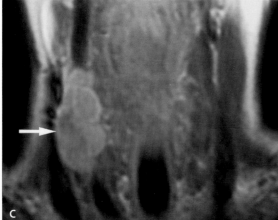

Neurofibromatosis

Plexiform Neurofibromatosis of the Neck

Clinical Presentation

A 9-year-old female presents with a painless swelling of the right lower neck.

Images (Fig. 9.5)

A. Axial T2-weighted image with fat suppression shows a multilobulated complex mass in the right lower neck extending across the midline (*arrow*). It is separating the common carotid artery and the jugular vein and abutting the spine posteriorly
B. Axial postcontrast T1-weighted image shows the enhancing mass separating the carotid and the jugular on the right (*arrow*)
C. Coronal contrast-enhanced T1 weighted image shows the multilobulated mass in the carotid sheath on the right (*arrow*)

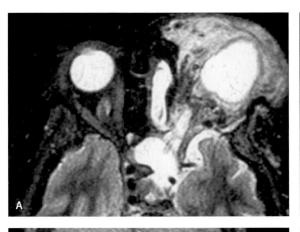

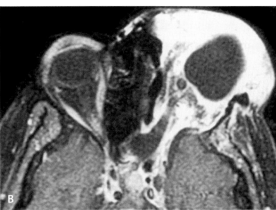

Figure 9.6

Neurofibromatosis of the orbit

Neurofibromatosis of the Orbit

Clinical Presentation

A 30-year-old presenting with a large periorbital mass on the left.

Images (Fig. 9.6)

A. Axial T2-weighted image shows a large expansible mass in the left orbit deforming the globe and extending into the retro-orbital area. There are large flow voids in this highly vascular mass
B. Contrast-enhanced T1-weighted fat-suppressed image demonstrates marked enhancement of the periorbital mass with compression and deformation of the globe
C. Coronal contrast-enhanced T1-weighted fat-suppressed image demonstrates the mass expanding the orbit and deforming the globe

Discussion

Neurofibromas and schwannomas are the most common nerve sheath tumors of the peripheral nerves in the head and neck. There are three types of neurofibromas, namely: localized, diffuse and plexiform. The vast majority of these lesions are localized and may not have association with NF1. Plexiform neurofibromas are associated with NF1. These lesions usually occur in early childhood. Plexiform neurofibromas involve a long nerve segment and its branches and tortuous expansion giving the appearance of a "bag of worms". Malignant transformation may be seen in 4% of cases.

On noncontrast-enhanced CT images, they are seen as large multilobulated masses of low attenuation related to the fat content of myelin from Schwann cells, water content of myxoid tissue, cystic areas of hemorrhage and necrosis. On T1-weighted images, plexiform neurofibromas show signal intensity similar to that of muscle. On T2-weighted images, the lesions may show the "target sign". This sign consists of low-to-intermediate signal intensity centrally, with a ring of high signal intensity peripherally. This may be due to a high collagen content located centrally and more myxoid tissue at the periphery. Contrast enhancement is variable. Irregular nodular enhancement with central necrosis is typical of malignant peripheral nerve sheath tumors.

Suggested Reading

Chung CJ, Armfield KB, Mukherji SK, Fordham LA, Krause WL (1999) Cervical neurofibromas in children with NF-1. Pediatr Radiol 29:353–356

Visrutaratna P, Oranratanachai K, Singhavejsakul J (2004) Clinics in diagnostic imaging (96). Plexiform neurofibromatosis. Singapore Med J 45:188–192

Weber AL, Montandon C, Robson CD (2000) Neurogenic tumors of the neck. Radiol Clin North Am 38:1077–1090

Kikuchi Disease

Clinical Presentation

An 18-year-old with renal failure and lupus presents with neck pain and swelling.

Images (Fig. 9.7)

A. Axial T2-weighted image shows bilateral cervical lymphadenopathy in the posterior triangles (*arrows*). There is also a large retropharyngeal/prevertebral fluid collection
B. Axial T1-weighted image after contrast and with fat suppression shows the bilateral cervical lymphadenopathy. The retropharyngeal/prevertebral fluid collection is not enhancing and there is no ring enhancement to suggest an abscess
C. Axial DW image shows the bilateral cervical lymphadenopathy with high signal intensity. The retropharyngeal/prevertebral fluid collection also has high signal intensity
D. Axial ADC map confirms restricted diffusion in the posterior lymphadenopathy bilaterally. The retropharyngeal/prevertebral fluid collection is not decreased and therefore does not have true restricted diffusion

Discussion

Kikuchi disease, also referred as Kikuchi-Fujimoto lymphadenopathy (KFL) or histiocytic necrotizing lymphadenitis, is a self-limiting benign lymphadenopathy with unknown etiology that predominantly affects young females. The cervical lymph nodes are usually involved, more commonly unilaterally, and may be associated with tenderness, fever, skin rashes, weight loss, chills, and sometimes splenomegaly.

Figure 9.7

Kikuchi disease

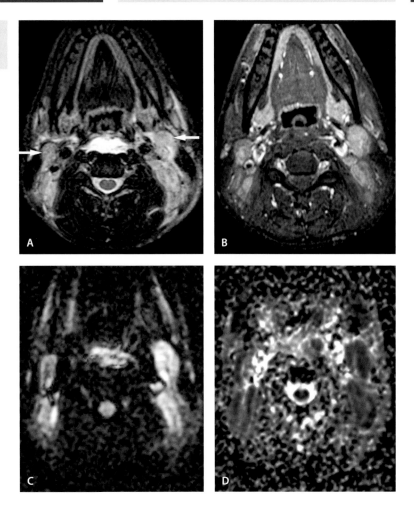

The CT imaging appearance of Kikuchi disease may be variable, mimicking various nodal diseases, such as lymphoma, metastasis, tuberculosis, and especially in children, Still's disease. However, the necrotic areas of the nodes emit relatively lower signal than the non-necrotic portion on T2-weighted MR images, different from the usual bright signal intensity of nodal necrosis seen in other nodal diseases. The speculated reason for this is restricted mobile protons within high protein content in fibrinoid material of necrotic focus. The high signal on DW images and the corresponding low signal on ADC images in the present case further support this.

Suggested Reading

Bennie MJ, Bowles KM, Rankin SC (2003) Necrotizing cervical lymphadenopathy caused by Kikuchi-Fujimoto disease. Br J Radiol 76:656–658

Lerosey Y, Lecler-Scarcella V, Francois A, Guitrancourt JA (1998) A pseudo-tumoral form of Kikuchi's disease in children: a case report and review of the literature. Int J Pediatr Otorhinolaryngol 45:1–6

Na DG, Chung TS, Byun HS, Kim HD, Ko YH, Yoon JH (1997) Kikuchi disease: CT and MR findings. AJNR Am J Neuroradiol 18:1729–1732

Dermoid

Clinical Presentation

An 18-year-old male presents with a doughy swelling of the floor of the mouth clinically resembling a thyroglossal duct cyst.

Images (Fig. 9.8)

A. Axial noncontrast T1-weighted image shows a well-circumscribed 5-cm oval lesion in the center of the floor of the mouth (*arrow*)
B. The lesion is intermediate to high signal on T2-weighted image (*arrow*)
C. On coronal T2-weighted image the lesion is high signal and is located in the sublingual space, depressing the mylohyoid muscles
D. Axial post-contrast T1-weighted image shows no enhancement
E. Coronal post-contrast fat-suppressed image confirms the lack of enhancement and the location to the sublingual space

Discussion

Dermoid cysts are the least common of the congenital neck lesions and account for about 7% of all cysts in the neck. The cystic lesions are classified as epidermoid, dermoid and teratoid. Dermoid cysts are commonly used in reference to all three types of lesions without regard to the differentiating histological types. Histologically it is important to distinguish between epidermoid and dermoid/teratoid cysts because the dermoid/teratoid has a malignant potential which the epidermoid does not.

It has been theorized that epithelial rests become enclaved during midline closure of the first and second branchial arteries. The dermoids are frequently located in the floor of the mouth (sublingual, submental or submandibular regions). They can also occur in other locations such as the tongue, lips and oral mucosa. The differential diagnosis is of a cystic mass in this region includes glossal duct cyst, abscess, ranula, and mucocele.

Suggested Reading

Fuchshuber S, Grevers G, Issing WJ (2002) Dermoid cyst of the floor of the mouth – a case report. Eur Arch Otorhinolaryngol 259:60–62

Ho MW, Crean SJ (2003) Simultaneous occurrence of sublingual dermoid cyst and oral alimentary tract cyst in an infant: a case report and review of the literature. Int J Paediatr Dent 13:441–446

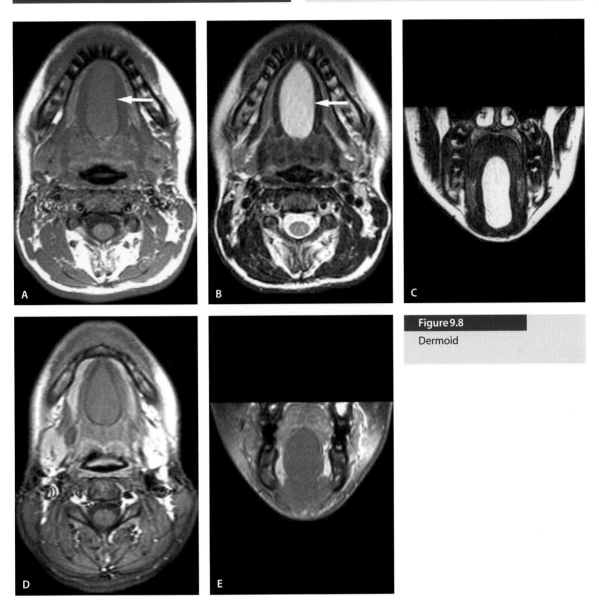

Figure 9.8
Dermoid

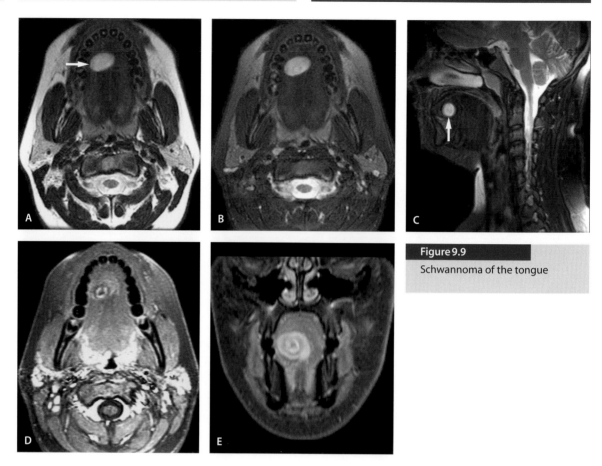

Figure 9.9

Schwannoma of the tongue

Schwannoma of the Tongue

Clinical Presentation

A 13-year-old presents with a slowly growing mass of the tongue.

Images (Fig. 9.9)

A. Axial T2-weighted image shows a high signal mass in the anterior tongue (*arrow*)
B. Axial T2-weighted image with fat suppression shows a well-defined high signal intensity lesion in the anterior aspect of the right body of the tongue. The signal is not decreased after fat suppression indicating that there is no significant fatty component in the lesion

C. Sagittal T2-weighted image with fat suppression demonstrates a high signal mass in the anterior tongue (*arrow*)
D. After contrast there is marked enhancement
E. Coronal fat-suppressed contrast-enhanced image shows the mass in the right anterior tongue

Discussion

Schwannomas are nervous tissue tumors that arise from Schwann cells. They are uncommon in peripheral nerves and they are rare in the tongue. They often present as a slowly growing mass producing no or few symptoms. Treatment for Schwannomas is exclusively surgical and usually enucleation of the mass is uncomplicated. Malignant transformation of Schwannomas is exceedingly rare.

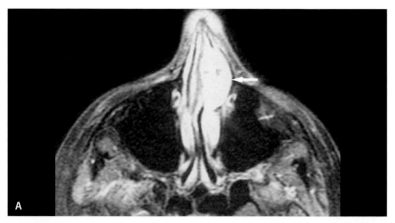

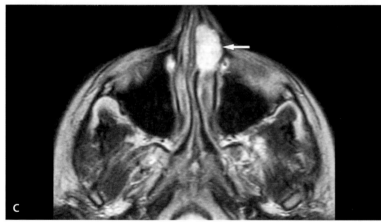

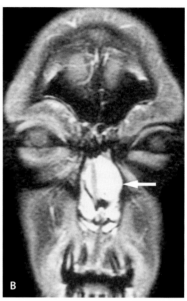

Figure 9.10

Pleomorphic adenoma
of the nose

Suggested Reading

Dreher A, Gutmann R, Grevers G (1997) Extracranial schwannoma of the ENT region. Review of the literature with a case report of benign schwannoma of the base of the tongue. HNO 45:468–471

Mevio E, Gorini E, Lenzi A, Migliorini L (2002) Schwannoma of the tongue: one case report. Rev Laryngol Otol Rhinol 123:259–261

Pfeifle R, Baur DA, Paulino A, Helman J (2001) Schwannoma of the tongue: report of 2 cases. J Oral Maxillofac Surg 59:802–804

Piatelli A, Angelone A, Pizzicannella G, Piatelli M (1984) Malignant schwannoma of the tongue. Report of a case and review of the literature. Acta Stomatol Belg 81:213–225

Pleomorphic Adenoma of the Nose

Clinical Presentation

A 13-year-old girl with a history of nasal obstruction and epistaxis. On clinical examination she has a mass in the left nasal cavity.

Images (Fig. 9.10)

A. Axial T1-weighted fat-suppressed MR image shows an overall enhancing mass lesion in the nasal cavity on the left side (*arrow*). This is contiguous with the turbinates

B. Coronal T1-weighted fat-suppressed image demonstrates the mass in the left nasal cavity (*arrow*)

C. Axial T2-weighted fat-suppressed image demonstrates the mass in the anterior of the left nasal cavity (*arrow*). It is a more intense signal than the adjacent nasal turbinates

Discussion

Pleomorphic adenomas (benign mixed tumors) are the most common benign glandular tumors of the oral cavity. They are characterized by the presence of both mesodermal and glandular tissue. The majority of pleomorphic adenomas occur in the parotid gland but 8% occur in the submandibular gland, 0.5% occur in the sublingual gland, and 6.5% occur in the minor salivary glands situated throughout the upper aerodigestive tract.

On imaging, pleomorphic adenomas are well-demarcated, homogeneous and slightly hyperdense to muscle on noncontrast-enhanced images. There is often significant enhancement.

Pleomorphic adenomas in the nose are unusual and the differential diagnosis would be polyp, lymphoma or just an asymmetric turbinate. Treatment is surgical resection.

Suggested Reading

Mirich DR, McArdle CB, Kulkarni MV (1987) Benign pleomorphic adenomas of the salivary glands: surface coil MR imaging versus CT. J Comput Assist Tomogr 11:620–623

Unlu HH, Celik O, Demir MA, Eskiizmir G (2003) Pleomorphic adenoma originated from the inferior nasal turbinate. Auris Nasus Larynx 30:417–420

Rhabdomyosarcoma

Clinical Presentation

A 5-week-old female with stridor and a posterior pharyngeal mass.

Images (Fig. 9.11)

A. Axial T1-weighted MR image shows a large mass in the nasopharynx (*arrow*)
B. Axial T2-weighted image shows the well-circumscribed mass (*arrow*) in the nasopharynx with linear and punctate areas of low attenuation presumed to be vascular structures
C. Contrast-enhanced T1-weighted image shows enhancement and flow voids (*arrow*)
D. Coronal contrast-enhanced T1-weighted image with fat suppression shows the large enhancing lesion in the nasopharynx (*arrow*)

Discussion

Rhabdomyosarcoma is the most common malignancy in the nasopharyngeal region in children and accounts for approximately 8% of childhood cancer. Rhabdomyosarcoma is divided into four histological types: embryonal, botryoid, alveolar and pleomorphic. The embryonal and botryoid types account for about 90% of primary head and neck lesions. The three common sites of predilection in head and neck region are: the orbit, the nasopharynx and paranasal cavities, and the temporal bone. Tumors in the nasopharynx region or sinuses more commonly manifest with airway obstruction, epistaxis, dysphagia, local pain and cranial nerve palsies.

Figure 9.11

Rhabdomyosarcoma

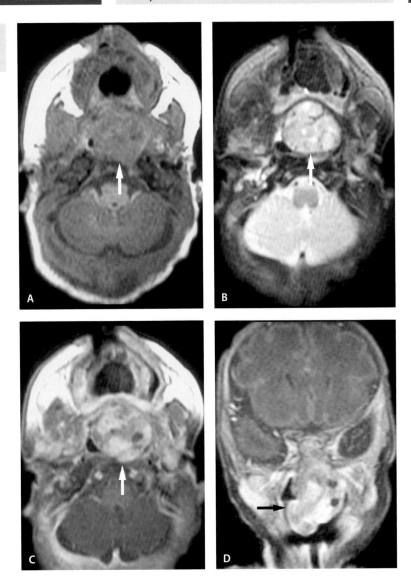

On CT, rhabdomyosarcomas are seen as ill-defined, inhomogeneous, large soft-tissue masses which may have erosion effects on the surrounding bones. Hemorrhage or calcification is uncommon. MR imaging is the technique of choice for evaluation of the tumor site because of superior ability to characterize the soft tissues. On T1-weighted images, the mass is of intermediate signal intensity, and on T2-weighted images the mass is hyperintense to adjacent muscle. The enhancement is variable. Lymphadenopathy when present, tends to be unilateral and small in comparison to nasopharyngeal carcinoma.

Suggested Reading

Hicks J, Flaitz C (2002) Rhabdomyosarcoma of the head and neck in children. Oral Oncol 38:450–459

Lee H, Lee MS, Choe DH, et al (1996) Rhabdomyosarcoma of the head and neck in adults: MR and CT findings. AJNR Am J Neuroradiol 17:1923–1928

Acinic Cell Carcinoma of the Parotid Gland

Clinical Presentation

An 11-year-old female presents with an asymptomatic swelling of the right parotid gland. This has not responded to antibiotic treatment.

Images (Fig. 9.12)

Ultrasound scan showed a multilobulated noncalcified mass in the right parotid gland (not shown)

A. Axial T1-weighted image shows a well-circumscribed intermediate to low attenuation mass (*arrow*) in the posterior portion of the right parotid gland

B. Sagittal T1-weighted image demonstrates the mass in the tail of the right parotid gland (*arrow*)

C. Coronal T1-weighted image demonstrates the mass occupying a large portion of the posterior aspect of the right parotid gland (*arrow*)

D. Contrast-enhanced axial T1-weighted MR image with fat suppression shows slight enhancement of the mass lesion (*arrow*)

E. Axial DW image demonstrates high diffusion signal from the mass (*arrow*)

F. Axial T2-weighted image demonstrates high heterogeneous signal from the mass lesion in the right parotid gland (*arrow*)

Discussion

Acinic cell carcinoma is a rare form of parotid cancer. It accounts for approximately 1% of parotid cancers. Acinic cell cancer usually grows relatively slowly. This type of cancer has a good prognosis with an almost 90% 10-year survival. It is considered a low-grade malignancy.

Masses in the tail of the parotid gland can be a source of consternation to the radiologist and the clinician. The most common lesion in the parotid gland is pleomorphic adenoma followed by Wharton's tumor, infectious processes, venous malformation, Sjögren's disease, lymphatic malformation, lipoma, and HIV related to epithelial lesions. The malignant lesions include non-Hodgkin's lymphoma, metastatic disease, mucoepidermoid carcinoma, acinic cell carcinoma and undifferentiated carcinomas. Parotid tumors are in general unusual in pediatric patients and acinic cell carcinomas in this patient group are exceedingly rare. The imaging findings are nonspecific and, based on the MR imaging, we would not be able to tell whether this lesion is malignant or benign, or whether it represents a specific type of parotid tumor. There are no soft tissue abnormalities around it to indicate an infection and therefore, from an imaging point of view, it is relatively clear that it represents a neoplasm benign or malignant.

Suggested Reading

Depowski PL, Setzen G, Chui A, Koltai PJ, Dollar J, Ross JS (1999) Familial occurrence of acinic cell carcinoma of the parotid gland. Arch Pathol Lab Med 123:1118–1120

Hamilton BE, Salzman KL, Wiggins RH 3rd, Harnsberger HR (2003) Earring lesions of the parotid tail. AJNR Am J Neuroradiol 24:1757–1764

Millar BG, Johnson PA, Leopard PJ (1989) Bilateral acinic cell carcinoma of the parotid. Br J Oral Maxillofac Surg 27:192–197

Sakai O, Nakashima N, Takata Y, Furuse M (1996) Acinic cell Carcinoma of the parotid gland: CT and MRI. Neuroradiology 38:675–679

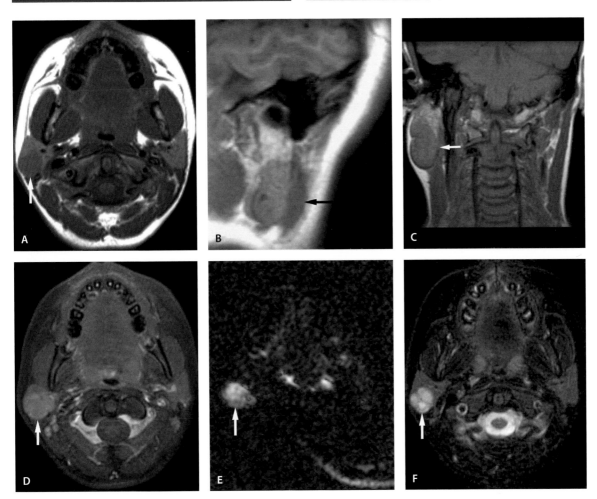

Figure 9.12

Acinic cell carcinoma of the parotid gland

Anophthalmos

Clinical Presentation

A 2-year-old female with congenital anophthalmos and seizures.

Images (Fig. 9.13)

A. Sagittal T1-weighted image demonstrates hypoplasia of the orbital region and absence of the orbit. The splenium of the corpus callosum is somewhat small
B. Axial T2-weighted image demonstrates the absence of both eyes
C. Sagittal T1-weighted image through the orbit shows anophthalmos with a malformed congenitally small globe
D. Axial T1-weighted image demonstrates bilateral anophthalmos with micro-optic features

Discussion

Anophthalmos, congenital absence of an eye or eyes, is a rare anomaly that occurs as a result of insults to the developing eye during first 8 weeks of life. Anophthalmos can be of three types: (1) primary anophthalmos which is usually bilateral and sporadic and occurs when the optic primordial does not develop, (2) secondary anophthalmos which is an extremely rare and lethal anomaly that occurs when the entire neural tube fails to develop, and (3) secondary anophthalmos that occurs when the optic vesicle forms but subsequently degenerates. The diagnosis of true anophthalmos can be made when there is complete absence of the ocular tissue within the orbit. Extreme microanophthalmos is seen more commonly in which a very small globe is present within the orbital soft tissue, which is not visible on initial examination. The orbital findings include small orbital rim with absence of extraocular muscles and lacrimal gland. The optic foramen is small and maldeveloped. The globe is completely absent in primary anophthalmos.

CT and MR imaging is performed to assess the presence of an extremely microanophthalmic globe. The optic chiasm and corpus callosum may show agenesis or dysgenesis. Craniofacial anomalies may also be associated.

Suggested Reading

Albernaz VS, Castillo M, Hudgins PA, Mukherji SK (1997) Imaging findings in patients with clinical anophthalmos. AJNR Am J Neuroradiol 18:555–561

Daxecker F, Felber S (1993) Magnetic resonance imaging features of congenital anophthalmia. Ophthalmologica 206:139–142

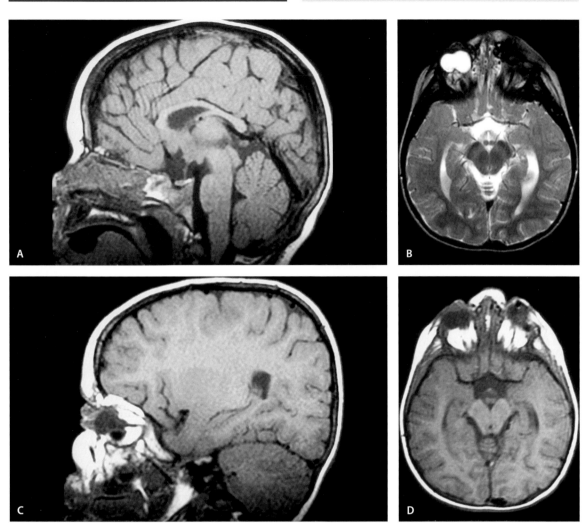

Figure 9.13

Anophthalmos

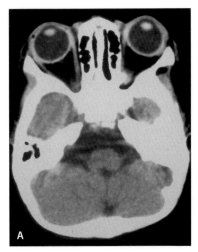
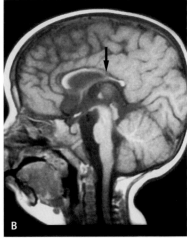
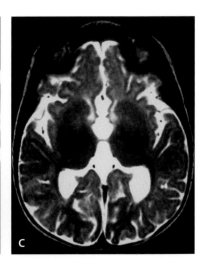

Figure 9.14

Wolf-Hirschhorn syndrome

Wolf-Hirschhorn Syndrome

Clinical Presentation

A 13-month-old male with seizures, developmental delay, sacral dimple and a clinical diagnosis of Wolf-Hirschhorn syndrome.

Images (Fig. 9.14)

A. CT scan through the orbits shows hypertelorism
B. Sagittal MR image shows absence of the posterior portion of the body of the corpus callosum (*arrow*). There is micrognathia with a small mandible and a relatively small maxilla
C. Axial T2-weighted image demonstrates low signal intensity in the basal ganglia bilaterally presumed to be secondary to early iron deposition. There is also decreased signal intensity in the cortical gyri presumed to be from the same etiology

Discussion

Wolf-Hirschhorn syndrome is caused by partial deletion of chromosome 4. Wolf-Hirschhorn syndrome has distinctive facial characteristics – prominent head, wide eyes, and broad beaked nose, collectively described as "Greek warrior helmet" features. Other clinical features include microcephaly, profound mental retardation, growth retardation, muscular hypotonia, seizures, congenital heart defects, coloboma of iris, genital and renal anomalies.

On imaging, findings of absent cavum septum pellucidum, agenesis of the corpus callosum, microgyria, migration defects and hydrocephalus may be seen. In addition, MR imaging shows multifocal white matter lesions.

Suggested Reading

De Keersmaecker B, Albert M, Hillion Y, Ville Y (2002) Prenatal diagnosis of brain abnormalities in Wolf-Hirschhorn syndrome(4p-). Prenat Diagn 22:366–370

Tutunculer F, Acunas B, Hicdonmez T, Deviren A, Pelitli V (2004) Wolf-Hirschhorn syndrome with posterior intraorbital coloboma cyst: an unusual case. Brain Dev 26:203–205

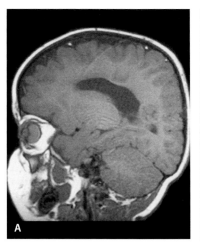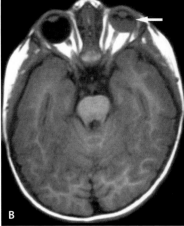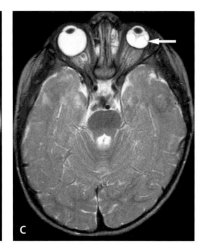

Figure 9.15

Retinopathy of prematurity

Retinopathy of Prematurity

Clinical Presentation

A 21-month-old ex-premature infant with a history of intraventricular hemorrhage and developmental delay. Impaired left sided vision.

Images (Fig. 9.15)

A. Sagittal T1-weighted image shows a small globe with intermediate signal
B. T1-weighted image shows a small globe on the left side with intermediate signal. The retina is displaced anteriorly and compressed (*arrow*)
C. T2-weighted axial image shows evidence of retinal detachment on the left side with a small globe (*arrow*)

Discussion

Retinopathy of prematurity is caused by the vasoconstrictive effect of high blood levels of oxygen used to treat hyaline membrane disease in premature infants. The vasoconstriction results in chronic retinal ischemia which secondarily causes neovascularization.

The neovascularization and its following regression cause subretinal exudation, hemorrhage and scarring. The scarring and the subretinal exudate often result in chronic retinal detachment and later on microophthalmia.

Most patients have bilateral imaging findings but often are asymmetrical. MR imaging of acute subretinal fluid will be high on CT images due to the presence of acute hemorrhage. MR imaging of the acute condition will show high signal on T1 and low signal on the T2 images. Chronic detachment will have low signal with no attenuation on CT images, intermediate to low signal on T1-weighted images, and often high or variable T2 signal.

More than 80% of infants weighing less than 1 kg at birth will develop retinopathy of prematurity. The main risk is administration of excessive oxygen. The diagnosis is generally made by ophthalmological examination. The treatment is mainly prophylactic, but severe cases can be treated with cryotherapy and laser to ablate the peripheral avascular retina.

Suggested Reading

Barkovich AJ (2000) Congenital malformations of the brain and skull. In: Barkovich AJ (ed) Pediatric neuroimaging, chap 5. Lippincott, Williams and Wilkins, Philadelphia, pp 251–381

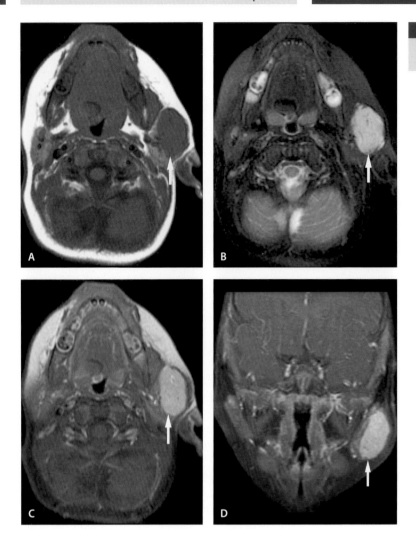

Figure 9.16

Hemangioma of the parotid gland

Images (Fig. 9.16)

A. Axial T1-weighted image shows a well-circumscribed mass in the left parotid gland (*arrow*). There is no reaction in the surrounding fat
B. Axial T2-weighted image with fat suppression shows the mass having high signal (*arrow*)
C. Axial T1-weighted image with contrast shows enhancement of the well-circumscribed mass (*arrow*). There is a rim of nonenhancing parotid gland tissue around the mass
D. Coronal T1-weighted image with contrast shows enhancement of the well-circumscribed mass. The rim of nonenhancing parotid gland tissue around the mass is well seen (*arrow*)

Hemangioma

Hemangioma of the Parotid Gland

Clinical presentation

A 9-month-old female presents with a soft asymptomatic swelling of the left parotid gland.

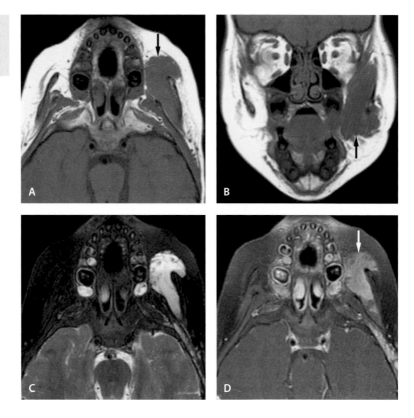

Figure 9.17
Hemangioma of the face and orbit

Hemangioma of the Face and Orbit

Clinical Presentation

A 4-month-old baby presents with a soft periorbital mass.

Images (Fig. 9.17)

A. Axial T1-weighted image shows a left periorbital and a cheek soft tissue mass (*arrow*)
B. Coronal T1-weighted image shows a soft tissue mass in the left face (*arrow*)
C. Axial T2-weighted image with fat suppression demonstrates the precise outline of the soft tissue hemangioma and the left facial structures
D. Axial contrast-enhanced T1-weighted fat-suppressed image shows enhancement of the left cheek mass (*arrow*)

Discussion

Hemangioma is the most common vascular tumor seen in infancy. The incidence is higher in females and in low-birth-weight babies. Hemangiomas are most prevalent in the head and neck region and constitute 18–38% of head and neck tumors. Approximately 20% of patients have multiple hemangiomas that involve sites such as skin, liver, gastrointestinal tract and brain. Intracranial and intraspinal hemangiomas may also be seen in association with multiple hemangiomas. Diagnosis of hemangiomas is made by a combination of the medical history, physical examination and ultrasound scan. Typical hemangiomas are red, raised and bosselated. Deep hemangiomas have normal overlying skin and may mimic other vascular malformations. Congenital hemangiomas typically show rapid growth and may involute completely.

On CT images, hemangiomas are seen as lobulated solid masses that are isodense with muscle and show intense enhancement. On MR images, they usually show intermediate signal intensity on T1-weighted images, high signal intensity on T2-weighted images, and diffuse intense enhancement. Areas of fatty replacement may also be seen. Hemangiomas need to be differentiated from arteriovascular malformations which are also associated with prominent vascularity. However, hemangiomas usually have a lobulated appearance and are not associated with reactive or trophic changes which are commonly associated with arteriovascular malformations.

Suggested Reading

Castellote A, Vazquez E, Vera J, et al (1999) Cervicothoracic lesions in infants and children.Radiographics.19:583–600

Tetsumura A, Yoshino N, Yamada I, Sasaki T (1999) Head and neck hemangiomas: contrast-enhanced three-dimensional MR angiography. Neuroradiology 41:140–143

Langerhans Cell Histiocytosis

Clinical Presentation

A 12-year-old with a history of Langerhans cell histiocytosis presents with decreased vision in the right eye.

Images (Fig. 9.18)

A. Axial CT scan shows a mass in the right orbital apex with erosion of the posterolateral wall of the right orbit (*arrow*)

B. Coronal reformatted CT scan demonstrates the mass filling the entire right orbital apex (*arrow*). The left orbit is normal

C. Coronal T1-weighted image demonstrates an intermediate to low signal intensity mass filling the right orbital apex (*arrow*). There is also expansion of the orbital apex

D. Sagittal T2-weighted fat-suppressed image demonstrates a high signal intensity well-demarcated mass in the right orbital apex. This is consistent with a Langerhans cell histiocytosis in a patient with a prior diagnosis of this condition

Discussion

Langerhans cell histiocytosis is an uncommon disease characterized by the idiopathic proliferation of Langerhans cells or their marrow precursors. Langerhans cell histiocytosis is classified according to sites of involvement into single or multisystem disease. Single system can be unifocal or multifocal. Bony involvement is seen in 78% of patients and often includes the skull (49%), innominate bone, femur, orbit (11%), and ribs. Extraskeletal involvement is well known. The lesions can be single or multiple. Orbital infiltration presents with pain, swelling and proptosis. Orbital soft tissue involvement without an obvious bony defect is rare. On CT images, they may be seen as a homogeneously hyperdense enhancing masses associated with bony erosion. On T1- and T2-weighted and proton density MR images, they are seen as isointense to gray matter and show enhancement.

Suggested Reading

Burton EM, Hickman M, Boulden TF, Joyner RE, Tierney MB (1989) Orbital sinus histiocytosis: MR appearance. J Comput Assist Tomogr 13:696–699

Stromberg JS, Wang AM, Huang FA, Vicini FA, Nowak PA (1995) Langerhans cell histiocytosis involving the sphenoid sinus and superior orbital fissure. AJNR Am J Neuroradiol 16:964–967

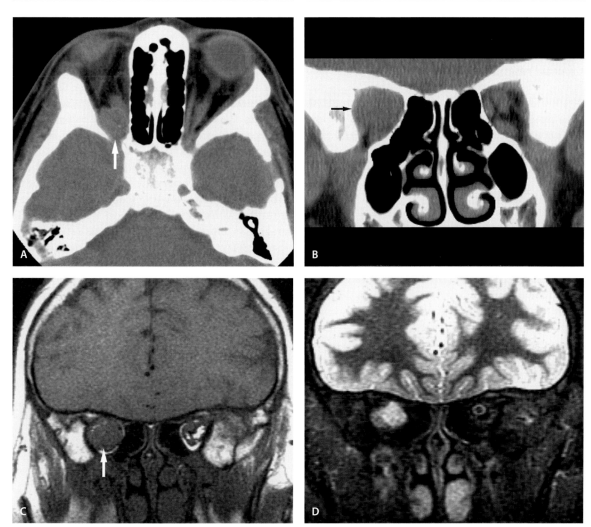

Figure 9.18

Langerhans cell histiocytosis

Osteosarcoma of the Cranium

Clinical Presentation

A 10-year-old presenting with a painless reddish swelling over the right periorbital zygoma region. The patient had a history of retinoblastoma and radiation.

Images (Fig. 9.19)

A. Axial CT image shows an expansile bony lesion in the right orbit
B. Coronal contrast-enhanced T1-weighted image shows the expansile lesion invading both the orbit and the brain
C. Sagittal contrast-enhanced T1-weighted image shows the invasion of the mass into the anterior and middle cranial fossae
D. Axial T2-weighted image shows an irregular low-intensity mass in the right periorbital region invading the orbit and infratemporal fossa. It also extends into the right middle cranial fossa.

Discussion

Osteosarcomas are malignant bone tumors, which commonly affect the long bones of young adults. Primary osteosarcomas of the skull are rare. Secondary osteosarcoma may be seen in patients with long-standing Paget's disease. The post-radiation osteosarcomas occur in portions of bones at the borders of the radiation field.

Cranial radiographs are of limited value in head and neck osteosarcomas due to superimposed bony structures. CT scanning provides excellent detection of tumor calcification, and cortical involvement. MR imaging is more sensitive in demonstration of intramedullary and extraosseous tumor components.

Suggested Reading

Chander B, Ralte AM, Dahiya S, et al (2003) Primary osteosarcoma of the skull. A report of 3 cases. J Neurosurg Sci 47:177–181

Kornreich L, Grunebaum M, Ziv N, Cohen Y (1988) Osteogenic sarcoma of the calvarium in children: CT manifestations. Neuroradiology 30:439–441

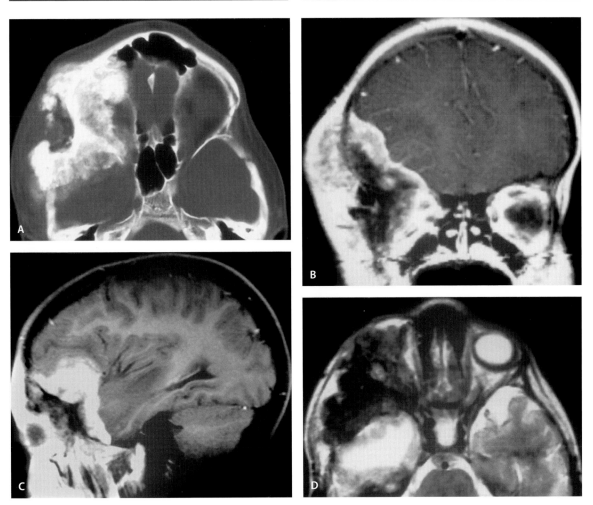

Figure 9.19

Osteosarcoma of the cranium

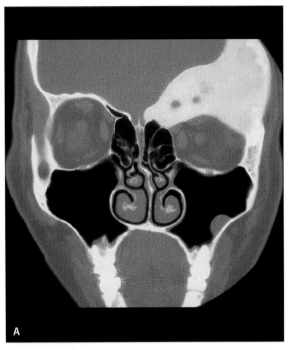

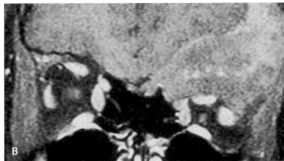

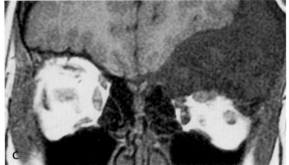

Figure 9.20

Fibrous Dysplasia

Fibrous Dysplasia

Clinical Presentation

A 17-year-old presents with asymmetry of the face and skull. There is a painless prominence in the left supraorbital region.

Images (Fig. 9.20)

A. Coronal CT scan shows a dense expansile greater wing of the sphenoid bone on the left side. There is decreased size of the left orbital cavity
B. Contrast-enhanced T1-weighted MR image shows an isointense lesion in the expanded greater wing of the sphenoid bone. The orbital cavity is compressed
C. T1-weighted image without contrast shows low signal intensity from the fibrous lesion in the greater wing of the sphenoid bone on the left side consistent with fibrous dysplasia

Discussion

Fibrous dysplasia is an idiopathic skeletal disorder in which the medulla bone is replaced by poorly organized, structurally, and sound fibro-osseous tissue. It most frequently affects children, teenagers and patients under the age of 30 years. The majority of the cases are mono-osteitic, and this condition affects the ribs, femur and craniofacial skeleton. Albright's syndrome is a variant that consists of poly-osteitic fibrous dysplasia, pigmented skin pigmentation and sexual precocity. Albright's syndrome is relatively rare and it has been stated that it occurs 40 times less than mono-osteitic fibrous dysplasia.

Malignant transformation of fibrous dysplasia is very rare (less than 1%). Fibrous dysplasia is typically painless but neurovascular compromise may cause symptoms. Craniofacial fibrous dysplasia is generally not functionally devastating unless in this case there is involvement of the orbit and skull base. There is a potential for optic nerve compression, pituitary dysfunction and compromise of other vital neurovascular structures. The disease is usually self-limiting and often does not progress after the third decade of life. Surgical treatment is limited to cosmetic debulking and re-contouring of the bone.

Suggested Reading

Daffner R, Kirks D, Gehweiler JJ, et al (1982) Computed tomography of fibrous dysplasia. AJR Am J Roentgenol 139:943–946

Fries J (1957) The roentgen features of fibrous dysplasia of the skull and facial bones. AJR Am J Roentgenol 77:71–75

Leeds N, Seaman W (1962) Fibrous dysplasia of the skull and its differential diagnosis. Radiology 78:570–582

Resnick D (1995) Diagnosis of bone and joint disorders, 3rd edn. Saunders, Philadelphia

Bilateral Coronoid Hyperplasia of the Mandible Causing Trismus

Clinical Presentation

A 16-year-old male presenting with gradually increasing trismus. He has no pain and he is able to move his jaw from left to right with a full range of motion, but he is not able to open more than 28 mm (normal 40 mm or more). There is no tenderness over the temporomandibular joints and no clinical suspicion of internal derangement.

Images (Fig. 9.21)

A. Three-dimensional CT scan with closed mouth shows elongation of the left coronoid process. The coronoid process is extending above the zygomatic arch

B. Three-dimensional CT scan with open mouth shows the coronoid process behind and interfering with the zygoma. There is normal range of motion in the temporomandibular joint

C. Axial CT scan with closed mouth demonstrates the prominent coronoid processes bilaterally

D. Coronal CT scan with closed mouth shows elongation of the coronoid processes bilaterally sticking up superior to the zygomatic arches

E. Axial CT scan with open mouth shows the coronoid processes close to the zygomatic arches

F. Coronal CT scan with open mouth demonstrates the close relationship between the zygomatic arches and the coronoid processes

Discussion

Hyperplasia and elongation of the coronoid process is one relatively unusual reason for limitation of jaw opening. It occurs most frequently in young males and one study has indicated that as many as 5% of all patients with TMJ symptoms and limitation of jaw opening have coronoid hyperplasia. This condition was described as long ago as the mid-1800s. Recent studies have indicated that CT scanning is the best imaging modality to document coronoid hyperplasia as the cause of limitation of opening.

If the coronoid process is significantly elongated, it can impact on the zygomatic process of the maxilla causing limitation of jaw opening. Surgical removal of the coronoid process usually results in improved opening with relatively few complications.

Suggested Reading

Isberg A, Isacsson G, Nah KS (1987) Mandibular coronoid process locking: a prospective study of frequency and association with internal derangement of the temporomandibular joint. Oral Surg Oral Med Oral Pathol 63:275–279

Langenbeck B (1860) Augeborene Kleinheit des Unterkiefers; Kiefersperre verbunden, geheilt durch Resection der processus coronoidei. Arch Klin Chir 1:30

Munk PL, Helms CA (1989) Coronoid process hyperplasia: CT studies. Radiology 171:783–784

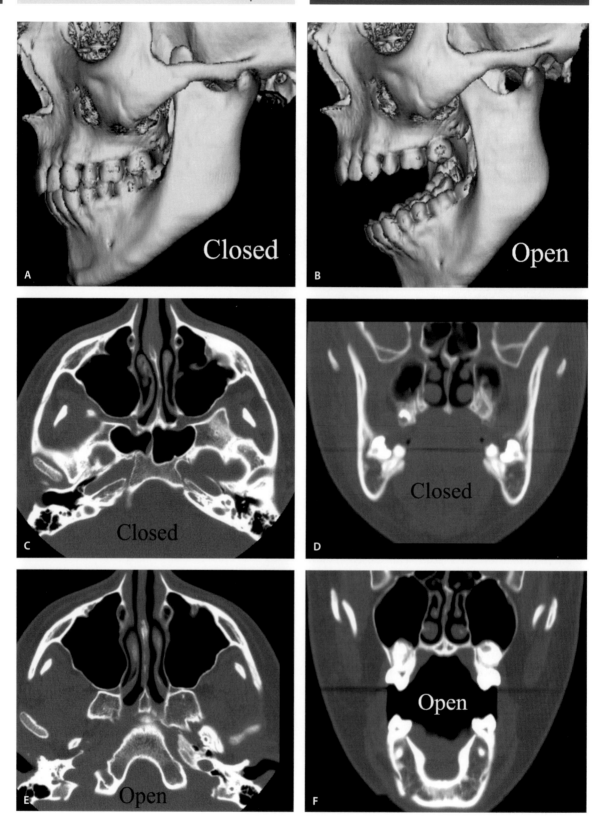

Figure 9.21

Bilateral coronoid hyperplasia of the mandible causing trismus

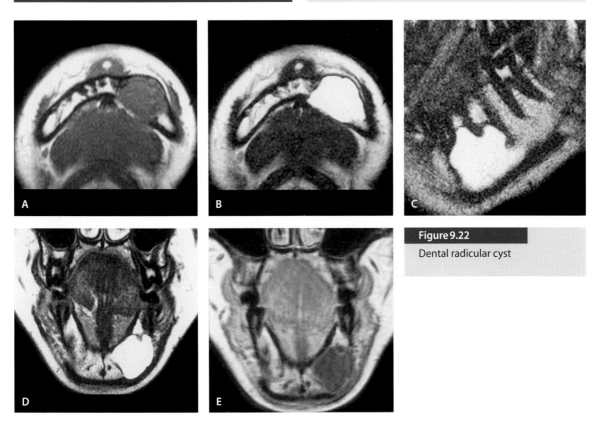

Figure 9.22
Dental radicular cyst

Dental Radicular Cyst

Clinical Presentation

A 13-year-old with an asymptomatic lucency on a panoramic radiograph was referred for MR imaging.

Images (Fig. 9.22)

A. T1-weighted axial image shows expansion of the left body of the mandible with a low signal intensity mass
B. T2-weighted image shows high signal in the expansile lesion in the left body of the mandible
C. Sagittal T2-weighted image with fat suppression demonstrates the lesion inferior to the first molar and premolar
D. Coronal T2-weighted image shows the expansion of the mandible on the left side with scalloping of the inner cortex
E. Coronal T1-weighted image post-contrast demonstrates no enhancement of the lesion but minimal enhancement of the wall of the cystic cavity

Discussion

Radicular cyst is the most common odontogenic cyst. The peak incidence is between 30 and 50 years of age, but it may occur in young individuals as in this 13-year-old patient. Caries leading to pulp infection and eventually necrosis is the most common cause of radicular cyst. Radiographically a radicular cyst is a well-circumscribed radiolucency arising from the apex of the tooth and is nearly always bounded by a thin rim of cortical bone. It is not uncommon to see expansion and scalloping of the cortical margins of the jaw. Radiographically a radicular cyst cannot be differentiated from a periapical granuloma. On MR imaging they typically have a low T1 and a high T2 signal intensity with no enhancement. A radicular cyst is usually treated endodontically or by extraction of the involved tooth and surgical enucleation of the cyst. There is no significant recurrence rate.

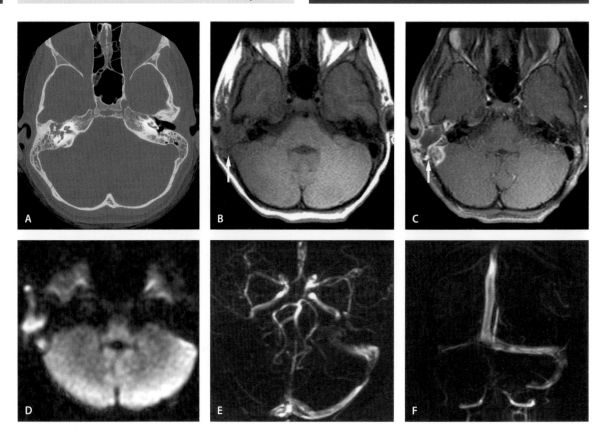

Figure 9.23

Mastoiditis with sigmoid sinus thrombosis

Suggested Reading

Kramer IRH, Pindborg JJ, Shar M (1992) Histological typing of odontogenic tumours. World Health Organization: International Histological Classification of Tumours, 2nd edn. Springer, Berlin Heidelberg New York, pp 1–42

Sciubba JJ, Fantasia JE, Kahn LB (2001) Tumors and cysts of the jaw. In: Rosai J (ed) Atlas of tumor pathology. Armed Forces Institute of Pathology, Washington DC

White SC, Pharoah MJ (2000) Oral radiology: principles and interpretation, 4th edn. Mosby, St Louis

Mastoiditis with Sigmoid Sinus Thrombosis

Clinical Presentation

A 7-year-old female with a chronic draining right ear.

Images (Fig. 9.23)

A. Axial CT scan demonstrates opacification of the entire right mastoid and the right middle ear cavity without appreciable bony erosions

B. Axial T1-weighted image without contrast shows a soft tissue mass in the right temporal bone (*arrow*). There is no flow void in the sigmoid sinus on this side

C. Axial contrast-enhanced T1-weighted image with fat suppression demonstrates abnormal contrast enhancement in the area of the right temporal bone (*arrow*). In the sigmoid sinus there is contrast enhancement in the periphery but a central filling defect suggesting a clot in the sigmoid sinus

D. Axial DW image shows high signal in the clot in the right sigmoid sinus suggesting restricted diffusion secondary to sigmoid sinus thrombosis

E. MR venogram in the axial plane demonstrates lack of flow in the right sigmoid and transverse sinus

F. Coronal venogram demonstrates no flow in the right sigmoid sinus

Discussion

Many predisposing factors have been implicated in the development of sinus thrombosis. Trauma, infection, tumors, dehydration, hypercoagulable states such as pregnancy, oral contraceptives and nephrotic syndrome are the most common causes. Approximately 20% of cases are idiopathic. Mastoiditis is a known cause of lateral venous sinus thrombosis. The sigmoid portion of the lateral venous runs on the inner aspect of the mastoid process. Diploic veins and small veins from the middle ear also drain into the lateral sinus. Patients presenting with lateral sinus thrombosis and mastoid congestion should be assessed for the presence of mastoiditis.

Dural sinus thrombosis manifests with diverse clinical findings. Early symptoms include headache, lethargy followed by seizures and focal neurological deficits. Strokes (hemorrhagic) may develop secondary to poor venous drainage. These strokes are often bilateral and outside the normal arterial distribution, reflecting the pattern of venous drainage.

MR venography is the modality of choice for venous thrombosis. The hyperacute thrombus has low signal intensity on both T1- and T2-weighted images. The effect is more pronounced on T2-weighted images. At about 3 weeks, the clot may have low signal on all sequences. Indirect signs of thrombosis include the presence of collateral flow.

Suggested Reading

Fink JN, McAuley DL (2002) Mastoid air sinus abnormalities associated with lateral venous thrombosis: cause or consequence? Stroke 33:290–292

Yuh WT, Simonson TM, Wang AM, et al (1994) Venous sinus occlusive disease: MR findings. AJNR Am J Neuroradiol 15:309–316

Arteriovenous Fistula of Vertebral Artery

Clinical Presentation

A 6-year-old male with right neck bruit.

Images (Fig. 9.24)

A. Sagittal T2-weighted image shows an intraspinal vascular malformation with abnormal vessels (*arrow*)

B. Axial T2-weighted image shows a large abnormal vascular connection between the right vertebral artery and the spinal canal (*arrow*). There is also an abnormal flow void in the anterior of the spinal canal

C. Contrast enhanced MR angiogram demonstrates the vascular malformation connecting the vertebral artery and the venous system on the right. There is a relatively broad and complex connection between the artery and the vein: arteriovenous fistula

D. FSPGR MR image shows the arterial and the venous side of the arteriovenous fistula but not the connection itself

Discussion

An arteriovenous fistula involving the cervical vertebral artery is rare. The etiologies of vertebral arteriovenous fistula include traumatic, iatrogenic, congenital, and spontaneous (neurofibromatosis). Traumatic and iatrogenic injuries appear to be the most common causes, with the greatest incidence arising from firearm and stab wounds. Symptoms include tinnitus and presence of a pulsatile mass with a thrill.

Color Doppler examination is a noninvasive modality which can be used as bedside screening investigation for detection of vertebral arteriovenous fistula. CT angiography and MR angiography demonstrate the anatomical relationship of the fistula accurately. Conventional angiography serves as a diagnostic as well as a therapeutic tool for interventional procedures. The current therapeutic management consists of direct closure of the fistula, either with surgical techniques or percutaneously with detachable balloon occlusion or coil embolization or stent grafts.

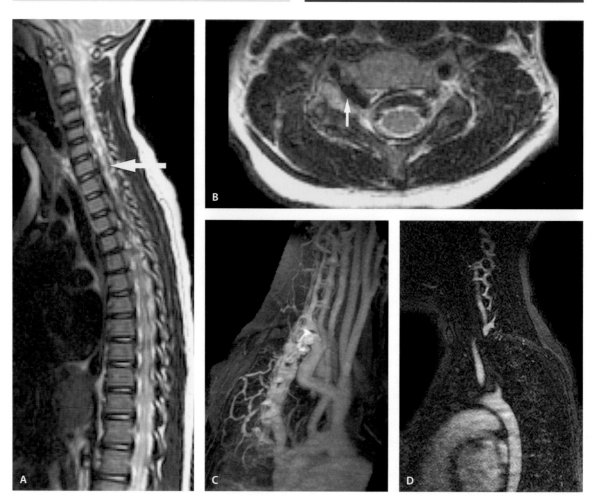

Figure 9.24

Arteriovenous fistula of vertebral artery

Suggested Reading

Friedman DP (1998) Neuroradiology case of the day. Vertebral
    arteriovenous fistula (AVF). Radiographics 18:527–529
Priestley R, Bray P, Bray A, Hunter J (2003) Iatrogenic vertebral
    arteriovenous fistula treated with a hemobahn stent-graft.
    J Endovasc Ther 10:657–663

Spine

Introduction

MR imaging has had a profound influence on our ability to accurately image the spine. The impact of MR imaging is much greater than the impact of CT imaging due better soft-tissue resolution. MR imaging is much better than CT imaging in demonstrating developmental anomalies, tumors and trauma. MR imaging opened our eyes to anatomic and pathological conditions that previously had only been seen by neurosurgeons and pathologists. From recognition of anatomic abnormalities, MR imaging now provides functional information such as CSF flow and pulsation and their effect on development of syringohydromyelia.

MR is the only imaging modality that demonstrates intrinsic cord signal abnormalities in both disease and trauma. Thus, MR imaging can be used as a predictor of neurological outcome in cases of acute spinal cord injury by separating hemorrhagic contusion from edema. Edema has a more favorable prognosis than hemorrhagic contusion. MR imaging is also able to separate posttraumatic myelomalacia from posttraumatic cystic lesions which may require surgical treatment.

Diffusion-weighted (DW) imaging of the brain is well established, but DW imaging of the spine has been more challenging. Preliminary studies with line scan DW imaging have shown great potential for evaluation of ischemic cord lesions, myelin loss, trauma, tumors and inflammatory processes of the spine. Similarly further development of MR spectroscopy might be as useful in the spine as in the brain, but

technical problems remain to be solved. Clinical application of MR angiography of the spine has lagged behind the use of MR angiography in the brain and neck. However, since the mid-1990s MR angiography has been used successfully to study the vascular anatomy and pathology of the spine. Spinal MR angiography is currently an active research area. Since its introduction in 1990, functional MR imaging has been widely used to study brain physiology. Using the same functional technique to study the spine, imaging has proven to be more challenging, but several recent studies on functional MR imaging of the spine have demonstrated motor activity in the human spinal cord.

As MR and CT imaging often provide complementary information, CT imaging is still useful in the evaluation of trauma to the spine and congenital anomalies of the pediatric spine, while MR imaging better detects soft-tissue malformations and pathology.

Suggested Reading

Madi S, Flanders AE, Vinitsky S, Herbison GJ, Nissanov J (2001) Functional MR imaging of the human cervical spinal cord. AJNR Am J Neuroradiol 22:1768–1774

Mascalchi M, Bianchi MC, Quilizi N, et al (1995) MR angiography of spinal vascular malformations. AJNR Am J Neuroradiol 16:289–297

Robertson RL, Maier SE, Mulkern RV, Bajapayam S, Robson CD, Barnes PD (2000) MR line-scan diffusion imaging of the spinal cord in children. AJNR Am J Neuroradiol 21:1344–1358

Sherman JL, Citrin CM (1986) Magnetic resonance demonstration of normal CSF flow. AJNR Am J Neuroradiol 7:4–6

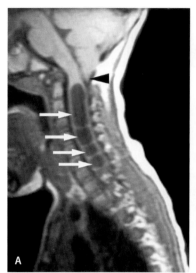 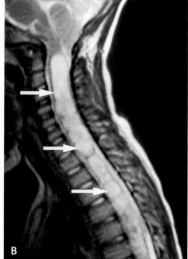 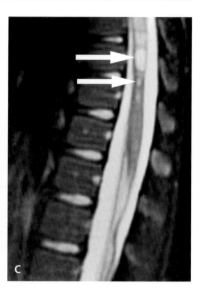

Figure 10.1

Chiari I malformation

Chiari I Malformation

Clinical Presentation

Asymptomatic 5-year-old male.

Images (Fig. 10.1)

A. Mid sagittal T1-weighted image demonstrates caudal displacement of the cerebellar tonsils (*arrowhead*). Dark signal hydromyelia with multiple loculations is seen (*arrows*)
B. Sagittal T2-weighted image of the cervical and upper thoracic spine reveals associated hydromyelia with multiple loculations (*arrows*)
C. Sagittal T2-weight image demonstrates the lower aspect of the hydromyelia cavity (*arrows*)

Discussion

Chiari I malformation is described as cerebellar dysgenesis with low-lying cerebellar tonsils into the upper spinal canal, occasionally as low as to C3–4 level. It is generally accepted that tonsillar herniation of 5 mm or more is diagnostic for the Chiari I malformation. The tonsils are pointed or peg-like. Associated hydrosyringomyelia is present in 30–50% of patients. Spinal anomalies involving the craniocervical junction are not uncommon. They include short clivus, atlanto-occipital assimilation, nonsegmentation of C2–3, cervical spine bifida occulta and basilar invagination. Abnormal CSF flow at the foramen magnum has been implicated in the clinical symptomatology associated with Chiari I malformation. CSF flow studies (cine) can be used to demonstrate possible CSF flow velocity changes caused by the low-lying tonsils. This may assist in the evaluation of the need for possible cranio-occiput decompression surgery.

Suggested Reading

Aboulezz AO, Sartor K, Gayer CA, et al (1985) Position of cerebellar tonsils in the normal population and in patients with Chiari malformation: a quantitative approach with MR imaging. J Comput Assist Tomogr 9:1033–1036
Elster AD, Chen MV (1992) Chiari I malformation: clinical and radiologic reappraisal. Radiology 183:347–353
Houghton VM, Korosec FR, Medow JE, Dolar MT, Iskaner BJ (2003) Peak systolic and diastolic CSF velocity in the foramen magnum in adult patients with chiari I malformations and in normal control participants. AJNR Am J Neuroradiol 24:169–176

Figure 10.2

Tethered cord with lipoma
(case 1)

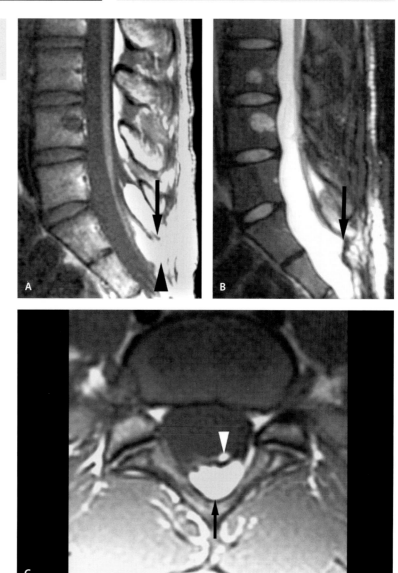

Tethered Cord with Lipoma

Case 1

Clinical Presentation

A 19-month-old male with walking difficulties.

Images (Fig. 10.2)

A. Sagittal T1-weighted image shows a tethered cord ending at the S2 region (*arrow*). The caudal spinal canal is wide and there is spine bifida. The subcutaneous lipid is continuous with the intraspinal lipoma (*arrowhead*)

B. T2-weighted image demonstrates neural placode where the caudal tip of the cord ends (*arrow*)

C. Axial T1-weighted image shows extension of the lipoma (*arrow*) inside the spinal canal. There is also lipid in the cord (*arrowhead*)

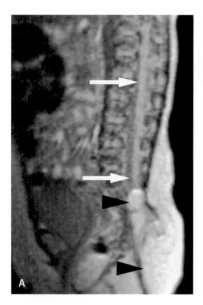 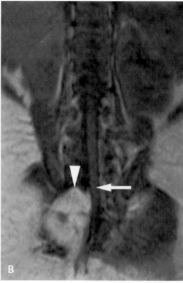

Figure 10.3
Tethered cord with lipoma
(case 2)

Case 2

Clinical Presentation

Newborn with soft mass in the back.

Images (Fig. 10.3)

A. Sagittal T1-weighted image shows a low-lying cord (*arrows*) that ends in a lipoma (*arrowheads*) at the S2 level
B. Coronal T1-weighted image shows a large extradural lipoma (*arrowhead*) that displaces the low-lying cord to the left (*arrow*)

Discussion

The tethered cord is classically defined as low-lying tip of cord below the L2 vertebra. This segment of tethered cord is stretched beyond its tolerance and damage to blood vessels, nerve cells, and nerve fibers occurs. Many conditions including bony protrusions or tough membranous bands as well as lipomas and tumors (mostly benign) prevent the cord from moving.

CSF cine study may be helpful in some ambiguous cases when the cord lies in a near-normal position. The tip of the conus normally moves freely in systole and diastole. This normal movement is absent in a case of tethered cord.

CT scan is more sensitive for detection of bony abnormalities that are often seen in patients with tethered cord. MR imaging is regarded as the imaging modality of choice since it not only identifies the spinal cord and dural sac abnormalities, but also helps in detection of associated other abnormalities. The normal filum terminale measures less than or equal to 2 mm in diameter at the L5-S1 level. A diagnosis of tethered cord is established when conus is seen below the bottom of L2 with a thickened filum terminale. The clinical symptoms are usually related to cord tethering such as bladder and bowel dysfunction, gait disturbance and scoliosis. The symptoms are usually most apparent during the rapid somatic growth, but can start even in late adulthood. Half of the patients have associated cutaneous stigmata such as hemangioma, tuft of hair or simple dimple.

T1-weight imaging without fat suppression is the best sequence to visualize the conus tip and the filum with lipoma. Axial T1-weighted imaging allows differentiation between the laterally located nerve roots of the cauda equina and the mid-line filum. In the sagittal image the filum and nerve roots merge into a single longitudinal band of intermediate signal in the posterior thecal sac. In most cases MR imaging alone is adequate and myelography and postmyelography CT are not needed. To differentiate lipoma and hematoma, fat-suppressed MR imaging is sometimes required.

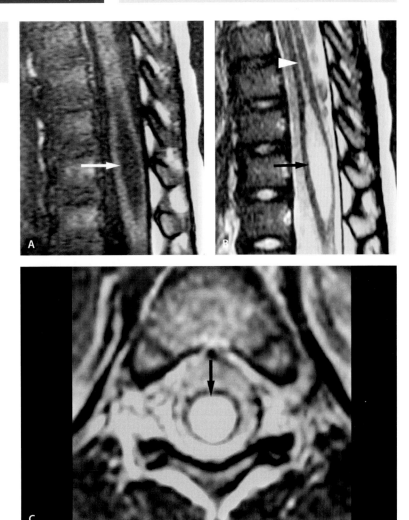

Figure 10.4

Ventriculus terminalis
of the conus medullaris

Suggested Reading

Khanna AJ, Wasserman BA, Sponseller PD (2003) Magnetic
    resonance imaging of the pediatric spine. J Am Acad Or-
    thop Surg 11:248–259

Schijiman E (2003) Split spinal cord malformations: report of
    22 cases and review of the literature. Childs Nerv Syst
    19:96–103

Selcuki M, Vatansever S, Inan S, Erdemli E, Bagdatoglu C, Polai
    A (2003) Is the filum terminale with a normal appearance
    really normal? Childs Nerv Syst 19:3–10

Witkamp TD, Vandertop WP, Beek FJ, et al (2001) Medullary
    cone movement in subjects with a normal spinal cord and
    in patients with a tethered spinal cord. Radiology 220:208–
    212

Ventriculus Terminalis of the Conus Medullaris

Clinical Presentation

A 2-year-old female with a history of dislocated hips.

Images (Fig. 10.4)

A. Sagittal T1-weighted image on the distal spinal
    cord shows an elongated CSF-containing cyst (*ar-
    row*)

B. T2-weighted sagittal image of the distal cord.
    There is an oval ventriculus terminalis of the
    conus medullaris (*arrow*) that is a distal continua-
    tion of a more rostral dilated central canal (*arrow-
    head*)

C. Axial T2-wieighted image shows the ventriculus terminalis as a high signal consistent with CSF (*arrow*). No associated mass lesion is seen

Discussion

The ventriculus terminalis is also known as "fifth ventricle". It is a small ependyma-lined cavity in the conus medullaris which is usually continuous with the central canal of the distal spinal cord. It was first described by Stilling in 1859 and a more detailed classification was given by Kernohan in 1924. Although originally thought to be present only in children, it has also been described in adults. It is present mainly in asymptomatic people; however, in rare cases it is considered to be the cause of back pain. It is formed during embryogenesis as a result of the differentiation between the canalization and regression of the spinal cord. The clinical significance of this normal structure is that it must be distinguished from syringohydromyelia and intramedullary cystic tumors. Syringohydromyelia that is limited only to lumbar segments is extremely uncommon. There is high incidence of associated birth defects with syringohydromyelia, most commonly spina bifida occulta, pes cavus and syndactylism. None of these features should be present in children with ventriculus terminalis.

Suggested Reading

Coleman LT, Zimmerman RA, Rorke LB (1995) Ventriculus terminus of the conus medullaris: MR findings in children. AJNR Am J Neuroradiol 16:1421–1426

Kernohan JW (1924) The ventricose terminalis: its growth and development. J Comp Neurol 38:10–125

Poser CM (1956) The relationship between syringomyelia and neoplasms. Thomas, Springfield

Sijal R, Denys A, Halimi P, Shapeero L, Doyon D, Voudghene F (1991) Ventriculus terminalis of the conus medullaris: MR imaging in four patients with congenital dilatation. AJNR Am J Neuroradiol 12:733–737

Diastematomyelia

Separate Thecal Sacs

Clinical Presentation

Female with known spina bifida and long history of bladder dysfunction and gait difficulties.

Images (Fig. 10.5)

A. Axial T2-weighted image through the lumbar spine demonstrates two hemicords (*arrows*) at the L2–3 level each surrounded by a separate thecal sac and divided by a fibrous band (*arrowhead*)

B. Sagittal T2-weighted image through the lumbar spine shows the distal widened spinal canal with a linear area of hypointense signal that represents the midline spur (*arrowhead*). One hemicord has syringohydromyelia (*arrow*)

C. AP view of the lumbar spine. Another patient. Irregular bony spur is present (*arrow*) at L2–3. There is also widening of the interpedicular distance with segmentation anomaly

Single Thecal Sac

Clinical Presentation

A 7-month-old male with dysraphism and dermal sinus over the right side of the sacrum.

Images (Fig. 10.6)

A. Sagittal T2-weighted image shows a wide distal spinal canal and thecal sac with spinal dysraphism and tethered cord at the S2 level. The cord bifurcates at L2 and both hemicords (*arrows*) extend inferiorly to the S2 level. No fibrous, cartilaginous or bony spur is seen

B. Axial T2-weighted image shows both hemicords inside the same thecal sac. This was also visualized in a myelogram study, where contrast was seen between the hemicords (not shown). The right hemicord is slightly larger and distally divides to anterior and posterior segment (see A). Both hemicords have anterior and posterior roots (*arrowheads*). The dermal sinus did not extend to the thecal sac

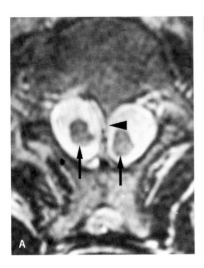
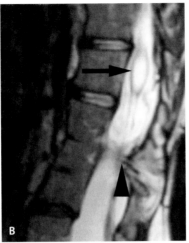
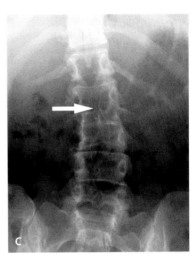

Figure 10.5

Diastematomyelia with separate thecal sacs

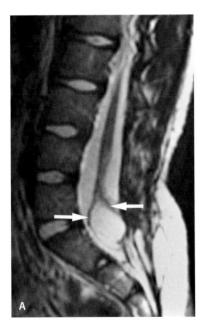
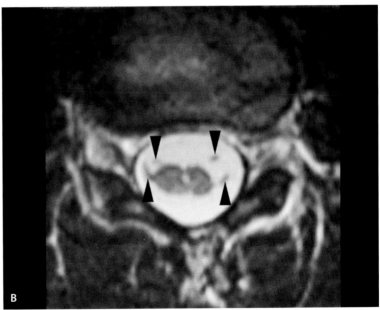

Figure 10.6

Diastematomyelia with single thecal sac

Discussion

Diastematomyelia is a rare entity in which some portion of the spinal cord is split into two symmetric or asymmetric hemicords by a midline septum. The septum may be fibrous bony or cartilaginous and may occur at any level with the thoracic spine being the commonest location. There are two types of diastematomyelia. The first type has a midsagittal bony osteocartilaginous spur separating the spinal cord into two parts, each with its own arachnoid and dural sheath. The second type has no spur, but has a split spinal cord that lies within a single arachnoid and dural sheath. Females are more often affected than males.

Plain films and CT scan show widening of the spinal canal with a bony septum. MR imaging is the modality of choice for diastematomyelia as it provides direct visualization of the split cord and helps in identifying other associated abnormalities. There is often a cutaneous stigma, most commonly a long silky patch of hair (Fawn's tail) or dermal sinus. There is also a high incidence of spinal segmentation anomalies, such as hemivertebrae and butterfly vertebrae. There are often associated orthopedic abnormalities. The symptoms are often those of tethered cord. Both cutaneous stigmata and segmentation anomalies occur at the same level as the split cord, thus representing an important clue to the level of the lesion.

Suggested Reading

Han JS, Benson JE, Kaufman B, et al (1985) Demonstration of diastematomyelia and associated abnormalities with MR imaging. AJNR Am J Neuroradiol.6:215–219

Pang D, Dias MS, Ahab-Barmada M (1992) Split cord malformation, part 1. A unified theory of embryogenesis for double spinal cord malformations. Neurosurgery 31:451–480

Dermal Sinus Tract

Clinical presentation

A 4-day-old full-term girl with a deep sacral dimple with yellow drainage. Ultrasonography showed a dermal sinus tract with air in it.

Images (Fig. 10.7)

A. Sagittal proton density image shows a sinus tract (*arrow*) extending from the sacral dimple through the subcutaneous fat to the tip of the coccyx. It is low signal in all pulse sequences compatible with an air-containing structure or a fibrous band. No connection is seen with the thecal sac

B. Axial T1-weighted image shows the low signal band (*arrow*) from the dimple to the coccyx. No fluid was seen on the T2-weighted image (not shown)

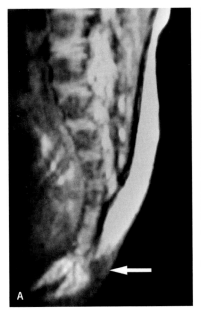
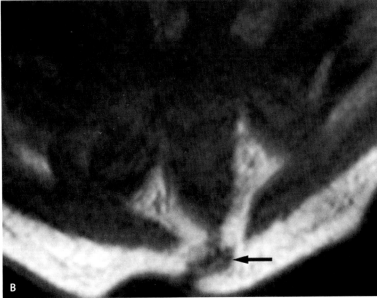

Figure 10.7

Dermal sinus tract

Discussion

Congenital dermal sinus (CDS) is an epithelium-lined tube extending from the skin inward to varying depths. The sinus may terminate in the subcutaneous tissue, paraspinal muscle, vertebrae, dura, or spinal cord. They can occur at any level along the spinal axis but are most commonly seen in the lower lumbosacral segment, followed by the occipital area. The hallmark of CDS is a midline cutaneous dimple overlying the spine. CDS may become symptomatic as a result of either infection, or associated mass lesions, which can be epidermoid, dermoid or teratoma.

Radiologically, MR imaging provides rapid and accurate identification of the extent of these lesions. It shows the extraspinal portion of the sinus tract and associated inclusion tumor, and defines the degree of spinal cord compression. The dermoid cyst is seen as hypointense lesion on T1-weighted and hyperintense on T2-weighted images with peripheral enhancement on contrast administration.

Suggested Reading

Ceddia A, Di Rocco C, Pastorelli G (1990) The congenital cervical dermal sinus. A clinical case report and review of literature. Minerva Pediatr 42:553–558

Lee J-K, Kim J-H, Kim J-S, et al (2001) Cervical dermal sinus associated with dermoid cyst. Childs Nerv Syst 17:491–493

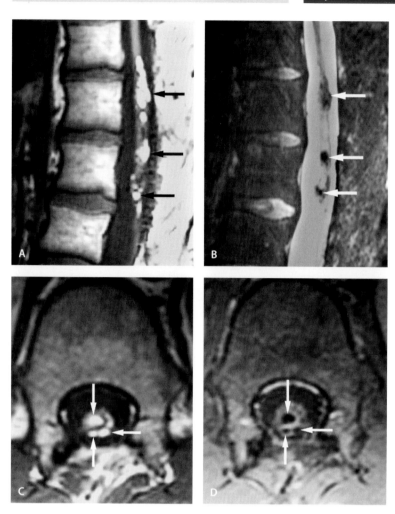

Figure 10.8

Intra- and extramedullary lipomas

Spinal Lipomas

Case 1. Intra- and Extramedullary Lipomas

Clinical Presentation

Young adult male with long-term symptoms of bladder dysfunction.

Images (Fig. 10.8)

A. Sagittal T1-weighted image shows small multiple round hyperintense foci on the surface of the distal thoracic cord and conus consistent with intradural and extramedullary lipomas (*arrows*)
B. The lipomas are hypointense on T2-weighted fat-saturated image (*arrows*)
C. Axial T1-weighted image shows the hyperintense lipomas to be intra- and extramedullary in location (*arrows*)
D. Contrast-enhanced T1-weighted image with fat suppression fails to demonstrate contrast enhancement in the hypointense lipomas (*arrows*)

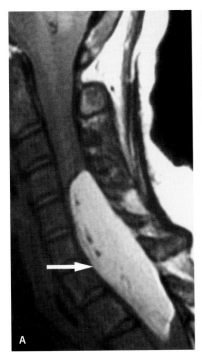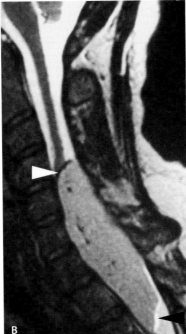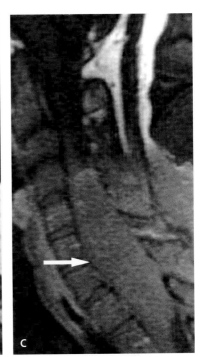

Figure 10.9

Extramedullary cervical lipoma with cord compression

Case 2. Extramedullary Cervical Lipoma with Cord Compression

Clinical Presentation

The patient has a long history of cord compression symptoms. Surgery confirmed the location and fatty nature of the encapsulated lesion.

Images (Fig. 10.9)

A. Sagittal proton density image through the cervical canal shows a large intradural lipoma (*arrow*). The canal is widened secondary to long-standing pressure by the lipoma
B. The lipoma is slightly hyperintense compared to the spinal cord on T2-weighted image. Note the chemical shift misregistration artifacts at the CSF/lipoma and lipoma/CSF borders (*arrowheads*)
C. T1-weighted fat-suppressed image shows the fatty nature of the lesion (*arrow*)

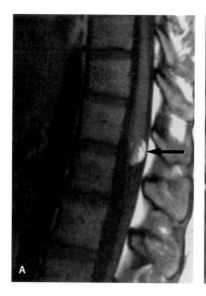
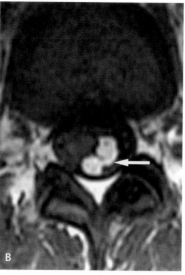

Figure 10.10

Intradural, extramedullary lipoma at the conus

Case 3. Intradural, Extramedullary Lipoma at the Conus

Clinical Presentation

Young adult with a 1-year history of back and leg pain.

Images (Fig. 10.10)

A. Sagittal T1-weighted image. A simple lipoma is attached to the surface of the distal conus (*arrow*), the T12–L1 level
B. The lipoma wraps around the conus on the left side (*arrow*)

Discussion

Lipomas are rare tumors most often found in relation to meninges and account for 1% of all intraspinal tumors. The majority of them are found in the thoracic region, although they can occur anywhere in the canal. Cutaneous stigmata are usually absent in patients with lipoma. The lipomas can be large enough to cause cord compression.

Spinal cord lipomas have been described as consisting of muscle (myolipoma), neuroglia (neurolipoma), fibrous tissue (fibroblastic lipoma), and proliferating vessels (angiolipoma). Frequently, they are intradural and extramedullary. Rarely, they may be intramedullary and intraosseous.

On CT, a lipoma is well defined and homogeneously hypodense with a fatty attenuation value (–15 to –100HU). On MR, lipoma is seen as a hyperintense signal on T1-weighted and hypointense on T2-weighted images. A T1-weighted image with fat suppression is helpful in doubtful cases to differentiate the lipid-containing lesion from methemoglobin in a hematoma.

Suggested Reading

Phillips WE II, Figueroa RE, Viloria J, Ransohoff J (1995) Lumbosacral spinal intradural extramedullary paciniomyolipoma: magnetic resonance imaging, computed tomography, and pathology findings. J Neuroimaging 5:130–132

Xenos C, Sgouros S, Walsh R, Hockley A (2000) Spinal lipomas in children. Pediatr Neurosurg 32:295–307

Figure 10.11

Caudal regression syndrome

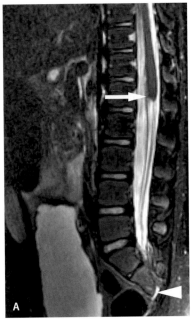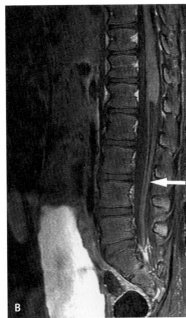

Caudal Regression Syndrome

Clinical Presentation

A 4-year-old male with urinary retention and sacral agenesis on radiographs.

Images (Fig. 10.11)

A. Sagittal T2-weighted image shows typical blunted appearance of conus medullaris (*arrow*). This is due to a decreased number of anterior horn cells. There is absence of the distal sacral segments (*arrowhead*). An enlarged and trabeculated bladder is seen

B. Sagittal contrast-enhanced T1-weighted image with fat suppression shows thickened posterior roots (*arrow*)

Discussion

Caudal regression syndrome (CRS) is a rare congenital anomaly of the lower vertebral column, frequently associated with orthopedic deformities, and genitourinary, gastrointestinal and neurological malformations. Maternal diabetes, genetic predisposition and vascular hypoperfusion have been suggested as possible causative factors.

Prenatal sonography is the diagnostic tool for fetal spine for the diagnosis of CRS that can be made by 20–22 weeks of gestation. Transvaginal sonography increases the sensitivity by diagnosing the syndrome at 11–12 weeks of gestation. MR imaging is the modality of choice, since it effectively demonstrates the level of vertebral agenesis, the position and configuration of the spinal cord and also associated anomalies of the spine. The conus is usually clubshaped and ends at an unusually high position.

It has been suggested that segmental spinal dysgenesis (SSD) and CRS may represent two manifestations of a single spectrum of segmental malformations of the spine and spinal cord. The only difference from an embryological standpoint is the location of the segmental derangement along the longitudinal axis of the developing embryo. There are, however, reasons to differentiate CRS from other forms of dysraphism, since patients with CRS suffer from congenital hypoplasia/aplasia of the nerve roots rather than cord tethering. There patients are less likely to benefit from untethering surgery.

Suggested Reading

Adra A, Cordero D, Mejides A, Yasin S, Salman F, O'Sullivan MJ (1994) Caudal regression syndrome: etiopathogenesis, prenatal diagnosis, and perinatal management. Obstet Gynecol Surv 49:508–516

Gonzalez-Quintero VH, Tolaymat L, Martin D, Romaguera RL, Rodriguez MM, Izquierdo LA (2002) Sonographic diagnosis of caudal regression in the first trimester of pregnancy. J Ultrasound Med 21:1175–1178

Tortori-Donati P, Fondelli MP, Rossi A, Raybaud CA, Cama A, Capra V (1999) Segmental spinal dysgenesis: neuroradiologic findings with clinical and embryologic correlation. AJNR Am J Neuroradiol 20:445–456

Unal O, Sakarya ME, Arslan H (1999) The club-shaped cord terminus in siblings with caudal agenesis: MRI. Neuroradiology 41:735–737

Congenital Spinal Scoliosis, Kyphosis and Kyphoscoliosis

Lumbar Hemivertebra

Clinical Presentation

A 3-year-old with developmental delay and scoliosis.

Images (Fig. 10.12)

A. Plain film shows incomplete separation of L3 and L4 vertebral bodies. L3 has two pedicles (*arrowheads*), right and left, while L4 has only a right pedicle (*arrow*). The L3-L4 complex is incompletely separated from the L5 vertebral body. T12 has a rudimentary rib on the right

B. Right lateral sagittal T2-weighted image shows two pedicles and laminae (*arrows*) at L3–4 leading to mild scoliosis

C. Midsagittal T2-weighted image shows the incompletely separated L3–4 complex from L5

D. Left-lateral sagittal T2-weighted image shows normal-appearing vertebral body separations

E. Axial T2-weighted image through the L3–4 hemivertebra reveals asymmetry of the pedicles

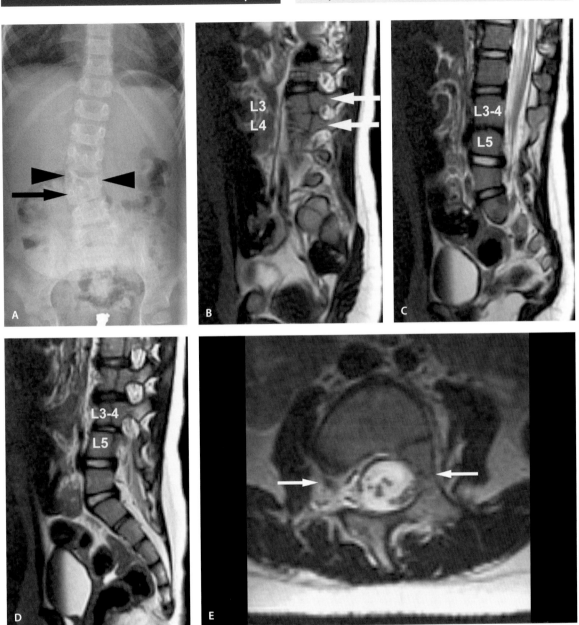

Figure 10.12
Lumbar hemivertebra

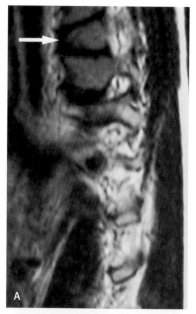

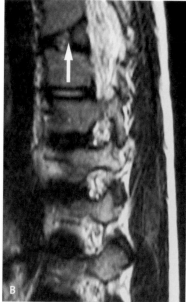

Figure 10.13

Thoracic hemivertebra

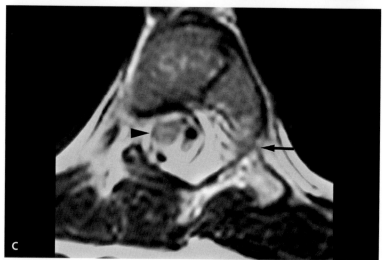

Thoracic Hemivertebra

Clinical Presentation

An 8-year-old asymptomatic male with scoliosis.

Images (Fig. 10.13)

A. Sagittal T2-weighted image through the left pedicles shows scoliosis and a hemivertebra of T8 (*arrow*). There is no lamina
B. Sagittal image through the right pedicles shows anterior wedging of the T8 hemivertebra (*arrow*)
C. Axial T2-weighted image shows the left hemivertebra with pedicle (*arrow*). Note that the cord takes the shortest course through the scoliotic canal (*arrowhead*)

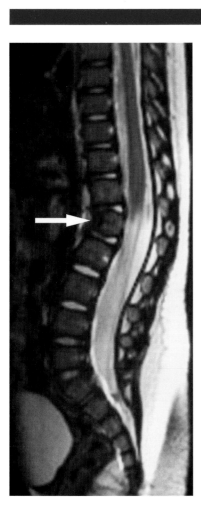

Figure 10.14

Kyphosis

Kyphosis

Clinical Presentation

A 12-month-old asymptomatic male with kyphosis since birth.

Images (Fig. 10.14)

A. Sagittal T2-weighted image shows failure in anterior vertebral body formation (type I kyphosis, subtype: anterior wedge formation) of L1 (*arrow*) with decreased anterior vertebral body height. The malformation is limited to the vertebral body, with normal-appearing cord

Discussion

Congenital scoliosis and kyphoscoliosis are present at birth, but the deformity might not become clinically apparent until later in childhood. Congenital kyphosis and kyphoscoliosis are more rare than congenital scoliosis. The most common type of kyphosis is due to failure of formation of the anterior segment (type I with various subtypes) of the vertebral body. Hemivertebra can also cause, in addition to scoliosis, canal compromise. In patients with scoliosis, the most common type of hemivertebra is fully segmented; semisegmented and incarcerated types are less common. The two latter types usually do not require treatment. Fully segmented nonincarcerated hemivertebra may require prophylactic treatment to prevent significant deformity. Additional cord abnormalities associated with hemivertebra are not common.

Suggested Reading

McMaster MJ, David CV (1986) Hemivertebra as a cause of scoliosis. A study of 104 patients. J Bone Joint Surg Br 68:588–595

McMaster MJ, Singh H (1999) Natural history of congenital kyphosis and kyphoscoliosis. A study of one hundred and twelve patients. J Bone Joint Surg Am 81:1367–1383

Winter RB, Lonstein JE, Heithoff KB, Kirkham JA (1997) Magnetic resonance imaging evaluation of the adolescent patient with idiopathic scoliosis before spinal instrumentation and fusion. A prospective, double-blinded study of 140 patients. Spine 15:855–858

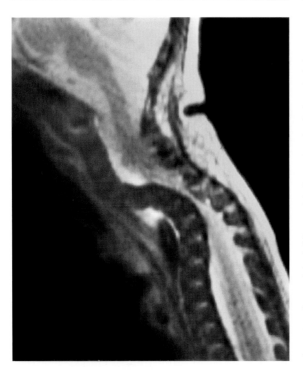

Figure 10.15

Arthrogryposis (Larsen's syndrome)

Arthrogryposis (Larsen's Syndrome)

Clinical Presentation

An 11-day-old male infant with arthrogryposis multiplex congenita (Larsen's syndrome).

Images (Fig. 10.15)

A. Sagittal T2-weighted image shows prominent kyphosis in cervicothoracic junction with severe narrowing of the canal at the T2 level with cord compression; otherwise the canal is capacious. The brain and cerebellum were normal

Discussion

Arthrogryposis is a congenital, nonprogressive limitation of movement in two or more joints in different body areas. Arthrogryposis is a rare condition, with an incidence of 1 in 5000–10,000 live births. It is of unknown etiology. Generally, the vast majority of these children are categorized under the diagnosis of arthrogryposis multiplex congenita. Larsen et al. in 1950 described the association of multiple congenital dislocations with a characteristic facial abnormality, known as Larsen's syndrome.

Larsen's syndrome is characterized by joint hypermobility, multiple joint dislocations, especially of the hips and knees, and talipes equinovarus. The midface is hypoplastic with a depressed nasal bridge and bossing of the forehead. Cleft palate may be present. Radiographs reveal under-mineralization of the long bones, a bifid calcaneus and advanced bone age in the carpal bones or extra carpal bones. The spine shows scoliosis, subluxation and coronal clefts of the vertebrae. Spinal anomalies may lead to major spinal instability and cord injury. The cervical cord is more affected than the rest of the spine. Since early surgical stabilization may be necessary to prevent cord injury, serial imaging may be necessary to avoid neurological sequelae.

Suggested Reading

Banks JT, Wellons JC III, Tubbs RS, Blount JP, Oakes WJ, Grabb PA (2003) Cervical spine involvement in Larsen's syndrome: a case illustration. Pediatrics 111:199–201

Larsen LJ, Schottstaedt ER, Bost FD (1950) Multiple congenital dislocations associated with characteristic facial abnormality. J Pediatr 37:574–581

Wong V (1997) The spectrum of arthrogryphosis in 33 Chinese children. Brain Dev 19:187–196

Mucopolysaccharidoses (MPS)

Hurler/Scheie Syndrome (MPS Type I H/S)

Clinical Presentation

A 22-year-old female with multiple genetic abnormalities and known MPS Type I H/S. The patient presents with new right leg weakness and left leg numbness and tingling and increasing weakness in both arms. Patient also has brain changes (see chapter 3).

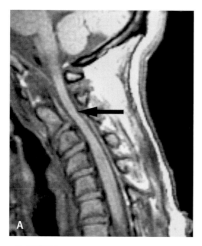

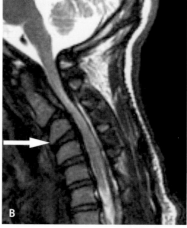

Figure 10.16

Hurler/Scheie syndrome
(MPS type I H/S)

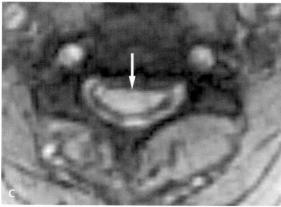

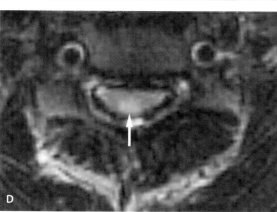

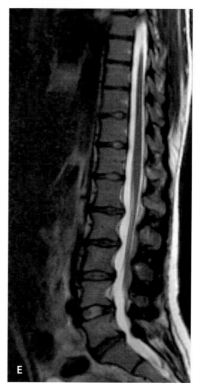

Images (Fig. 10.16)

A. Sagittal T1-weighted image demonstrates increased kyphosis with marked narrowing of the spinal canal from the foramen magnum to the upper border of C5. Additionally, there is evidence of cord compression at the C2–3 and C3–4 levels with flattening of the cord (*arrow*)

B. Sagittal T2-weighted image demonstrates increased signal intensity within the cord suggesting myelopathy. Inferior beaking of the vertebral body is seen at C3 (*arrow*)

C. Axial gradient echo image through the narrowed area demonstrates cord flattening (*arrow*)

D. Axial T2-weighted image through the same area demonstrates cord edema (*arrow*)

E. Sagittal T2-weighted image demonstrates multi-level degenerative disc disease with posterior disc/osteophyte complexes

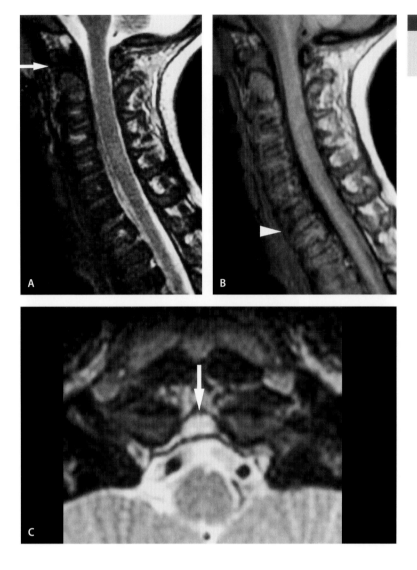

Figure 10.17

Morquio's syndrome
(MPS type IV-A)

Morquio's Syndrome (MPS Type IV-A)

Clinical Presentation

A 4-year-old girl with clinical suspicion of craniocervical instability.

Images (Fig. 10.17)

A. Sagittal T2-weighted image shows a hypoplastic dens (*arrow*). No spinal canal narrowing is seen
B. Sagittal proton density image shows platyspondyly with prominent beaking of the anterior portions of the lower vertebral bodies (*arrowhead*)

C. Axial T2-weighted image shows the absent dens (*arrow*)

Discussion

MPS are inherited metabolic disorders due to deficiency of lysosomal enzymes required for the catabolism of mucopolysaccharides or glycosaminoglycans. Based on the type of enzyme deficiency, ten MPS types have been classified with different clinical manifestations. The group comprises progressive multisystemic disorders mainly affecting the skeleton, eyes and internal organs. The CNS is affected to a variable degree.

Hurler/Scheie Syndrome: The typical skeletal findings in classical MPS (Hunter's disease) seen in the cervical spine include thickening of the soft tissue posterior to the odontoid process, disc dehydration with anteroinferior beaking of the vertebral bodies. In contrast to the classical form of MPS I, skeletal changes of the spine are usually minimal in Hurler/ Scheie syndrome. Soft tissue compression of the cervical cord has been described in Hurler disease.

Morquio's Syndrome: MPS IV (MPS Type IVa-c) is an uncommon autosomal recessive disorder. It is characterized by excessive excretion of keratin sulfate in the urine. In addition to chest wall and spinal deformities, the children with Morquio's syndrome have hypoplasia of the dens (odontoid process) as a consistent finding causing cervical myelopathy. This particular finding of hypoplasia of the dens also puts them at a considerable risk of anterior dislocation of the vertebral axis with resultant spinal cord compression.

Suggested Reading

Hughes DG, Chadderton RD, Cowie RA, Wraith JE, Jenkins JP (1997) MRI of the brain and craniocervical junction in Morquio's disease. Neuroradiology 39:381–385

Kachur E, del Maestro R (2000) Mucopolysaccharidoses and spinal cord compression: case report and review of the literature with implications of bone marrow transplantation. Neurosurgery 47:223–228

Parsons VJ, Hughes DG, Wraith JE (1996) Magnetic resonance imaging of the brain, neck and cervical spine in mild Hunter's syndrome (mucopolysaccharidoses type II). Clin Radiol 5:719–723

Rigante D, Antuzzi D, Ricci R, Segni G (1999) Cervical myelopathy in mucopolysaccharidosis type IV. Clin Neuropathol 18:84–86

Schmidt H, Ullrich K, von Lengerke HJ, Kleine M, Bramswig J (1987) Radiological findings in patients with mucopolysaccharidosis I H/S (Hurler-Scheie syndrome). Pediatr Radiol 17:409–414

Tandon V, Williamson JB, Cowie RA, Wraith JE (1996) Spinal problems in mucopolysaccharidosis I (Hurler syndrome). J Bone Joint Surg Br 78:938–944

Spinal Cord Astrocytoma

Clinical Presentation

An 8-year-old female with known low-grade astrocytoma in the cervical cord since the age of 18 months when she presented with breathing and swallowing difficulties.

Images (Fig. 10.18)

A. Sagittal T2-weighted image reveals intramedullary slightly heterogeneous tumor (*white arrow*) in the upper spinal cord extending to the medulla (*black arrow*) and lower pons. Cord edema is evident inferior to the mass (*black arrowhead*). Congenital fusion of C2–3 vertebral bodies is seen (*white arrowhead*). Decompression surgery has been performed
B. Sagittal T1-weighted image shows intramedullary slightly hyperintense tumor mass (*arrow*) posteriorly with low signal edema inferior to the mass (*arrowhead*)
C. Sagittal STIR better outlines the full extent of the tumor (*arrow*) and edema (*arrowhead*)
D. Sagittal contrast-enhanced T1-weighted image shows intense contrast enhancement in the tumor (*arrow*)
E. Axial T2-weighted image shows expansion of the cord with slightly eccentric mass along the posterior margin of the cord (*arrow*)
F. Axial contrast-enhanced T1-weighted image with fat suppression shows the eccentric location of the tumor and homogeneous enhancement (*arrow*)

Discussion

Astrocytomas are most common intramedullary spinal cord tumors in children. Male patients are more commonly involved. The cervical spine is the most common site, closely followed by the thoracic cord. Multisegmental involvement is the rule. The involvement of the entire cord (holocord presentation) is common in children. Astrocytomas are rare in the region of the filum terminale. Tumor cysts and syrinx formation are common, especially in grade I tumors. In the WHO classification, four grades are recognized (grade I to IV), where grade I corresponds to pilocytic astrocytoma, grade II fibrillary type, grade III

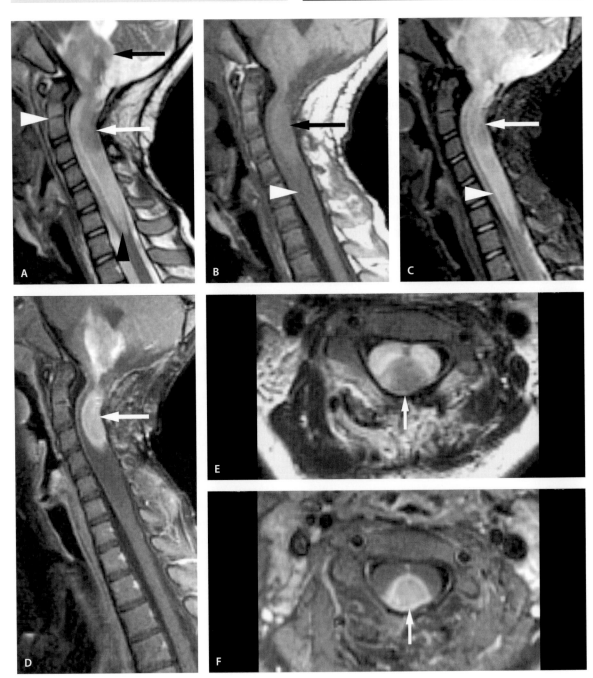

Figure 10.18

Spinal cord astrocytoma

anaplastic astrocytomas, and grade IV glioblastoma multiforme. Although grade IV tumors make up half of the brain astrocytomas, they are uncommon in the spinal cord. The well-differentiated grade I astrocytoma accounts for 75% of spinal cord astrocytomas.

On plain films and CT, mild scoliosis, widened interpedicular distance and bone erosions are commonly seen. These signs are less common in astrocytomas than in ependymomas. On MR imaging, astrocytomas are iso- to slightly hypointense on T1-weighted images and hyperintense on T2-weighted images. They are ill-defined and show patchy enhancement. Cysts are a common feature, with both polar and intratumoral types being commonly observed. Intramedullary astrocytomas are usually eccentric since they arise from cord parenchyma.

Suggested Reading

Koeller KY, Rosenblum RS, Morrison AL (2000) Neoplasms of the spinal cord and filum terminale: radiologic-pathologic correlation. Radiographics 20:1721–1749

Lowe GM (2000) Magnetic resonance imaging of intramedullary spinal cord tumors. J Neurooncol 47:195–210

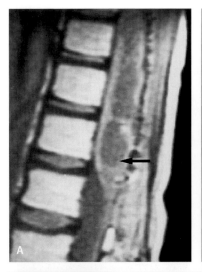

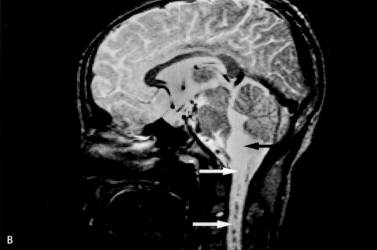

Figure 10.19

Holocord ependymoma

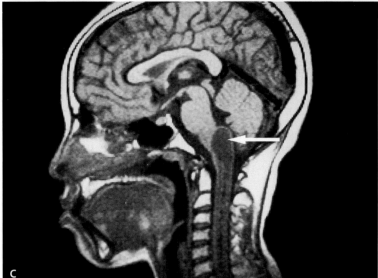

Intraspinal Ependymoma

Holocord Ependymoma

Clinical Presentation

A 13-year-old boy with gradual onset of motor and sensory deficits and leg pain.

Images (Fig. 10.19)

A. Sagittal contrast-enhanced T1-weighted image shows expanded conus with a cystic intramedullary tumor (*arrow*) and with associated multilocular cavities throughout the cord
B. T2-weighted image reveals a septate syringohydromyelia up to the medulla oblongata (*arrows*)
C. T1-weighted image shows diffuse expansion of the medulla and cervical cord with a large cyst (*arrow*) in the medulla. This patient has a holocord extension of the lesion

Figure 10.20

Conus ependymoma

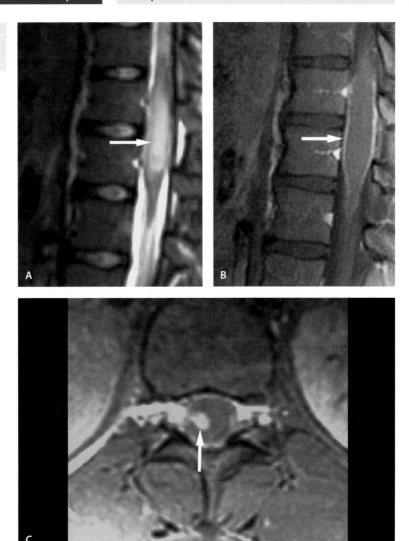

Conus Ependymoma

Clinical Presentation

A 15-year-old female with back and leg pain and walking difficulties.

Images (Fig. 10.20)

A. Sagittal T2-weighted image reveals expansion of the conus (*arrow*). The mass is hyperintense to the normal cord
B. Sagittal contrast-enhanced T1-weighted image with fat suppression reveals peripheral enhancement of the lesion (*arrow*)

C. Axial contrast-enhanced T1-weighted image with fat suppression demonstrates focal enhancement of the mass (*arrow*) with eccentric location of the mass

Discussion

Spinal intramedullary neoplasms account for 4–10% of all CNS tumors. Spinal cord ependymomas are the most common type of intraspinal gliomas in adults whereas astrocytomas are most common in children. Both entities constitute up to 70% of all intramedullary intraspinal gliomas. Ependymomas commonly involve the lower thoracic cord, conus, and the filum terminale. Myxopapillary ependymoma, a histological variant, is virtually always located along the filum terminale with occasional extension to the conus medullaris. The symptoms often mimic those of a discogenic pathology. They are characteristically sausage-shaped masses with hyperintense T2 signal and intense enhancement.

Ependymomas tend to arise centrally and expand the cord in a centrifugal pattern, reflecting the origin of ependymal cells lining the central canal. Localized involvement is the most common presentation, although holocord involvement is seen. Cysts are a common feature, with three-quarters having at least one cyst. Associated syringohydromyelia is also seen often. The majority of ependymomas show heterogeneous contrast enhancement. Multifocal ependymomas are generally found in teenagers and people with neurofibromatosis type 2.

On noncontrast MR imaging, ependymomas are usually isointense to cord on T1-weighted images and hyperintense on T2-weighted images. Foci of hemorrhage are frequently associated with ependymoma, especially capping the superior and inferior borders of the tumor. After contrast administration, ependymomas usually show intense, homogeneous sharply marginated enhancement. In about 20–33% of ependymomas, a rim of extreme hypointensity (hemosiderin) suggestive of the "cap sign" may be seen at the poles of the tumor on T2-weighted images. Ependymomas need to be differentiated from astrocytomas. A central location within the cord, the presence of a cleavage plane and intense homogeneous enhancement are imaging features that favor ependymoma.

Suggested Reading

Do-Dai DD, Rovira MJ, Ho VB, Gomez RR (1995) Childhood onset of myxopapillary ependymomatosis: MR features. AJNR Am J Neuroradiol 16:835–839

Miyazawa N, Hida K, Iwasaki Y, Koyanagi I, Abe H (2000) MRI at 1.5 T of intramedullary ependymoma and classification of pattern of contrast enhancement. Neuroradiology 42:828–832

Sun B, Wang C, Wang J, Liu A (2003) MRI features of intramedullary spinal cord ependymomas. J Neuroimaging 13:346–351

Sze G (1992) MR imaging of the spinal cord: current status and future advances. Review. AJR Am J Roentgenol 159:149–159

Sze G, Stimac GK, Bartlett C, Dillon WP, Haughton VM, Orrison W, Kashanian F, Goldstein H (1990) Multicenter study of gadopentetate dimeglumine as an MR contrast agent: evaluation in patients with spinal tumors. AJNR Am J Neuroradiol 11:967–974

Neurofibromatosis Type 1 (NF-1)

Clinical Presentation

A 16-year-old girl with known NF-I. She presents with balance and coordination problems.

Images (Fig. 10.21)

A. Sagittal T2-weighted image with fat suppression of the cervical and upper thoracic spine shows enlargement of the neural foramina with multiple rounded neurofibromas (*arrows*)

B. Axial T2-weighted image through a cervical canal reveals large soft-tissue masses extending out of the neural foramina (*arrows*). The cord is compressed by these masses (*arrowheads*). Numerous soft-tissue neurofibromas are seen

C. Sagittal contrast-enhanced T1-weighted image with fat suppression through the lumbosacral spine shows many tiny enhancing neurofibromas in the cauda equina (*arrows*)

D. T2-weighted image shows hypointensity of the cauda equina neurofibromas (*arrows*)

E. Enhanced coronal T1-weighted image with fat suppression of the cervical spine (another patient) better shows the extent of bilateral neurofibromas that enhance with contrast

Discussion

Neurofibromas are almost always associated with neurofibromatosis type 1 (NF-1, Von Recklinghausen's Disease). NF-1 is the most common neurocutaneous syndrome. Manifestations can arise from almost any system of the body. In the spine, the lesions can be best detected by MRI. These lesions include dural dysplasias, such as dural ectasia and lateral meningocele and spinal tumors, most commonly benign neurofibromas. These tumors typically demonstrate bone expansion: expansion of the spinal canal and neural foramina. There is often erosion of pedicles, laminar thinning and scalloping of the vertebral body. In addition to spinal neurofibromas, intramedullary neurofibromas have been described in association with NF-1. Neurofibromas appear isointense to the neural tissue on CT imaging and they rarely calcify. They demonstrate variable contrast enhancement. On MR imaging neurofibromas are usu-

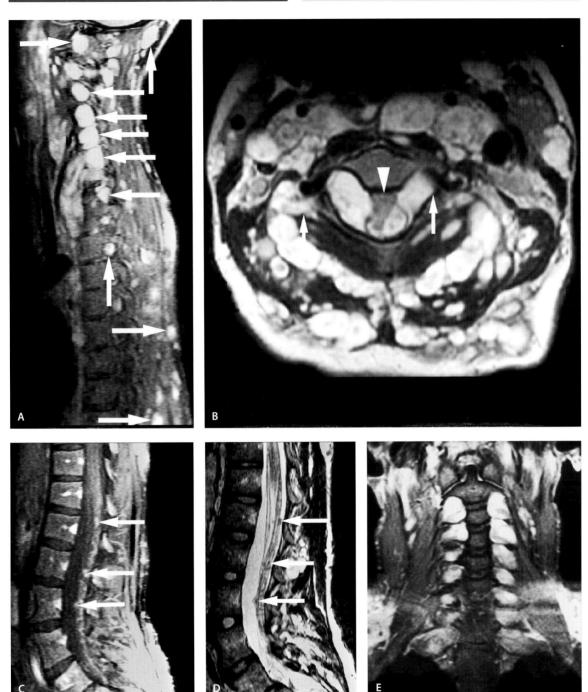

Figure 10.21

Neurofibromatosis type 1 (NF-1)

ally hypointense or isointense in both T1- and T2-weighted images with variable enhancement. Plexiform neurofibromas are composed of Schwann cells and fibroblasts and have more variable appearance on MRI. These are usually larger and can be associated with extensive spinal masses and erosion of the spinal bones. Most malignant peripheral nerve sheath tumors are believed to arise from plexiform neurofibromas, although the risk of malignant transformation is low.

Suggested Reading

Conti P, Pansini G, Mouchaty H, Capuano C, Conti R (2004) Spinal neurinomas: retrospective analysis and long-term outcome of 179 consecutively operated cases and review of the literature. Surg Neurol 61:34–43

Faro SH, Higginson SN, Koenigsberg R, Poon CM, Swidryk JP, Mohammed FB, Zimmerman RA, Chen CY (2000) Phakomatoses, part I. Neurofibromatosis type 1: common and uncommon neuroimaging findings. Review. J Neuroimaging 10:138–146

Khong PL, Goh WH, Wong VC, Fung CW, Ooi GC (2003) MR imaging of spinal tumors in children with neurofibromatosis 1. AJR Am J Roentgenol 180:413–417

Neurofibromatosis Type 2 (NF-2)

Clinical Presentation

A 14-year-old female with known NF-2.

Images (Fig. 10.22)

A. Sagittal T2-wighted image shows multiple intramedullary high signal lesions (*arrows*) with localized cord engorgement

B. Sagittal contrast-enhanced T1-weighted image shows multiple enhancing intramedullary tumors within the cord parenchyma (*arrows*) throughout the cervical and upper thoracic cord

C. Axial T2-weigted image at C3 shows an intramedullary high-signal lesion (*arrow*). The left neural foramen is enlarged by a schwannoma (*arrowhead*)

D. Axial T1-weighted postgadolinium image at C3 shows intense enhancement in the left neural foramen schwannoma (*arrowhead*). Note the bony remodeling at the same level. Part of the intramedullary lesion shows enhancement (*arrow*)

E. Sagittal T2-weighted image with fat suppression through the lumbar spine shows numerous small nodules in the cauda equina (*arrows*) consistent with small nerve sheath tumors (NSTs)

F. Sagittal contrast-enhanced T1-weighted image with fat suppression through the lumbar area shows strong enhancement in the cauda equina NSTs (*arrows*)

G. Axial contrast-enhanced T1-weighted image with fat suppression at T11 shows enhancement of the cauda equina NSTs (*arrows*)

Discussion

NF-2 is an autosomal dominant disorder characterized by the occurrence of bilateral vestibular schwannomas. The NF-2 gene was cloned from chromosome 22q in 1993. A patient is considered to have NF-2 if there is a first-degree relative with NF-2 and either a single eighth nerve mass or any two of the following: schwannoma, neurofibroma, meningioma, glioma, or juvenile posterior subcapsular lens opacity. Although NF-2 is considered to be an adult-onset disease, about 10–18% of children presenting with a meningioma or schwannoma are likely to have NF-2. Unlike NF-1 in which glial tumors are common, the tumors associated with NF-2 generally arise from Schwann and meningothelial cells.

Spinal cord involvement in NF-2 may be seen in 85–90% of cases. Multiple intradural, extramedullary soft-tissue masses of meningiomas or Schwannomas are usually seen. Intramedullary tumors such as ependymoma and astrocytoma are common. These intramedullary tumors are commonly located in the cervicomedullary, cervical and thoracic regions. Osseous abnormalities are common in NF-2 patients.

MR imaging is the modality of choice. Schwannomas are seen as well-delineated masses that are iso- to hypointense compared to brain on T1-weighted sequences and iso- to hyperintense on T2-weighted sequences. Postgadolinium images show strong but heterogeneous enhancement. Solid intramedullary tumors appear hyperintense on T2-weighted images with respect to the normal cord parenchyma. Intramedullary tumors usually enhance with contrast. In the setting of NF-2, the intramedullary tumors show more indolent behavior than tumors in the general population, making frequent follow-up studies necessary. In contrast to intramedullary tumors, the extramedullary tumors may necessitate surgical intervention more often.

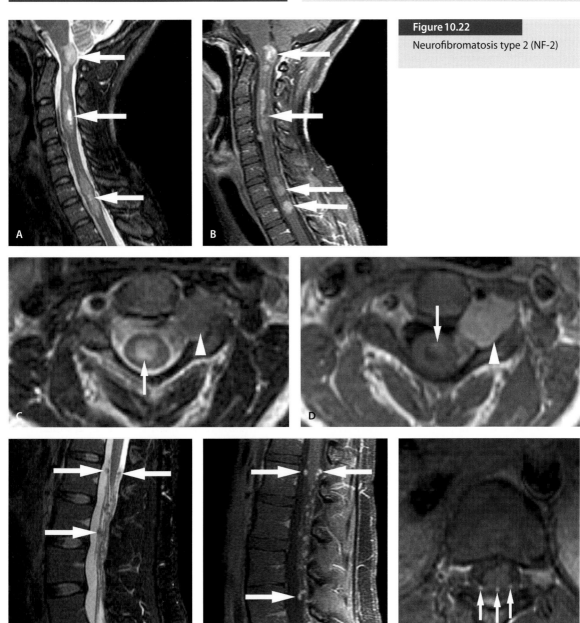

Figure 10.22
Neurofibromatosis type 2 (NF-2)

Suggested Reading

Evans DG, Birch JM, Ramsden RT (1999) Paediatric presentation of type 2 neurofibromatosis. Arch Dis Child 81:496–499

Lee M, Rezai AR, Freed D, Epstein FJ (1996) Intramedullary spinal cord tumors in neurofibromatosis. Neurosurgery 38:32–37

Nunes F, MacCollin M (2003) Neurofibromatosis 2 in the pediatric population. J Child Neurol 18:718–724

Patronas NJ, Courcoutsakis N, Bromley CM, Katzman GL, MacCollin M, Parry DM (2001) Intramedullary and spinal canal tumors in patients with neurofibromatosis 2: MR imaging findings and correlation with genotype. Radiology 218:434–442

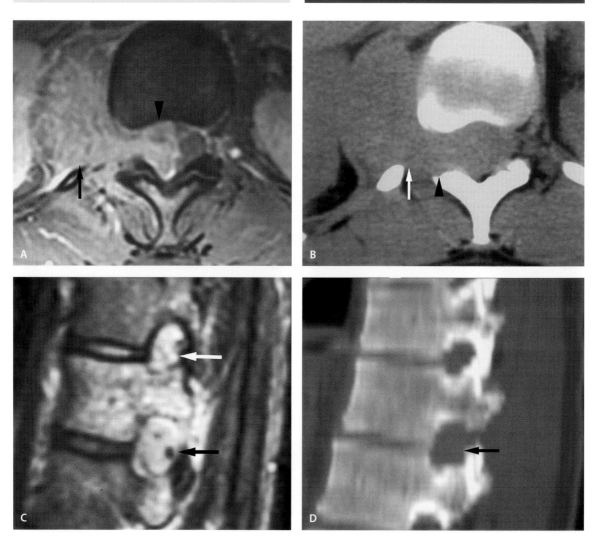

Figure 10.23

Neurofibroma

Neurofibroma

Clinical Presentation

A young adult female with worsening back pain.

Images (Fig. 10.23)

A. Axial contrast-enhanced T1-weighted image through lower the thoracic spine shows an enhancing paraspinal mass lesion (*arrow*) extending to the epidural space (*arrowhead*) through the enlarged neural foramen. The cord is displaced to the left. A diagnosis of neurofibroma was confirmed histopathologically

B. CT scan at the same level as A shows the lesion to be homogeneous and well defined (*arrow*). Bone erosion (*arrowhead*) is better appreciated with CT

C. Sagittal contrast-enhanced T1-weighted image shows the enhancing mass to occupy two neural foramina (*arrows*)

D. Sagittal reconstructed CT scan at the same location as C shows enlargement of only one neural foramen (*arrow*)

Discussion

Tumors of nerve sheath origin include neurilemmoma (schwannoma), neurofibroma, neurofibromatosis and neurogenic sarcoma (malignant schwannoma). More than 90% of these tumors are benign. The benign lesions are seen usually in young and middle-aged adults. Neurilemmoma is more common than neurofibroma. Neurofibromas can present as a solitary tumor or as a component of neurofibromatosis. Although both neurilemmomas and neurofibromas are tumors of nerve sheath origin, each has a characteristic histological appearance and occur in different clinical settings. The microscopic appearance is different: in neurofibromas the nerve fibers run through the lesion, whereas in neurilemmomas the nerve fibers course over the surface of the tumor. Neurofibromas are usually solid tumors without cystic degeneration; however, they may present with myxoid degeneration. Malignant transformation is rare in solitary neurofibroma; it is more common in tumors associated with NF-1.

On CT images neurofibromas appear as homogeneous, round lesions with distinct borders. They demonstrate significant enhancement. If the tumor is located in the paraspinal area, it can have both intra- and extradural components. Neurofibromas have the tendency to be hyperintense on T2-weighted images. Myxoid degeneration can cause the presence of multiple small cystic spaces of various sizes. On CT and MR imaging, neurofibromas occasionally demonstrate a target-like enhancement pattern. There is different enhancement and signal intensity in the central portion than at the periphery of the lesion due to myxoid degeneration peripherally.

Suggested Reading

Faro SH, Higginson SN, Koenigsberg R, Poon CM, Swidryk JP, Mohammed FB, Zimmerman RA, Chen CY (2000) Phakomatoses, part I. Neurofibromatosis type 1: common and uncommon neuroimaging findings. J Neuroimaging 10: 138–146

Rha SE, Byun JY, Jung SE, Chun HJ, Lee HG, Lee JM (2003) Neurogenic tumors in the abdomen: tumor types and imaging characteristics. Radiographics 23:29–43

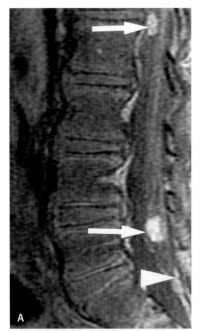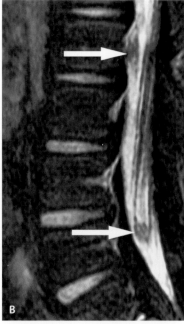

Figure 10.24

Intradural, extramedullary metastases (drop metastases)

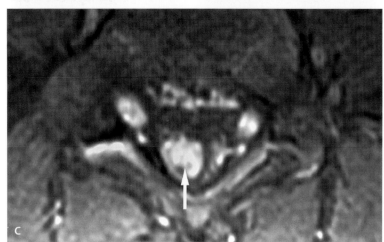

Metastatic Disease from CNS Primary Tumor

Intradural, Extramedullary Metastases (Drop Metastases)

Clinical Presentation

A 4-year-old male with posterior fossa ependymoma and drop metastases in the spinal canal.

Images (Fig. 10.24)

A. Sagittal contrast-enhanced T1-weighted fat-suppressed image demonstrates multiple enhancing nodules (*arrows*) with dural enhancement in the distal conus (*arrowhead*)
B. The metastatic nodules are isointense to the cord in the T2-weighted fat-suppressed image (*arrows*)
C. Axial contrast-enhanced T1-weighted fat-suppressed image shows intense enhancement in the sacral lesion (*arrow*)

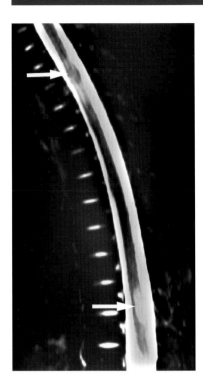

Figure 10.25

Intramedullary metastases

Intramedullary Metastases

Clinical Presentation

A 3-year-old female with posterior fossa medulloblastoma.

Images (Fig. 10.25)

A. Sagittal T2-weighted fat-suppressed image shows multiple hyperintense intramedullary lesions (*arrows*). The lesions enhanced with contrast (not shown)

Discussion

Metastatic tumor spread to the subarachnoid space from another CNS tumor is more common in children than in adults. These metastases can be present already at the time of diagnosis or they can occur later during the treatment without recurrence of the primary tumor. The dropped metastases are most commonly found in the thoracic and lumbar sacral area. The most common CNS neoplasms that present with metastatic CSF disease are primitive neuroectodermal tumor (PNET), pineoblastoma, ependymoma, germinoma, glioblastoma multiforme, lymphoma and choroid plexus tumors. Some uncommon lesions presenting with drop metastases include neuroblastoma, retinoblastoma, rhabdomyosarcoma, oligodendroglioma and leukemia. T1-weighted imaging with contrast enhancement is the most sensitive method for detecting metastatic disease since the nodules may be isointense to the spinal cord on T2-weighted images but they usually present with intense enhancement. They may be also difficult to distinguish from adjacent CSF signal in T2-weighted images. Occasionally diffuse enhancement may be seen in the thecal sac.

Intramedullary metastases are rare. Cerebellar medulloblastoma has been reported to be a causative source. MR imaging is the method of choice to visualize intramedullary lesions. Mild cord expansion is usually present. The lesions are of low signal intensity on T1-weighted images and high signal intensity on T2-weighted images. Cysts are rare in contrast to primary cord tumors. Intramedullary metastases usually demonstrate extensive enhancement.

Suggested Reading

Bradley WG (1999) Use of contrast in MR imaging of the lumbar spine. Magn Reson Imaging Clin North Am 7:439–457

Schick U, Marquardt G, Lorenz R (2001) Intradural and extradural spinal metastases. Neurosurg Rev 24:1–5

Schuknecht B, Huber P, Buller B, Nadjmi M (1992) spinal leptomeningeal neoplastic disease. Eur Neurol 32:11–16

Zumpano BJ (1978) Spinal intramedullary metastatic medulloblastoma. Case report. J Neurosurg 48:632–635

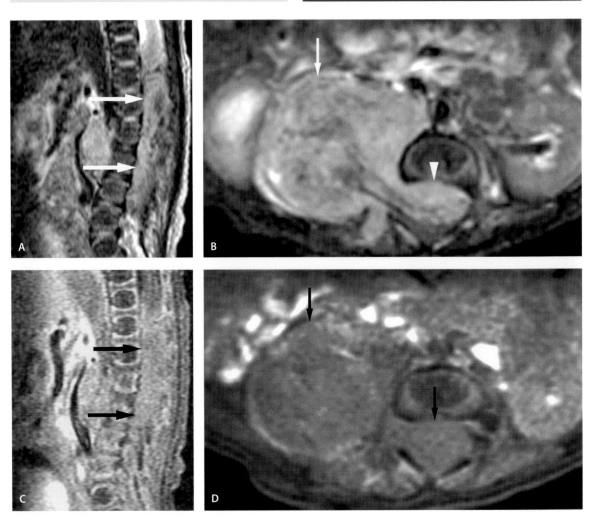

Figure 10.26

Neuroblastoma

Neuroblastoma

Clinical Presentation

A 22-month-old infant with a paraspinal mass.

Images (Fig. 10.26)

A. Sagittal T2-weighted image demonstrates a mixed but mainly hypointense lesion in the lumbar spine. The whole lumbar spinal canal is filled by this hypointense mass
B. Axial T2-weighted image demonstrates a large mixed signal intensity paraspinal mass (*arrow*) with neural foraminal enlargement and spinal canal extension (*arrowhead*)
C. Contrast-enhanced T1-weighted image with fat suppression demonstrates heterogeneous enhancement of the mass (*arrows*)

D. Axial contrast-enhanced T1-weighted image reveals a large paraspinal mass with intraspinal extension (*arrows*). The mass is better appreciated in the fat-suppressed image (C)

Discussion

Neuroblastoma is a malignant tumor of primitive neuroblasts arising within the paravertebral sympathetic chain and adrenal medulla. It can extend from the paraspinal structures into the spinal canal and they are irregular in shape. Most children present before the age of 5 years with two-thirds of the tumors arising in the abdomen. The tumors can arise also in the chest, neck and pelvis. Neuroblastoma tends to metastasize to bone, bone marrow, liver, lymph nodes, and skin. On CT images neuroblastomas demonstrate heterogeneous soft tissue mass with areas of necrosis, hemorrhage, and calcification. MRI is the method of choice for evaluating epidural involvement and cord compression. T1- and T2-weighted images demonstrate heterogeneous signal intensities due to the presence of necrosis, calcifications and hemorrhage. The hyperintensity on T2 images makes it difficult to differentiate intraspinal tumor from CSF. Secondary erosive bony changes and foraminal enlargement can be seen in both CT and MRI.

Suggested Reading

Bousvaros A, Kirks DR, Grossman H (1886) Imaging of neuroblastoma: an overview. Pediatr Radiol 16:89–106

Meyer JS, Harty MP, Khademian Z (2002) Imaging of neuroblastoma and Wilms' tumor. Review. Magn Reson Imaging Clin North Am 10:275–302

Rha SE, Byun JY, Jung SE, Chun HJ, Lee HG, Lee JM (2003) Neurogenic tumors in the abdomen: tumor types and imaging characteristics. Review. Radiographics 23:29–43

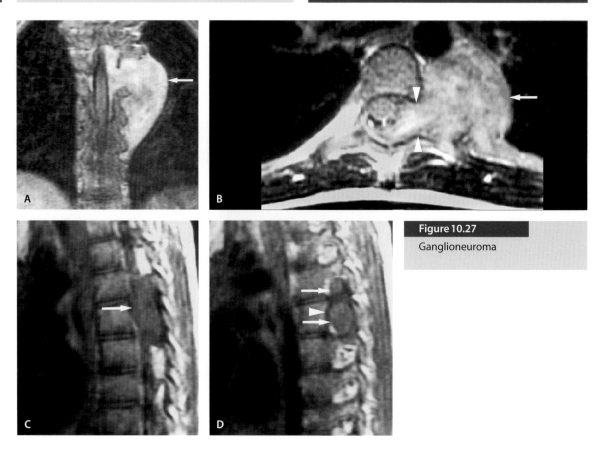

Figure 10.27
Ganglioneuroma

Ganglioneuroma

Clinical Presentation

An 8-year-old female with back pain.

Images (Fig. 10.27)

A. Coronal contrast-enhanced T1-weighted image shows a large retromediastinal mass that extends into the spinal canal through neural foramina (*arrow*). The cord is displaced to the right. The mass demonstrates relatively homogeneous enhancement

B. Axial contrast-enhanced T1-weighted image shows the large retromediastinal mass (*arrows*) with extension through the neural foramen (*arrowheads*) into the spinal canal. The cord is displaced anteriorly and to the right

C. Midsagittal noncontrast T1-weighted image shows hypointense lesion (*arrow*)

D. Sagittal noncontrast T1-weighted image through the neural foramina. The hypointense lesion is seen in two neural foramina (*arrows*) causing bone erosion in the posterior vertebral body (*arrowhead*) and lamina

Discussion

Ganglioneuromas (benign) and ganglioneuroblastomas (intermediate malignancy) are rare types of neural crest tumors that show the same imaging appearance as neuroblastomas (malignant), but have less-aggressive metastatic spread. Neuroblastomas and ganglioneuroblastomas most often occur in infants and younger children, whereas ganglioneuromas tend to occur in older children and young adults. They are composed of mature ganglion cells, nerve fibers and Schwann cells and present as a calcified paraspinal or posterior mediastinal mass with low signal on the T1-weighted image. The T2-weighted signal depends on the proportion of the myxoid stroma to cellular components and the amount of colla-

Figure 10.28

Ependymoblastoma

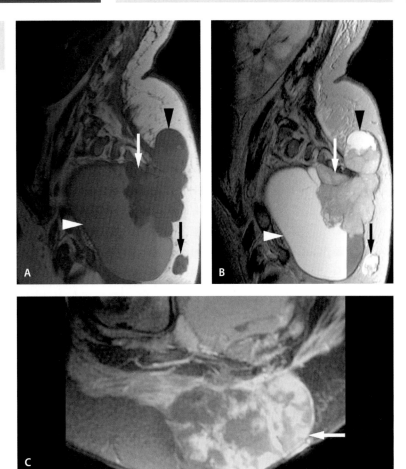

gen fibers in the tumor. The high-signal lesions are rich on myxoid material. The tumor often has characteristic curvilinear bands of low signal intensity. Following contrast injection there is gradual increasing enhancement.

Suggested Reading

Holgersen LO, Santulli TV, Schullinger JN, Berdon WE (1983) Neuroblastoma with intraspinal (dumbbell) extension. J Pediatr Surg 18:406–411

Lonergan GJ, Schwab CM, Suarez ES, Carlson CL (2002) Neuroblastoma, ganglioneuroblastoma, and ganglioneuroma: radiologic-pathologic correlation. Radiographics 22:911–934

Sofka CM, Semelka RC, Kelekis NL, et al (1999) Magnetic resonance imaging of neuroblastoma using current techniques. Magn Reson Imaging 17:193–198

Ependymoblastoma

Clinical Presentation

A 3-year-old female with profound developmental delay presents with acute urinary retention.

Images (Fig. 10.28)

A. Sagittal T1-weighted image shows a large infiltrating mass lesion in the sacrococcygeal area. This well-demarcated mass has solid (*arrow*) and cystic (*arrowheads*) parts and no fat infiltration is seen

B. Sagittal T2-weighted image shows heterogeneous but intermediate intensity in the solid part (*arrow*). Cystic parts show homogeneous hyperintensity (*arrowheads*)

C. Axial contrast-enhanced T1-weighted image with fat suppression shows heterogeneous enhancement in the solid part (*arrow*)

Discussion

Ependymoblastoma is a rare, highly malignant tumor with distinct ependymal differentiation. It is considered to be a subtype of PNETs with clear histological characteristics, which allow its differentiation from medulloblastomas and other PNETs. Ependymoblastoma is seen in young children including neonates with no sex predilection. These tumors are usually massive at the time of diagnosis, yet well circumscribed.

On CT and MR imaging, they are seen as a large, heterogeneous, well-circumscribed mass with no surrounding edema. Mild central enhancement may be seen. Calcification or hemorrhage may be associated. MRI is helpful in demonstrating total absence of peritumoral edema. Ependymoblastoma can be distinguished from PNETs histologically; there is no clear distinction by imaging criteria. All case reports until now have been in the brain in the near proximity of the ventricles; however, the absence of proximity does not exclude the diagnosis.

Suggested Reading

Dorsay TA, Rovira MJ, Ho VB, Kelley J (1995) Ependymoblastoma: MR presentation. A case report and review of the literature. Pediatr Radiol 22:433–435

Ng SH, Ko SF, Chen YL, Wong HF, Wai YY (2002) Ependymoblastoma: CT and MRI demonstration. Chin J Radiol 27:21–25

Meningioma

Clinical Presentation

A 17-year-old male with cauda equina syndrome.

Images (Fig. 10.29)

A. Sagittal T2-weighted image demonstrates a well-outlined mixed signal lesion (*arrow*) in the intradural space displacing the nerve roots (*arrowheads*)
B. Sagittal contrast-enhanced T1-weighted image with fat suppression demonstrates intense and near-homogeneous enhancement (*arrow*)
C. Axial contrast-enhanced T1-weighted image with fat suppression demonstrates heterogeneous enhancement of the lesion (*arrow*)

Discussion

Meningiomas of the spinal canal are rare in childhood outside neurofibromatosis, but they do occur in children as well. In children and adolescents there is often a comorbid diagnosis. Patients with NF-2 can have multiple meningiomas and they occur both intracranially as well as along the spinal axis. Meningiomas originate from meningothelial cells which may be found in the spinal arachnoid membranes. Meningiomas usually have similar characteristics to schwannomas, being isointense to the cord on T1-weighted image and dark on T2-weighted image. Calcification is not uncommon. Homogeneous and significant contrast enhancement is a characteristic appearance.

Suggested Reading

Cohen-Gadol AA, Zikel OM, Koch CA, Scheithauer BW, Krauss WE (2003) Spinal meningiomas in patients younger than 50 years of age: a 21-year experience. J Neurosurg 98:258–263

Solero CL, Fornari M, Giombini S, et al (1989) Spinal meningiomas: review of 174 operated cases. Neurosugery 25:153–160

Zwerdling T, Dothage J (2002) Meningiomas in children and adolescents. J Pediatr Hematol Oncol 24:199–204

Figure 10.29

Meningioma

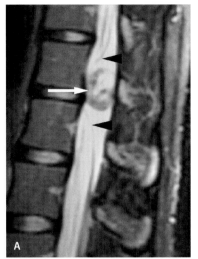
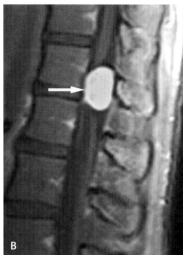
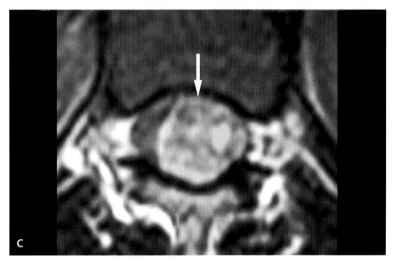

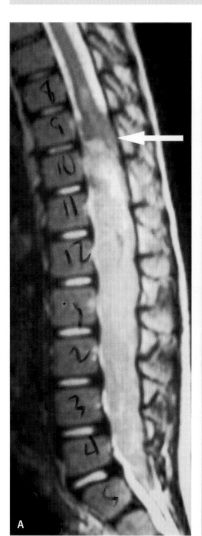
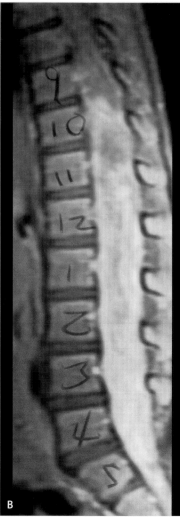

Figure 10.30

Meningeal sarcoma

Meningeal Sarcoma

Clinical Presentation

A 4-year-old female with urinary retention, bowel incontinence and bilateral leg pain with absent reflexes.

Images (Fig. 10.30)

A. Sagittal T2-weighted image demonstrates a slightly heterogeneous mass lesion in the thecal sac from T9 to S1. This mass is predominantly intramedullary. Significant cord compression (*arrow*) is present. The spinal canal is dilated

B. Sagittal contrast-enhanced T1-weighted image shows diffuse enhancement

Discussion

Primary meningeal sarcoma is a rare and highly aggressive tumor primarily affecting children. Primary meningeal sarcoma with leiomyoblastic and meningothelial differentiation has also been reported. CT and MR imaging findings are nonspecific, although both tests allow full visualization of the disease process. There are no imaging criteria that will allow differentiation of meningeal sarcoma from other solid tumors, or tumorous or inflammatory meningeal disease. Biopsy is needed to confirm the diagnosis in unclear cases.

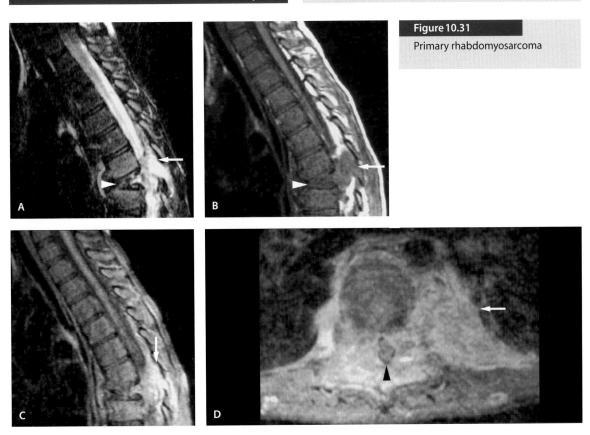

Figure 10.31

Primary rhabdomyosarcoma

Suggested Reading

Buttner A, Pfluger T, Weis S (2001) Primary meningeal sarcomas in two children. Review. J Neurooncol 52:181–188

Sugita Y, Shigemori M, Harada H, Wada Y, Hayashi I, Morimastu M, Okamoto Y, Kajiwara K (2000) Primary meningeal sarcomas with leiomyoblastic differentiation: a proposal for a new subtype of primary meningeal sarcomas. Am J Surg Pathol 24:1273–1278

Rhabdomyosarcoma

Primary Rhabdomyosarcoma

Clinical Presentation

An 8-year-old boy with severe back pain.

Images (Fig. 10.31)

A. Sagittal T2-weighted image with fat suppression shows near complete destruction of the T8 vertebral body (*arrowhead*) with loss of vertebral body height leading to acute kyphosis. An irregular mass is seen in the spinal canal (*arrow*)

B. Sagittal T1-weighted image better outlines the isointense spinal canal tumor (*arrow*). The mass is continuous with the collapsed T8 vertebral body (*arrowhead*)

C. Sagittal contrast-enhanced T1-weighted image with fat suppression demonstrates the full extent of the enhancing tumor (*arrow*)

D. Axial contrast-enhanced T1-weighted image with fat suppression shows the left paraspinal enhancing tumor (*arrow*) that is invading the spinal canal and encircling the spinal cord (*arrowhead*). The mass erodes both pedicles as well as the posterior elements.

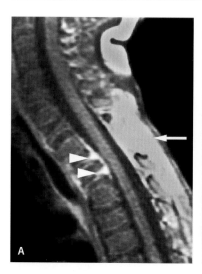
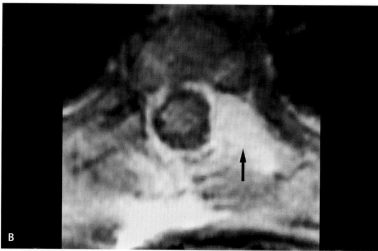

Figure 10.32

Metastatic rhabdomyosarcoma

Metastatic Rhabdomyosarcoma

Clinical Presentation

A 3-year-old female with metastatic rhabdomyosarcoma. The primary lesion is in the pelvis.

Images (Fig. 10.32)

A. Sagittal contrast-enhanced T1-weighted image demonstrates enhancement in the posterior spinal soft tissues extending from T2 to the top of T6 (*arrow*). There is also enhancing soft tissue in the spinal canal the epidural space at the T2–4 levels (*arrowheads*). No significant cord compression is present. There is partial collapse of T3 and T4 vertebral bodies with increased kyphosis at the same level. Partial clumps of the T1 vertebral body without abnormal enhancement are present

B. Axial contrast-enhanced T1-weighted image demonstrates abnormal enhancement within the left lateral aspect of the T4 vertebral body consistent a metastatic focus (*arrow*)

Discussion

Rhabdomyosarcoma is a malignant neoplasm of embryonic mesenchyma with rhabdoid differentiation. Rhabdomyosarcoma is an aggressive tumor that erodes and destroys the adjacent bone, but it can also metastasize into the spinal canal, especially into the epidural space. On T2-weighted images they demonstrate variable signal intensity with intense enhancement.

Suggested Reading

Curless RG, Toledano SR, Ragheb J, Cleveland WW, Falcone S (2002) Hematogenous brain metastasis in children. Pediatr Neurol 26:219–221

Spunt SL, Anderson JR, Teot LA, Breneman JC, Meyer WH, Pappo AS (2001) Routine brain imaging is unwarranted in asymptomatic patients with rhabdomyosarcoma arising outside of the head and neck region that is metastatic at diagnosis: a report from the Intergroup Rhabdomyosarcoma Study Group. Cancer 92:121–125

Figure 10.33
Teratoma

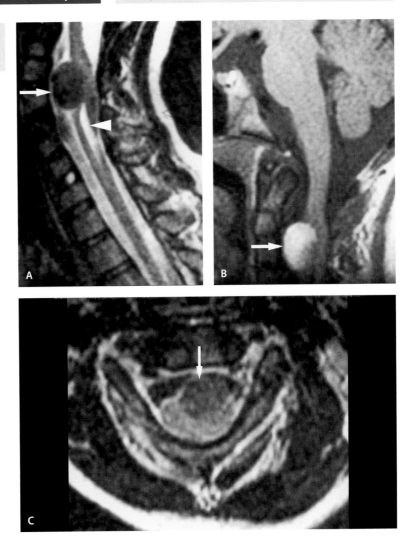

Teratoma

Clinical Presentation

A 7-year-old female with right hemiparesis.

Images (Fig. 10.33)

A. Sagittal T2-weighted image shows enlargement of the upper cervical canal. Anterior to the cord there is a hypointense mass lesion displacing the cord (*arrow*). The lesion largely fills the spinal canal with almost complete obliteration of the CSF space. This mass appears to be exophytic. Only the posterior margin appears to infiltrate the cord. Syrinx is seen below the mass (*arrowheads*)

B. Sagittal contrast-enhanced T1-weighted image shows near-homogeneous enhancement of the lesion (*arrow*). There is no cord enhancement

C. Axial T2-weighted image through the lesion (*arrow*). The cord is compressed and displaced posteriorly by the mass

Discussion

The most common intradural, extramedullary tumors in childhood are neurofibroma/schwannoma, drop metastases, congenital lipomas and epidermoids/dermoids. Teratomas are rare tumors. Teratoma is a true neoplasm and it consists of all three embryonic layers, none of which is native to the spinal area. Plain films and CT images often demonstrate enlargement of the bony spinal canal with bone

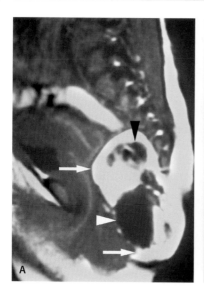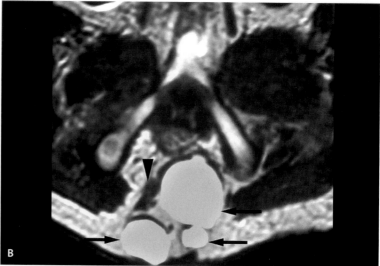

Figure 10.34

Sacrococcygeal teratoma

erosion or remodeling or spinal dysraphism. The appearance of these tumors on MRI is variable depending on the composition of the tumor. The solid portion usually enhances with contrast. It can exist at any spinal level.

Suggested Reading

Cohen MD, Edwards MK (eds) (1990) Magnetic resonance imaging of children (Teratoma of the spine). Decker, Philadelphia

Sacrococcygeal Teratoma

Clinical Presentation

A 1-day-old female with a sacrococcygeal mass.

Images (Fig. 10.34)

A. Sagittal T1-weighted image shows a mixed signal intensity mass in the sacrococcygeal region. This mass has hyperintense areas representing fat (*arrows*) and hypointense lesions (*arrowheads*)
B. Axial T1-weighted image also shows hyperintense (*arrows*) and hypointense areas (*arrowhead*) in the teratoma

Discussion

Sacrococcygeal teratomas are rare tumors: approximately 1 in 40,000 live births with a female preponderance. The tumor is derived from the pluripotent cell line originating in Hansen's node which migrate caudally to rest in the coccyx. They contain components arising from all three germ layers. Sacrococcygeal teratomas are classified into four types based on their external and internal extent: type I is predominantly exterior, with only a minimal presacral component; type II is predominantly exterior, but with a significant intrapelvic component; type III is predominantly internal, with intraabdominal extension; and type IV is entirely internal, with no external component.

CT and MR imaging are the most important investigations for characterization of the mass, evaluation of its intrapelvic extension, and relationship to other structures as well as for detection of other associated spinal abnormalities. Most commonly, teratomas appear as a complex heterogeneous mass with solid and cystic areas along with areas of fat. Calcification is seen in more than 50% of cases. CT is the most sensitive method for detection of calcification. MRI better depicts cystic elements, the contents of which might be inferred from signal intensity patterns on different sequences. Fat components can be identified by either CT or MR imaging.

Suggested Reading

Avni FE, Nicaise N, Hall M, et al (2002) MR imaging of fetal sacrococcygeal teratoma: diagnosis and assessment. AJR Am J Roentgenol 178:179–183

Monteiro M, Cunha TM, Catarino A, Tome V (2002) Case report: sacrococcygeal teratoma with malignant transformation in an adult female: CT and MRI findings. Br J Radiol 75:620–623

Okamura M, Kurauchi O, Itakura A, Naganawa S, Watanabe Y, Mizutani S (1999) Fetal sacrococcygeal teratoma visualized by ultra-fast T2 weighted magnetic resonance imaging. Int J Gynecol Obstet 65:191–193

Osteochondroma

Clinical Presentation

A young male with a painless lump in the neck since the age of 18 years.

Images (Fig. 10.35)

A. Axial CT scan of the neck demonstrates a pedunculated, irregularly ossified mass arising from the facet joint of a cervical vertebral body (*arrow*)
B. Coronal T1-weighted image of the neck shows a mixed signal intensity mass lesion (*arrow*)
C. Axial T2-weighted image shows a mixed signal lesion in the region in the right paraspinal area. The lesion fills and dilates the neural foramen (*arrow*)

Discussion

Osteochondromas are benign subperiosteal cartilaginous exostoses composed of mature cancellous, cortical and cartilaginous bone. These tumors usually occur in the cervical and thoracic spine as a solitary mass lesion involving the spinous or transfer process. They usually present before the age of 20 years and they have a slight male predominance. Malignant degeneration is rare. They are usually asymptomatic unless they reach a large size. CT findings are characteristic.

Suggested Reading

Murphey MD, Choi JJ, Kransdorf MJ, Flemming DJ, Gannon FH (2000) Imaging of osteochondroma: variants and complications with radiologic-pathologic correlation. Radiographics 20:1407–1434

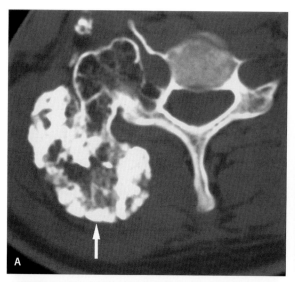

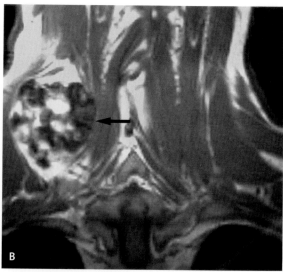

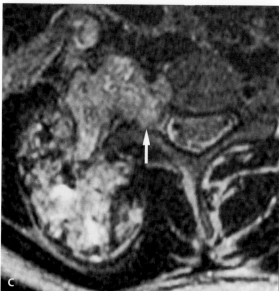

Figure 10.35

Osteochondroma

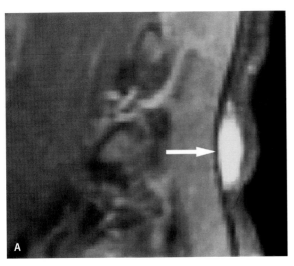
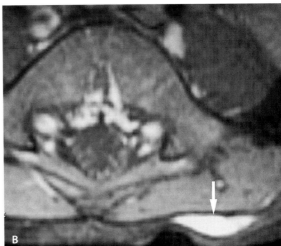

Figure 10.36

Hemangioma

Hemangioma

Clinical Presentation

A 2-year-old female with a palpable mass in the lower back near the midline.

Images (Fig. 10.36)

A. Sagittal contrast-enhanced T1-weighted image with fat suppression shows an enhancing mass overlying the sacral region (*arrow*). It is superficial to the deep fascia and does not invade the deeper structures

B. Axial contrast-enhanced T1-weighted image with fat suppression shows the superficial nature of the lesion (*arrow*) without connection to the deeper structures

Discussion

Hemangiomas are benign neoplasms of endothelial cells and are the most common childhood tumor, occurring in approximately 12% of infants. Hemangiomas are more commonly found in girls, whites, premature infants, and twins. They undergo a char-

acteristic two-stage process of proliferation and regression. Hemangiomas can have deep, superficial, or mixed components. The clinical appearance of hemangiomas varies with the degree of dermal involvement and depth of the lesions. A characteristic strawberry appearance is present when the lesions involve the skin. Deep hemangiomas, which do not involve the subcutaneous tissues, may have a blue appearance.

Imaging is performed to characterize the lesion and examine the extent of disease. On MRI, proliferating hemangiomas are seen as a discrete lobulated isointense mass on T1-weighted images as compared to muscle and a hyperintense mass on T2-weighted images. Hemangiomas usually enhance diffusely with gadolinium. Involuting hemangiomas are seen as high signal intensity on T1-weighted images suggestive of areas of fibrous/fatty tissue and show less contrast enhancement than proliferating hemangiomas.

Suggested Reading

Donnelly LF, Adams DM, Bisset GS III (2000) Vascular malformations and hemangioma a practical approach in a multidisciplinary clinic. AJR Am J Roentgenol 174:597–608

Wild AT, Raab P, Krauspe R (2000) Hemangioma of skeletal muscle. Arch Orthop Trauma Surg 120:139–143

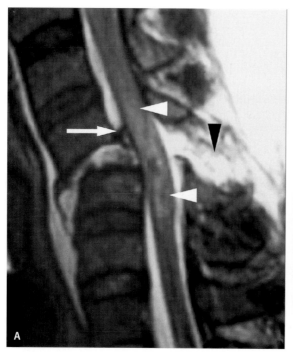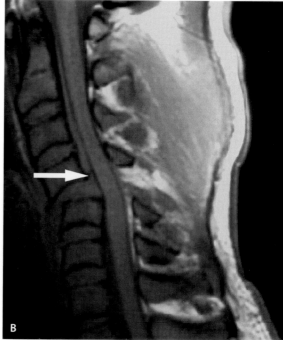

Figure 10.37

Ligament injury and subluxation with acute cord edema

Spinal Trauma

Ligament Injury and Subluxation with Acute Cord Edema

Clinical Presentation

A patient with acute quadriparesis following a trampoline accident.

Images (Fig. 10.37)

A. Sagittal T2-weighted image shows anterior subluxation of C4 on C5. There is retropulsion of a small bone fragment. The posterior longitudinal ligament is disrupted (*arrow*). Severe spinal cord swelling and edema (*white arrowheads*) are seen. Hyperintense interspinous ligament injury between the spinous processes (*black arrowhead*) is present
B. Sagittal T1-weighted image demonstrates again ligament disruption (*arrow*). Edema and cord swelling are better appreciated on T2-weighted image (A)

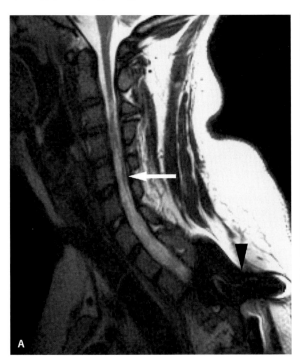 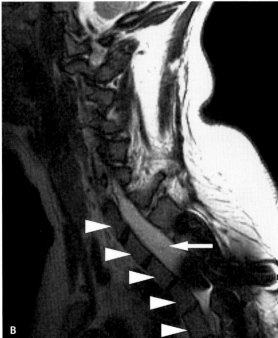

Figure 10.38
Myelomalacia

Myelomalacia

Clinical Presentation

A 16-year-old female with history of C3 quadripare-sis since birth; developmental anomaly or intrauter-ine event is suspected. Patient presents with headache and neck stiffness.

Images (Fig. 10.38)

A. Sagittal T2-weighted image shows very thin upper cervical cord from the craniocervical junction down to the C5 level (*arrow*). The spinal canal is narrow. Note the abnormally elongated and nar-row vertebral bodies of C6–T3. A metallic hard-ware artifact is present (*arrowhead*)
B. Sagittal T2-weighted image shows again elongated vertebral bodies (*arrowheads*). They were present throughout thoracic spine. The thoracic spinal canal is widened, but no cord is visualized (*arrow*)

Discussion

Traumatic injuries observed in the cervical spine in-clude burst fractures, ligament trauma and fractures with anterior subluxation. Instability of the fracture implies that physiological motion of the spine may result in serious deformity and/or place neurological structures in danger or result in significant pain. Al-though CT scan shows better the fracture fragments and their location, MRI is more useful in detecting soft-tissue injuries including the cord injury and lig-ament trauma. MR imaging provides information in acute cervical spine trauma that cannot be obtained with any other modality. It is the only modality that directly demonstrates cervical cord injury. Vascular injury has been reported to play an important role in the injury mechanism that causes damage to the traumatized spinal cord. Diffusion imaging with ap-parent diffusion coefficient has proven to be useful in evaluation of spinal cord injury and development myelomalacia that presents as T2 hyperintensity and cord atrophy in late MR imaging. MR imaging also plays an important role in detection of acute epidural hematomas. MR imaging is also the most sensitive method for detecting ligamentous injury. Disruption of the anterior and posterior longitudinal ligaments manifests as discontinuity in the normal dark signal intensity of the intact ligament. The ruptured area can contain edema or hemorrhage as well. Interspinous ligament injuries produce T2 hyperintensity within the spinous processes.

Suggested Reading

Beers GJ, Raque GH, Wagner CG, et al (1988) MR imaging in acute cervical spine trauma. J Comput Assist Tomogr 12: 755–761

Katzberg RW, Benedetti PF, Drake CM, et al (1999) Acute cervical spine injuries: prospective MR imaging assessment at a level 1 trauma center. Radiology 213:203–212

Sagiuchi T, Tachibana S, Endo M, Hayakawa K (2002) Diffusion-weighted MRI of the cervical cord in acute spinal cord injury with type II odontoid fracture. J Comput Assist Tomogr 26:654–656

Tator CH, Koyanagi H (1997) I Vascular mechanisms in the pathophysiology of human spinal cord injury. J Neurosurg 86:483–492

Figure 10.39

Nerve root avulsion from accident

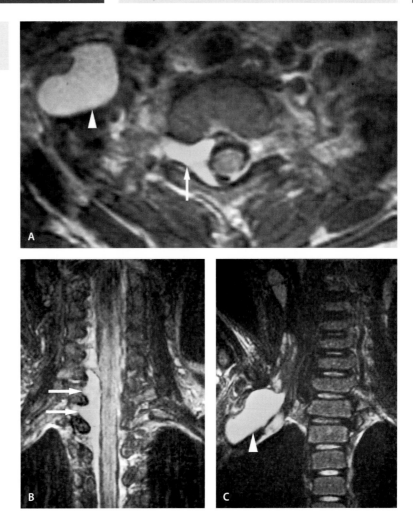

Brachial Plexus Trauma

Nerve Root Avulsion from Accident

Clinical Presentation

An 8-year-old girl who was struck by a car while walking. Following the accident she was not able to move her arm.

Images (Fig. 10.39)

A. Axial T2-weighted image shows traumatic meningocele. There is marked asymmetry of the CSF space with an extradural CSF collection pushing the cord to the left. The avulsed nerve root sleeve (*arrow*) with CSF collection extends through the neural foramen into the middle cervical triangle. Another CSF collection is seen along the distal brachial plexus (*arrowhead*)

B. Coronal T2-weighted image shows the cord displacement to the left by multiple pseudomeningoceles. Avulsion of C7 and C8 nerve roots from the cord is present with "empty sleeves" (*arrows*)

C. Coronal T2-weighted image demonstrates a CSF collection (*arrowhead*) along the peripheral brachial plexus in the neck, not uncommonly seen in this condition

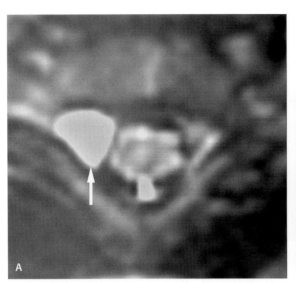
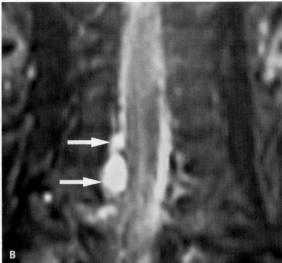

Figure 10.40

Obstetric brachial plexus injury

Obstetric Brachial Plexus Injury

Clinical Presentation

A newborn with obstetric brachial plexus injury.

Images (Fig. 10.40)

A. Axial T2-weighted image shows a traumatic pseudomeningocele (*arrow*) along the nerve root sleeve in the spinal canal extending through the neural foramen. The cord is not displaced
B. Coronal T2-weighted image reveals two pseudo-meningoceles (*arrows*) without cord displacement

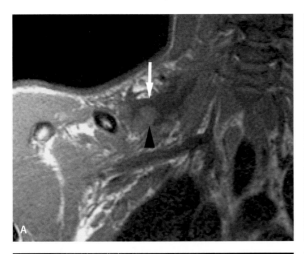

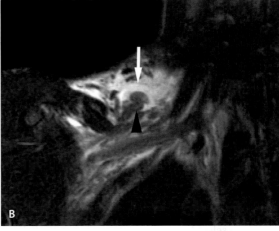

Figure 10.41

Blunt trauma to the brachial plexus

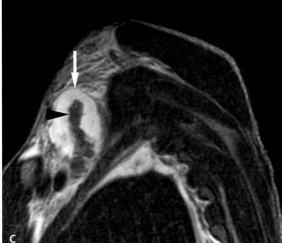

Blunt Trauma to the Brachial Plexus

Clinical Presentation

A 15-year-old male involved in a snowmobile accident has right arm weakness.

Images (Fig. 10.41)

A. Coronal T1-weighted image shows a large supraclavicular fluid collection surrounding the brachial plexus (*arrow*). There is transection and retraction of the upper trunk (*arrowhead*)

B. T2-weighted image with fat suppression at the same level as A. The retracted trunk (*arrowhead*) and fluid collection (*arrow*) are better visualized in A because of the better contrast

C. Sagittal T2-weighted image shows fluid collection (*arrow*) around the brachial plexus and avulsed upper trunk (*arrowhead*)

Discussion

Complete or partial nerve root avulsion results from traction trauma when nerve roots are stretched beyond their elastic limit. The nerve roots usually separate at their weakest point at the site of their attachment to the cord. Although this injury most commonly involves the brachial plexus, it may also involve the lumbar sacral nerve roots. Duchenne-Erb's syndrome is the most common presentation of obstetric brachial plexus injury. Usually multiple nerve roots are involved and the level of avulsion is most commonly from C5 to C6 (Erb's palsy), but obstetric nerve injury can happen from C5 to C7 (intermediate severity) or C5 to T1 (severe trauma). Rupture of the dura allows CSF to leak through the neural foramina into the paraspinal soft tissues along the course of the nerve roots with pseudomeningocele formation. This usually causes a fibrotic response and the leak closes spontaneously. Before MR imaging was introduced, cervical myelography and/or postmyelographic CT with intrathecal contrast were the best methods to visualize brachial plexus injuries. Currently MR imaging is the method of choice in evaluating the brachial plexus after trauma, although also ultrasonography has been used for brachial plexus lesion diagnosis. A careful assessment of the nerve root lesions is vital to be able to select the correct root avulsions for microsurgical treatment. In the intradural avulsions the prognosis is invariable. Heavily T2-weighted images ("MR myelograms") are able to visualize the cord, CSF spaces and preganglionic nerve roots traversing through it. They are also able to reveal the "empty sleeves" following avulsion.

Suggested Reading

Francel PC, Koby M, Park TS, Lee BC, Noetzel MJ, Mackinnon SE, Henegar MM, Kaufman BA (1995) Fast spin-echo magnetic resonance imaging for radiological assessment of neonatal brachial plexus injury. J Neurosurg 83:461–466

Lindell-Iwan HL, Partanen VS, Makkonen ML (1996) Obstetric brachial plexus palsy. J Pediatr Orthop B 5:210–215

Miller SF, Glasier CM, Griebel ML, Boop FA. Miller SF, Glasier CM, Griebel ML, Boop FA (1993) Brachial plexopathy in infants after traumatic delivery: evaluation with MR imaging. Radiology 189:481–484

Valanne L, Ketonen L, Barsotti J, Peterson P, Pilcher W (1995) Interesting images: posttraumatic nonfunctioning arm. Case report. J Child Neurol 1:30–31

Figure 10.42

Epidural hematoma

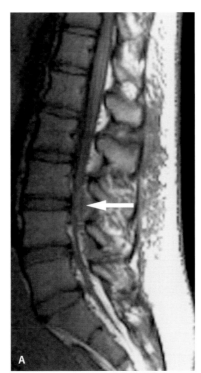
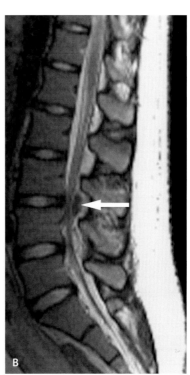

Epidural Hematoma

Clinical Presentation

A 15-year-old post-partum patient with eclampsia had epidural anesthesia and presented with sudden-onset right lower extremity weakness.

Images (Fig. 10.42)

A. Sagittal T1-weighted image of lumbar spine shows a focal isointense lesion of approximately 1×1 cm size posteriorly at the L3–4 level. The lesion causes compression upon the cauda equina (*arrow*)

B. Sagittal T2-weighted MR image reveals the lesion to be hypointense (*arrow*)

Discussion

Spinal epidural hematoma is a rare condition, which can present with acute spinal cord compression. Spinal hematoma may be spontaneous or related to trauma, anticoagulant therapy, blood dyscrasias, vascular malformations, epidural anesthesia, surgery or lumbar puncture. The incidence of spinal epidural hematoma following epidural anesthesia is 1 in 220,000 cases.

MR imaging is considered the modality of choice to evaluate spinal epidural hematoma. Sagittal MR typically shows hematoma in the posterior epidural space with well-defined borders tapering superiorly and inferiorly. The dura mater separates the hematoma from the spinal cord on T1- and T2-weighted images. In the acute stage (within 24 h of onset), the hematoma is usually isointense on T1-weighted images. On T2-weighted images, there may be homogeneous high signal or inhomogeneous areas of mixed high and low signal. After 24 h, there is usually high signal on T1-weighted images; T2-weighted images in most cases give the same signal as that of CSF.

Suggested Reading

Dorsay TA, Helms CA (2002) MR imaging of epidural hematoma in the lumbar spine. Skeletal Radiol 31:677–685

Ng WH, Lim CC, Ng PY, Tan KK (2002) Spinal epidural hematoma: MRI-aided diagnosis. J Clin Neurosci 9:92–94

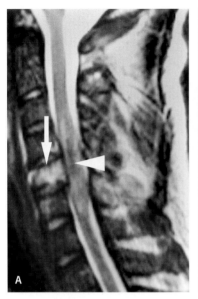
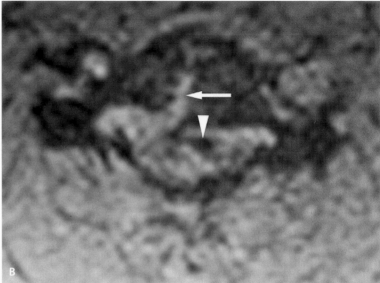

Figure 10.43

Cervical spine burst fracture

Spine Fractures

Cervical Spine Burst Fracture

Clinical Presentation

A 22-year-old male who was the unrestrained driver of a vehicle accident involved in an accident.

Images (Fig. 10.43)

A. Sagittal T2-weighted image demonstrates burst fracture involving the C5 vertebral body with minor retropulsion of the posterior vertebral body. The vertebra body demonstrates abnormal hyperintensity (*arrow*). This is secondary to bone edema. Some edematous changes are also seen in the neighboring vertebral bodies. There is significant cord edema from C4–5 down to C6–7 with heterogeneous cord signal. The linear decreased signal inside the cord (*arrowhead*) most likely represents hemorrhage. Some edema is also seen at the posterior aspect of the neck between the spinous processes

B. T2-weighted image with fat suppression clearly demonstrates a linear fracture through the vertebral body (*arrow*). The cord is swollen with hemorrhagic foci (*arrowhead*)

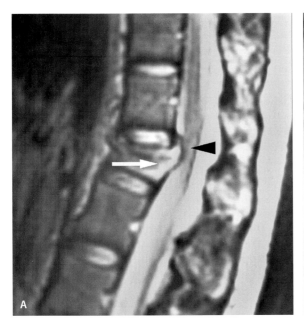 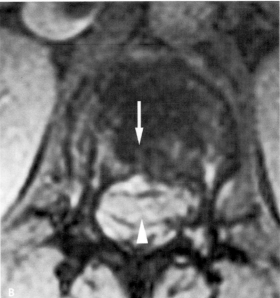

Figure 10.44

Lumbar spine burst fracture

Lumbar Spine Burst Fracture

Clinical Presentation

An 8-year-old female with trauma.

Images (Fig. 10.44)

A. Sagittal T2-weighted image shows burst fracture involving the L1 vertebral body with retropulsion of the posterior vertebral body which compresses the conus. The vertebra body demonstrates abnormal hyperintensity (*arrow*). Hyperintensity in the conus is seen (*arrowhead*)

B. T2-weighted image with fat suppression clearly shows a linear fracture through the vertebral body (*arrow*). Hyperintensity in the conus is seen (*arrowhead*)

Lumbar Spine Compression Fracture

Clinical Presentation

A 16-year-old female fell from a horse.

Images (Fig. 10.45)

A. Plain film (AP and lateral) shows compression fracture of L3 vertebral body (*arrow*)
B. Axial CT scan shows the anterior vertebral body fracture (*arrows*) with sparing of the posterior body
C and D. Sagittal (C) and coronal (D) reconstructed CT images better define the L3 compression fracture with an anterior bone fragment (*arrowheads*)
E. Sagittal T2-weighted image shows vague edema involving L3 and L4 vertebral bodies (*arrows*)
F. Sagittal STIR image better defines the bone marrow edema (*arrows*)
G. The bone marrow edema is seen as a hypointense area on the sagittal T1-weighted image (*arrows*)
H. Axial T2-weighted image shows the fracture line (*arrows*) without canal compromise

Discussion

Burst fracture results from axial compression forces and in this type of fracture the vertebral body fractures in to multiple fragments resulting anterior wedge deformity and retropulsion of the posterior aspect of the vertebral body into the spinal canal. Burst fracture can extend to one or both laminae. The neurological symptoms depend on the amount of retropulsion, size of the canal and level of the lesion. Although thin section CT scan shows better the fracture fragments, MRI is the method of choice for demonstrating the extent of cord involvement and possible epidural hematoma. MRI also better delineates the extent of the trauma by demonstrating the marrow edema.

Compression fracture results from a combination of vertical loading and flexion leading to anterior wedge deformity of the vertebral body. They are most common in the lower thoracic and upper lumbar regions.

Suggested Reading

Atlas SW, Regenbogen V, Rogers LF, et al (1986) The radiographic characterization of burst fractures of the spine. AJNR Am J Neurol 7:675–682

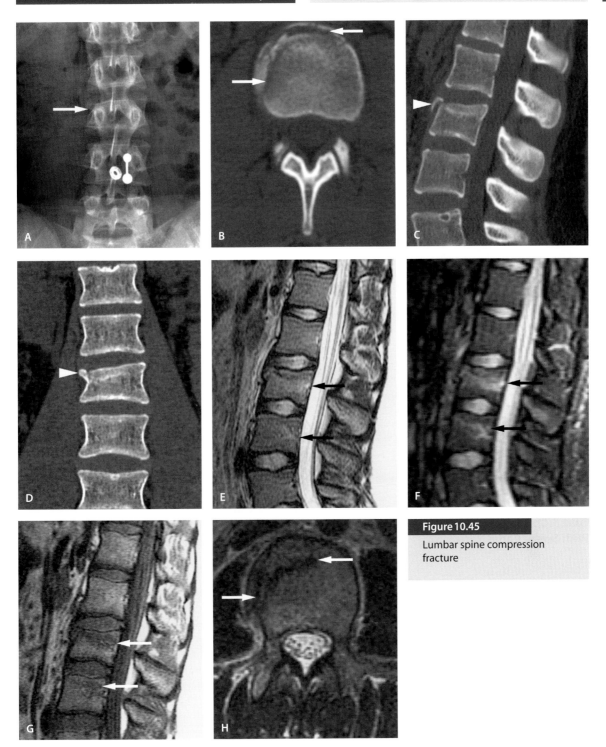

Figure 10.45

Lumbar spine compression
fracture

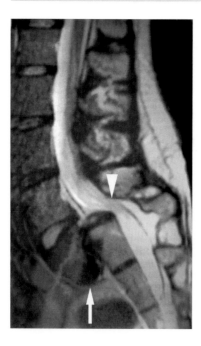

Figure 10.46

Spondylolisthesis with spinal canal narrowing

Spondylolisthesis

Case 1. Spondylolisthesis With Spinal Canal Narrowing

Clinical Presentation

A 17-year-old cheerleader with chronic back pain which is exacerbated during sports activities. She has had the symptoms since childhood, but has no neurological dysfunction. Patient has known bilateral pars interarticularis defects on plain films.

Images (Fig. 10.46)

A. Sagittal T2-weighted image reveals severe (grade 4) spondylolisthesis (*arrow*) of the L5 vertebral body with respect to the S1 vertebral body. There is overriding of the L5 vertebral body anterior the S1 vertebra. There is focal spinal stenosis at the center of the canal (*arrowhead*). Note the degenerated dark disk (*arrow*) adhering to the parent L5 vertebra

Case 2. Spondylolisthesis Without Spinal Canal Narrowing

Clinical Presentation

A young adult female with chronic low back pain related to sports activity. She has no neurological dysfunction. Bilateral pars defects are present in plain films. The symptoms were persistent in spite of fusion.

Images (Fig. 10.47)

A. Sagittal T2-weighted image through the midline shows grade 2 spondylolisthesis (*arrow*) of the L5 vertebral body with respect to the S1 vertebral body. There is no canal narrowing at the site of spondylolisthesis. The dark signal overlapping the thecal sac is artifact from fusion hardware
B. Axial T1-weighted image through the spondylolisthesis reveals a normal-sized canal without nerve root displacement

Discussion

Spondylolysis refers to a lesion in the pars interarticularis region. This is likely to represent chronic stress fracture of the bone caused by accumulative effect of repetitive stress imposed by physical activity. This commonly occurs at L5 and less frequently at L4, but involvement of the upper lumbar spine is rare.

Spondylolisthesis refers to anterior or posterior displacement of one vertebra on another, usually in the lumbar region. Spondylolisthesis occurs in a significant number of patients with spondylolysis. Spondylolisthesis can be of five types: dysplastic, isthmus, degenerative, traumatic, and pathological. However, two common types of spondylolisthesis in children include dysplastic and isthmic. The dysplastic type is secondary to underdeveloped facet joints (dysplastic joints). The isthmic type is usually due to a fatigue fracture of the pars interarticularis but there is also a hereditary element in this type. Most children are asymptomatic (80%). They may become symptomatic due to overstress, aggressive sports activities, and injury. Pain may be the presenting symptom.

Standard radiographic examinations (AP, lateral, oblique) are helpful in diagnosis. The value of an oblique radiograph of the lumbosacral spine in a pars defect is unproven. The severity of the slip can be

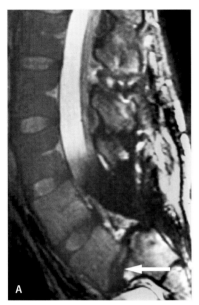
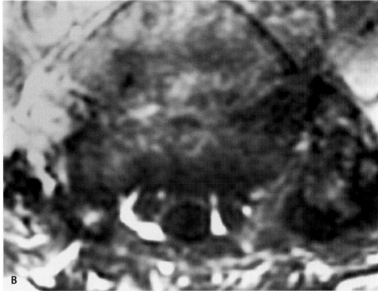

Figure 10.47

Spondylolisthesis without spinal canal narrowing

estimated on the lateral view of the radiograph. Grade 1 indicates more than 75% contact, grade 2 indicates 50–75% contact, grade 3 indicates 25–50% contact, and grade 4 indicates less than 25% contact.

Planar bone scintigraphy (PBS) and single-photon emission computed tomography (SPECT) are more sensitive than plain radiographs and show increased uptake in the pedicles of the affected segment suggestive of pars fractures. CT performed with a reverse gantry angle and thin sections is the investigation of choice for identifying radiographically occult lyses. MR imaging is a valuable technique for demonstrating pars and nerve root compression. T1-weighted images in coronal plane are helpful in demonstrating the pars defect as a hypointense area. Sagittal midline T2-weighted images reveal best the degree of the contact area (degree). MR imaging also helps rule out other causes associated with lower back pain.

Suggested Reading

Harvey CJ, Richenberg JL, Saifuddin A, Wolman RL (1998) The radiological investigation of lumbar spondylolysis. Clin Radiol 53:723–728

Logroscino G, Mazza O, Aulisa G, Pitta L, Pola E, Aulisa L (2001) Spondylolysis and spondylolisthesis in the pediatric and adolescent population. Childs Nerv Syst 17:644–655

Rosenblum BR, Rothman AS (1991) Low back pain in children. Mt Sinai J Med 58:115–120

Ulmer JL, Elster AD, Mathews VP, King JC (1994) Distinction between degenerative and isthmic spondylolisthesis on sagittal MR images: importance of increased anteroposterior diameter of the spinal canal ("wide canal sign"). AJR Am J Roentgenol 163:411–416

Yamane T, Yoshida T, Mimatsu K (1993) Early diagnosis of lumbar spondylolysis by MRI. J Bone Joint Surg Br 75:764–768

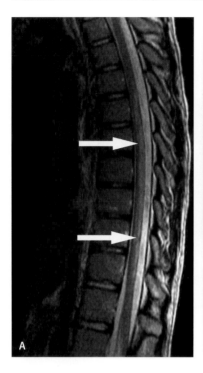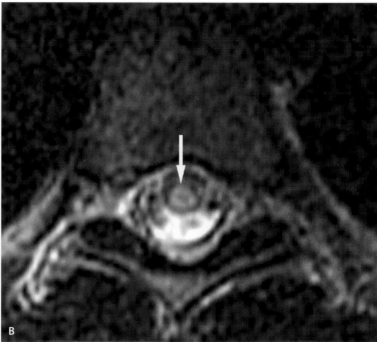

Figure 10.48

Acute disseminated encephalomyelitis of thoracic cord

Acute Disseminated Encephalomyelitis (ADEM)

ADEM of Thoracic Cord

Clinical Presentation

A 12-year-old female with sudden onset of numbness and weakness in both legs. She also has urinary incontinence.

Images (Fig. 10.48)

A. Sagittal T2-weighted image shows an area of hyperintensity within the thoracic spinal cord from T6 to T12 posteriorly (*arrows*). Minimal enhancement of this lesion is noted in the post-contrast scan

B. Axial T2-weighted image shows cord hyperintensity (*arrow*).

Figure 10.49

Acute disseminated encephalomyelitis of cervical cord

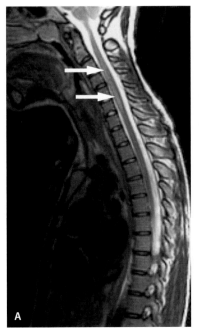
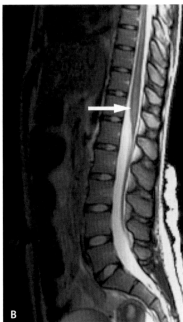

ADEM of Cervical Cord

Clinical Presentation

A 15-year-old female with a 2-day history of extremity weakness and confusion. Patient has also brain lesions (see also page 110, chapter 3).

Images (Fig. 10.49)

A. Sagittal T2-weighted image shows swelling of the cervical cord with a hyperintense lesion extending from C3 to C7 (*arrows*)
B. Sagittal T2-weighted image shows mild swelling of the conus medullaris and a hyperintense lesion (*arrow*)

Discussion

ADEM is a monophasic, autoimmune inflammatory demyelinating disease of the CNS. ADEM has been observed following viral infections, immunization, and *Mycoplasma* infections. Most cases are seen in children and young adults. The pathological hallmark of ADEM is perivenular inflammation and demyelination.

MR imaging is sensitive in the detection of lesions, but it lacks specificity because of the similarity in radiological appearance between ADEM and other demyelinating diseases, especially multiple sclerosis and its variants, but also leukodystrophies and mitochondrial diseases. However, in ADEM, the lesions are usually more extensive than in multiple sclerosis, with involvement of subcortical white matter, brain stem, cerebellum, spinal cord, and possibly basal ganglia. There is typically no mass effect. Enhancement is variable.

The frequency of concurrent spinal cord involvement is unknown. Spinal cord involvement may be suspected when there are signs of myelopathy. The spinal cord may show a hyperintense signal with or without cord widening on T2-weighted images.

Suggested Reading

Bizzi A, Ulug AM, Crawford TO, Passe T, Bugiani M, Bryan RN, Barker PB (2001) Quantitative proton MR spectroscopic imaging in acute disseminated encephalomyelitis. AJNR Am J Neuroradiol 22:1125–1130

Khong PL, Ho HK, Cheng PW, Wong VC, Goh W, Chan FL (2002) Childhood acute disseminated encephalomyelitis: the role of brain and spinal cord MRI. Pediatr Radiol 32:59–66

Singh S, Alexander M, Korah IP (1999) acute disseminated encephalomyelitis: MR imaging features. AJR Am J Roentgenol 173:1101–1107

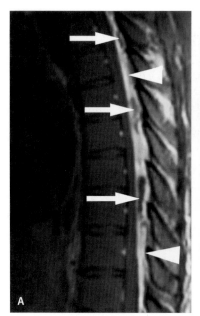 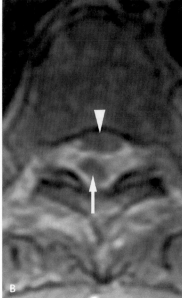

Figure 10.50

Epidural abscess

Epidural Abscess

Clinical Presentation

A 20-year-old male with back pain, bilateral leg weakness and fever. History of spider bite at the back 5 days previously with local inflammatory reaction and subcutaneous abscess formation.

Images (Fig. 10.50)

A. Sagittal contrast-enhanced T1-weighted image with fat suppression shows extensive epidural enhancement (*arrowheads*) from T2 to T11 with loculated fluid collections (*arrows*). The cord is displaced anteriorly
B. Axial contrast-enhanced T1-weighted image with fat suppression shows a localized fluid collection (*arrow*). The aspiration was positive for pus. Cord displacement is seen (*arrowhead*)

Discussion

The overall incidence of spinal epidural abscess varies from 0.2 to 1.2 patients per 10,000 hospital admissions, but only a few percent of these have been seen in children. Diabetes, recent surgical spinal procedures, overlying skin abscesses and furuncles, and intravenous drug use may be common sources of infection in adults. However, only one –third of pediatric patients may have associated underlying diseases. The immunocompromised states of patients with sickle cell anemia and leukemia may be associated with spinal epidural abscess. *Staphylococcal aureus* is the predominant organism.

MR imaging displays the greatest diagnostic accuracy and is the modality of choice. On MR images, low to intermediate signal is seen on T1-weighted images and high or intermediate signal is seen on T2-weighted images. A markedly increased signal on T2-weighted images is consistent with the fluid portion of an abscess. Postgadolinium images show an enhancing rim, which may represent granulation tissue surrounding the collection of pus.

Suggested Reading

Auletta JJ, John CC (2001) Spinal epidural abscesses in children: a 15-year experience and review of the literature. Clin Infect Dis 32:9–16

Parkinson JF, Sekhon LH (2004) Surgical management of spinal epidural abscess: selection of approach based on MRI appearance. J Clin Neurosci 11:130–133

Quach C, Tapiero B, Noya F (2002) Group a streptococcus spinal epidural abscess during varicella. Pediatrics 109:E14

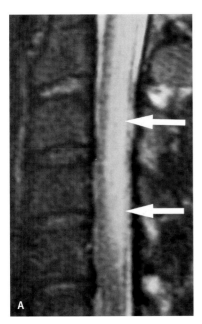
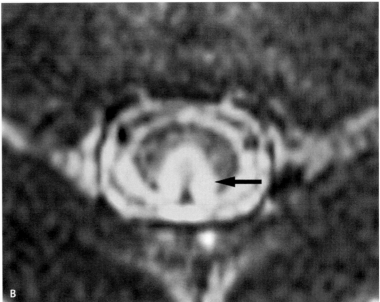

Figure 10.51

Subacute combined degeneration of spinal cord (B12 deficiency)

Subacute Combined Degeneration of Spinal Cord (B12 Deficiency)

Clinical Presentation

A 19-year-old with macrocytic anemia and B12 deficiency presents with paresthesias in hands and leg weakness. The patient has decreased vibration sense and a wide-based gait. The symptoms were relieved with vitamin B12 supplements and the MRI findings in the follow-up study 2 months later showed improvement.

Images (Fig. 10.51)

A. Sagittal T2-weighted image shows a hyperintense lesion along the posterior columns from the foramen magnum to C4 (*arrows*). Mild cord swelling is seen

B. Axial T2-weighted image shows a high-signal lesion in the posterior column (*arrow*)

Discussion

Subacute combined degeneration (SCD) of the spinal cord is a neurological complication of vitamin B12 deficiency. There is degeneration of myelin and axonal loss in the posterior and lateral columns of the spinal cord, typically beginning in the thoracic region and subsequently ascending or descending. The clinical presentation is dominated by dorsal column dysfunction, typically manifested as sensory ataxia.

Although diagnosis is based on the clinical features and laboratory estimation of vitamin B12 levels, MR imaging is the method of choice for showing the demyelination of the spinal cord, seen as high-signal lesions along the posterior columns on T2-weighted images predominantly in the upper and mid-thoracic regions, best seen on axial and sagittal sections. The brain stem, brain and cerebellum may also show changes in the form of hyperintense signal in periventricular white matter. MR imaging is also used to assess the therapeutic response as these changes tend to resolve with administration of vitamin B12.

Suggested Reading

Karantanas AH, Markonis A, Bisbiyiannis G (2000) Subacute combined degeneration of the spinal cord with involvement of the anterior columns: new MRI findings. Neuroradiology 42:115–117

Scherer K (2003) Images in clinical medicine. Neurologic manifestations of vitamin B12 deficiency. N Engl J Med 348:2208

Timms SR, Cure JK, Kurent JE (1993) Subacute combined degeneration of the spinal cord: MR findings. AJNR Am J Neuroradiol 14:1224–1227

Yamada K, Shrier DA, Tanaka H, Numaguchi Y (1998) A case of subacute combined degeneration: MRI findings. Neuroradiology 40:398–400

Fetal Imaging

In collaboration with Susan Blaser, MD

Introduction

Ultrasonography (US) is the screening method of choice for evaluation of fetal CNS anatomy, development, maturation and well being. The results of fetal US are of great value when counseling parents in cases with CNS anomalies. Fetal MR imaging is complementary to fetal US. Thus, MR imaging should not be performed without a preceding US scan and should be interpreted in conjunction with the US scan. Fetal MR imaging has a great potential for accurate evaluation of normal brain development, maturation and fetal structural anomalies. Antenatal diagnosis as early as possible in pregnancy is mandatory if intrauterine therapy is considered, for obstetric management and counseling of the parents. Prenatal detection of fetal anomalies has been shown to reduce perinatal mortality. Although current US equipment allows antenatal identification of many CNS anomalies early in gestation, it also has frequent limitations. MR imaging is currently a standard clinical service in many medical centers for prenatal evaluation when US examination is inconclusive. When intrauterine surgery is contemplated, MR imaging provides valuable anatomical information for planning and management of the procedure.

Single-shot fast spin-echo (SSFSE) T2-weighted imaging is the principal imaging sequence used for fetal MR imaging. Fetal sedation is not needed if ultrafast single slice imaging techniques are available. T2-weighted images are preferred over T1-weighted images because of better tissue contrast. DW imaging and MR spectroscopy have been performed on the fetus, but tend to be sensitive to motion and work better in late pregnancy with decreased fetal motion.

With ultra fast technique, fetal motion is almost "frozen" without sedation. Maternal fasting 4 hours prior to MR imaging also decreases fetal motion. Imaging is performed with a surface coil placed over the maternal abdomen. Although T2-weighted images are high contrast images, spatial resolution is a limiting factor in fetal imaging because a large field of view and relatively thick slices are used.

Classification of fetal CNS anomalies is often difficult and an entire fetus should always be examined to detect multiple anomalies constituting a syndrome rather than an isolated anomaly.

MR spectroscopy has been successfully used in evaluation of metabolic alterations in children. Although some metabolic disorders can be correctly diagnosed antenatally by MR imaging, the diagnoses are usually based on morphological changes, such as cortical dysgenesis seen in Zellweger syndrome rather than MR spectroscopy findings. Antenatal MR spectroscopy is difficult to perform because of the length of the acquisition and patient motion, although case reports of successful use of MR spectroscopy in the fetus have been published.

In addition to general safety issues involved in clinical MR imaging, some special issues have to be taken into account when examining a pregnant patient. They are mainly related to the concerns about the uncertain effect of a strong static magnetic field on the fetus. However, there is no reproducible evidence that MR imaging during pregnancy produces harmful effects on the fetus.

Suggested Reading

Levine D, Hatabu H, Gaa J, Atkinson MW, Edelman RR (1996) Fetal anatomy revealed with fast MR sequences. AJR Am J Roentgenol 167:905–908

Levine D, Barnes PD, Robertson RR, Wong G, Mehta TS (2003) Fast MR imaging of fetal central nervous system abnormalities. Radiology 229:51–61

Righini A, Bianchini E, Parazzini C, et al (2003) Apparent diffusion coefficient determination in normal fetal brain: a prenatal MR imaging study. AJNR Am J Neuroradiol 24:799–804

Zand DJ, Simon EM, Pulitzer SB, et al (2003) In vivo pyruvate detected by MR spectroscopy in neonatal pyruvate dehydrogenase deficiency. AJNR Am J Neuroradiol 24:1471–1474

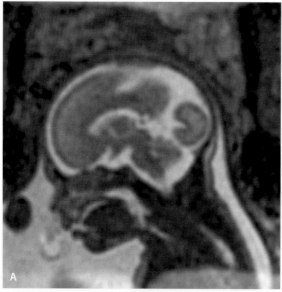

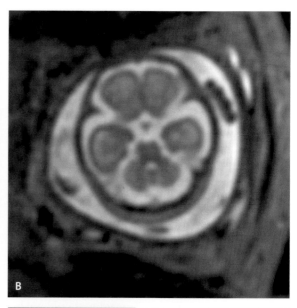

Figure 11.1

Normal fetus

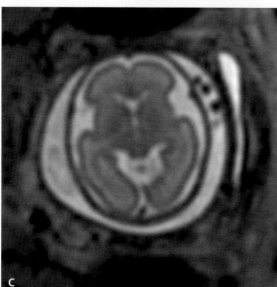

Normal MR Images of Fetus

Normal Fetus

Clinical Presentation

A normal MR image at 26-weeks gestation. The study was obtained because of suspected posterior fossa malformation on US.

Images (Fig. 11.1)

A. Sagittal image allows fetal face imaging. It permits assessment of frontal and nasal bones, hard palate, tongue and mandible. Abnormal facial morphology will be seen in sagittal images. Midline anomalies are also visualized in sagittal image. The parieto-occipital sulcus is visible

B. Lower axial image shows cerebellum and midbrain structures

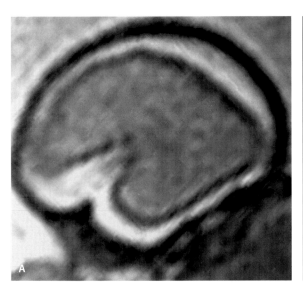
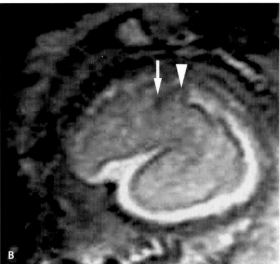

Figure 11.2

Parasagittal images of normal development

C. Brain parenchyma, basal ganglia and CSF spaces are visualized in the higher cuts. The sylvian fissures are wide open. Anterior coronal image is useful in evaluating the facial and orbital structures including cleft lip and palate. Images through the brain show the CNS midline and possible anomalies within it

Parasagittal Images of Normal Development

Clinical Presentation

Images of two different patients with normal MR imaging findings.

Images (Fig. 11.2)

A. Normal parasagittal SSFSE T2-weighted image at 24 weeks gestation shows wide sylvian fissure. At this age the brain is essentially agyric, the cortex is thin and hypointense compared to white matter in the T2 image
B. Between 25 and 28 weeks, the cortex shows development of rolandic fissure (*arrow*) and shallow gyri (*arrowhead*)

Discussion

The normal brain development and maturation in infants proceeds in an organized and predetermined pattern. MR imaging allows deviation of the normal development to be imaged. Before the development of modern neuroimaging it was not possible to visualize normal brain development in vivo. Current neuroimaging allows the development of the sulci and gyri to be visualized, and neuronal maturation and changes in water diffusion to be followed. Brain vessels and changes in blood velocity can be imaged as well. US has been used for more than 30 years in many European countries as an essential part of prenatal care. US can be used to establish gestational age, to document fetal number and lie, to evaluate the uterine environment and to assess fetal growth and well being. Brain imaging often requires a more sophisticated technique than US if abnormalities are suspected in the US scan. Normal development and fetal dysmorphism can be better diagnosed with MR imaging. Assessment of fetal gestational age is essential for the evaluation of normal fetal stage of development. MR imaging is superior to US in demonstrating blood products, cortical structures such as polymicrogyria or lissencephaly, ventricle shape and midline structures. When analyzing newborn brain images it is important to know the post-conceptional age of the child before assessing the brain anatomy.

In the early weeks of gestation, the surfaces of the cerebral hemispheres are small. The fetal sulci appear in an orderly sequence. The primitive sylvian fissure is the earliest fetal sulcus and it is usually present when the fetus is imaged in the 4th gestational month. The rolandic, interparietal and supratemporal sulci appear by the 25th week. The precentral, postcentral and middle temporal sulci appear during weeks 24 to 28. Basal ganglia and thalami are better seen at this age by MR imaging. On T2-weighted images the cortex is thin and not nearly as hypointense on T2-weighted images as before 24 weeks. By 31–32 weeks an increased number of gyri and shallow sulci become visible in the cortex. The sylvian fissures retain their immature appearance until late pregnancy. They may remain prominent in the immediate newborn period. The cavum vergae and cavum septi pellucidi are usually present at birth but they disappear rapidly as the septal leaves fuse. The cisterna magna and basal cisterns are relatively large throughout infancy.

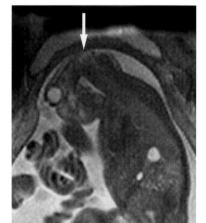

Figure 11.3

Anencephaly

Suggested Reading

Barkovich AJ (2000) Pediatric neuroimaging, 3rd edn. Lippincott, Williams and Wilkins, Philadelphia

Anencephaly

Clinical Presentation

Patient was referred to MR examination following abnormal findings in fetal US scan.

Image (Fig. 11.3)

A. Anencephaly results from failure of the rostral neuropore to close leading to lack of cranial vault (*arrow*) and normal appearing brain.

Discussion

Anencephaly is a defect in the closure of the neural tube during fetal development. The brain tissue is disorganized and most structures incompletely formed. The large defect in the vault of the calvaria, meninges, and scalp exposes a soft angiomatous mass of neural tissue covered with a thin membrane continuous with the skin. The optic globes may protrude due to inadequately formed bony orbits. The incidence of anencephaly is 1/1000 live births. It is associated with folic acid deficiency, environmental and toxic factors and nutritional/vitamin deficiencies. Polyhydramnios may be seen in 50% of cases. Other associated anomalies such as congenital heart disease, cleft palate and folded ears may be seen in 10–20% of cases. The maternal alpha-fetoprotein is elevated.

US performed between 14 and 16 weeks helps in detection of the anomaly. MR imaging serves as a complementary modality for detection of other associated anomalies.

Suggested Reading

Davies BR, Duran M (2003) Malformations of the cranium, vertebral column, and related central nervous system: morphological heterogeneity may indicate biological diversity. Birth Defects Res Clin Mol Teratol 67:563–571

Shakudo M, Inoune Y, Mochizuki K, et al (2001) Fast MR imaging and ultrafast MR imaging of fetal central nervous abnormalities. Osaka City Med J 47:127–135

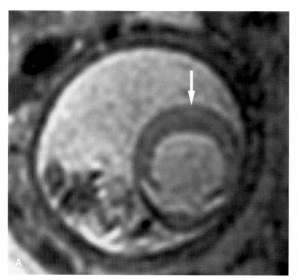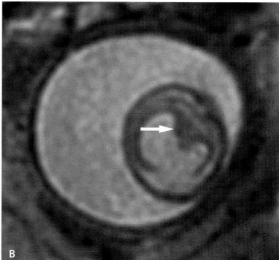

Figure 11.4
Alobar holoprosencephaly

Holoprosencephaly

Alobar Holoprosencephaly

Clinical Presentation

An 18-week gestational age fetus with suspected fetal CNS abnormality on a routine US examination.

Images (Fig. 11.4)

A and B.

SSFSE axial T2-weighted images through the fetal head reveal a large single monoventricle filling most of the intracranial cavity with fused frontal lobes (A, *arrow*) and basal ganglia (B, *arrow*). The falx cerebri and interhemispheric fissure are absent

Alobar Holoprosencephaly

Clinical Presentation

A patient was referred for MR evaluation because of abnormal fetal US and polyhydramnios.

Image (Fig. 11.5)

A. Coronal image through fetal brain demonstrates absence of cleavage of the embryonic forebrain (*arrow*) into discrete hemispheres

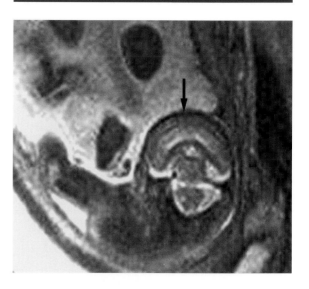

Figure 11.5
Alobar holoprosencephaly

Discussion

Incomplete or abnormal cleavage of the forebrain structures results in the holoprosencephaly spectrum. In holoprosencephaly, there is failure of lateral cleavage into distinct cerebral hemispheres and failure of transverse cleavage into diencephalon and telencephalon. The differentiation of the telencephalon from the diencephalon and the separation of the telencephalon into two cerebral hemispheres are in progress by the end of the 5th week of gestation.

Holoprosencephalies can be divided into three subcategories: alobar, semilobar and lobar. These categories are useful for classifying holoprosencephalies of different severities with the alobar type as the most severe and lobar type as the mildest form. Additionally, at the mildest end of the spectrum is septo-optic dysplasia.

Holoprosencephaly is caused by teratogens, and chromosomal and genetic factors, although most cases are sporadic. The most common teratogen in humans is maternal diabetes.

Although alobar holoprosencephaly is the most common form of holoprosencephaly diagnosed by prenatal US, affected patients are rarely imaged postnatally by CT or MR imaging. This rarity stems from the fact that most affected infants are still-born or have a very short life span.

Imaging studies in alobar holoprosencephaly show a completely unsegmented rim of brain that surrounds a largely undifferentiated central CSF-filled cavity. There is no interhemispheric fissure, falx cerebri or corpus callosum. A large posterior midline cyst is usually present. Usually there are associated severe craniofacial anomalies, such as cyclopia or hypotelorism.

Suggested Reading

Barkovich AJ (2000) Pediatric neuroimaging, 3rd edn. Lippincott Williams and Wilkins, Philadelphia, pp 318–320

Byrd SE, Osborn RE, Rodkowski MA, et al (1988) Disorders of midline structures: holoprosencephaly, absence of corpus callosum, and Chiari malformations. Semin Ultrasound CT MR 99:201–215

Septo-Optic Dysplasia

Clinical Presentation

Septo-optic dysplasia in a fetus at 21 weeks gestation.

Image (Fig. 11.6)

A. Coronal image shows complete absence of septum pellucidum (*arrow*) with enlarged ventricles

Discussion

Septo-optic dysplasia is an anterior midline congenital anomaly that consists of hypoplasia of the optic nerves, along with absence or hypoplasia of the septum pellucidum. The absent septum pellucidum causes a box-like configuration of the frontal horns of the lateral ventricles. Hypothalamic hypopituitarism is associated in more than half of cases. Migrational abnormalities and agenesis or hypoplasia of the corpus callosum may also be seen.

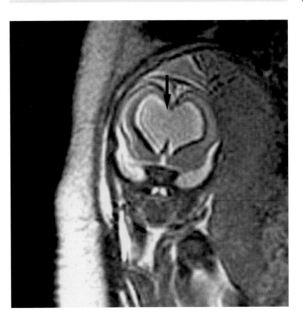

Figure 11.6
Septo-optic dysplasia

Suggested Reading

Barkovich AJ, Fram EK, Norman D (1989) Septo-optic dysplasia: MR imaging. Radiology 171:189–192

Righini A, Zirpoli S, Mrakic F, Parazzinin C, et al (2004) Early prenatal MR imaging diagnosis of polymicrogyria. AJNR Am J Neuroradiol 25:343–346

Aplasia of the Corpus Callosum

Clinical Presentation

Abnormal fetal US in late pregnancy.

Image (Fig. 11.7)

A. Axial fetal MR image demonstrates parallel configuration of the lateral ventricles with colpocephaly. This is the typical appearance in an absent corpus callosum

Discussion

Agenesis or hypoplasia of the corpus callosum are common developmental disorders. They may occur in isolation or as part of other midline anomalies, including hemispheric cysts, pericallosal lipoma, midline cleft lip and/or palate. They may be associated with X-linked hydrocephalus. This diagnosis is suggested in the male fetus with abducted thumbs and dilated lateral and third ventricles. Some other syndromes may be associated with corpus callosum malformations, including Chiari II malformation, Aicardi's syndrome and Dandy-Walker spectrum.

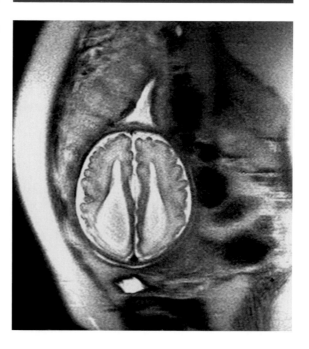

Figure 11.7

Aplasia of the corpus callosum

Suggested Reading

D'Ercole C, Girard N, Cravello L, Boubli L, Potier A, Raybaud C, Blanc B (1998) Prenatal diagnosis of fetal corpus callosum agenesis by ultrasonography and magnetic resonance imaging. Prenat Diagn 3:247–253

Rypens F, Sonigo P, Aubry MC, Delezoide AL, Cessot F, Brunelle F (1996) Prenatal MR diagnosis of a thick corpus callosum. AJNR Am J Neuroradiol 10:1918–1920

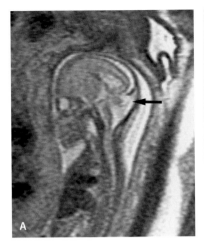 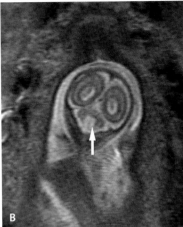 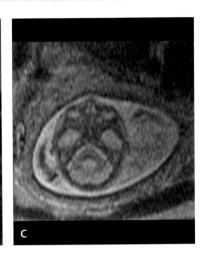

Figure 11.8

Dandy-Walker malformation

Dandy-Walker Malformation

Clinical Presentation

Dandy-Walker malformation at 22 weeks gestation.

Images (Fig. 11.8)

A. Sagittal image demonstrates a large posterior fossa cyst with wide communication with fourth ventricle (*arrow*). The torcula is elevated

B. Coronal image confirms the wide communication with the fourth ventricle (*arrow*)

C. Axial image reveals a large posterior fossa cyst

Discussion

Advances in MR imaging now allow routine visualization of fetal CNS if prenatal US is abnormal or fails to completely visualize the brain structures. Fetal MR imaging is being used routinely to evaluate posterior fossa cystic malformations. The Dandy-Walker spectrum of developmental anomalies are documented and any associated CNS anomalies searched. The Dandy-Walker variant is defined as vermian hypoplasia with cystic dilatation of the fourth ventricle without enlarged posterior fossa. The Dandy-Walker malformation is considered to be present when there is absence of the vermis, or at least a major part of it, and a dilated fourth ventricle communicates with a retrocerebellar cyst. The posterior fossa is enlarged and torcula elevated.

Suggested Reading

Sonigo PC, Rypens FF, Carteret M, Delezoide AL, Brunelle FO (1998) MR imaging of fetal cerebral anomalies. Pediatric Radiol 28:212–222

Stazzone MM, Hubbard AM, Bilaniuk LT, et al (2000) Ultrafast MR imaging of the normal posterior fossa in fetuses. AJR Am J Roentgenol 175:835–839

Fetal Hydrops

Clinical Presentation

Fetal hydrops at 16 weeks gestation.

Images (Fig. 11.9)

A. Sagittal single-shot T2-weighted image at 16 weeks gestation shows severe fetal hydrops, with diffuse abnormal thickening and lucency of the subcutaneous tissues (*arrow*)
B. Sagittal FLAIR image shows the abnormal subcutaneous tissue as black (*arrow*)
C. On coronal image severe hydrops fetalis is seen as lucency around the head and body (*arrows*)
D. Axial T2-weighted image through the brain shows normal ventricles and brain for gestational age

Discussion

Fetal hydrops (hydrops fetalis) usually is defined as the presence of fetal subcutaneous tissue edema accompanied by serous effusion in one or more body cavities. Placental edema invariably accompanies fetal edema, and hydramnios is usually present. Fetal hydrops can be of an immune (10%) or nonimmune (90%) etiology. Immune hydrops can be antibody-mediated hemolytic anemia or Rho/ABO incompatibility. Nonimmune hydrops can be caused by diseases namely primary heart failure, high output failure (twin-twin transfusion, vascular malformations, and hemoglobinopathies), decreased plasma oncotic pressure, lymphatic obstruction and congenital infections. A significant proportion of fetal hydrops is caused by chromosomal abnormalities.

Neonatal US is the screening modality of choice. However, technical factors and late gestation may hamper the detection of various anomalies. Fetal MR imaging is a complementary imaging technique which helps in the detection of abnormalities missed by ultrasound. On imaging, the fetus shows skin thickening which is especially prominent around the scalp ("helmet sign"), ascites, and pleural and pericardial effusions. When a central nervous system anomaly is detected on US, MR imaging may demonstrate additional findings that may alter patient counseling and case management.

Suggested Reading

Guo WY, Wong TT (2003) Screening of fetal CNS anomalies by MR imaging. Childs Nerv Syst 19:410–411

Levine D, Barnes PD, Robertson RR, Wong G, Mehta TS (2003) Fast MR imaging of fetal central nervous system abnormalities. Radiology 229:51–61

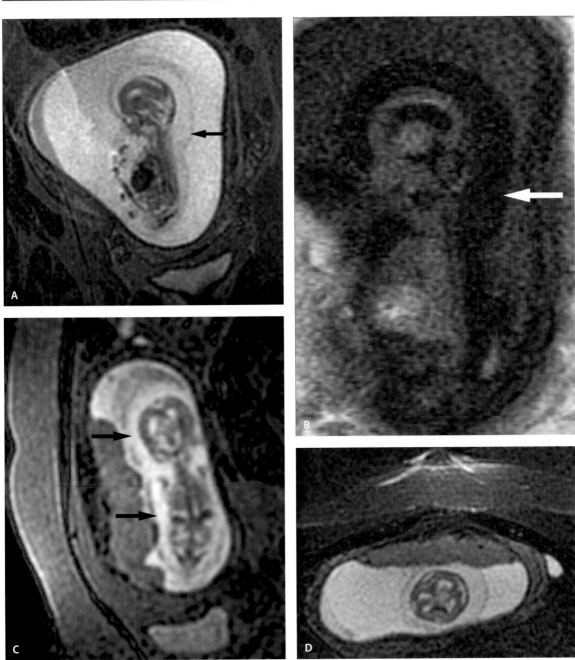

Figure 11.9

Fetal hydrops

Fetal Sacrococcygeal Teratoma

Clinical Presentation

Fetal US obtained because of maternal polyhydramnion at the end of the second trimester revealed sacral abnormality that was later confirmed with MR imaging.

Image (Fig. 11.10)

A. Prenatal sagittal SSFSE image at 20 weeks reveals a bright signal intensity mass over the sacrum

Discussion

Sacrococcygeal teratomas are the most common neonatal tumor with an incidence of 1 in 40,000 live births. They are diagnosed commonly in the prenatal period, and complications may occur in utero or during birth. There is a 4:1 female to male preponderance. The usual time of presentation is between 22 and 34 weeks of gestation when the size of the gravid uterus is more than the period of gestation. Polyhydramnios may be associated. Sacrococcygeal teratomas may be classified as benign (mature) and malignant or immature. Mature teratomas are most common in neonates (68%) and older children (73%). Immature teratomas are cystic, whereas malignant tumors are solid. Sacrococcygeal teratomas need to be differentiated from neural tube defects, epidermoid cysts, anal duct cyst, and lymphangioma. The prenatal diagnosis should lead to the decision regarding the individualization of the method of the delivery depending upon the size of the tumor.

Fast MR imaging has changed our ability to image the fetus. Although US remains the primary screening technique for evaluating the fetus, significant limitations still exists in the complex prenatal US diagnoses. Using the single-shot rapid acquisition technique, individual images are obtained in 300–400 ms, allowing imaging of the fetus without sedation. When a CNS anomaly is detected or suspected at US, MR imaging may demonstrate additional findings that can alter the diagnosis and case management. It may also confirm an equivocal US diagnosis. This is especially important when fetal surgery is considered, but it can also influence the selection of the level of the birth hospital or method of delivery.

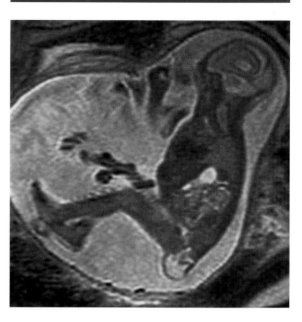

Figure 11.10

Fetal sacrococcygeal teratoma

Suggested Reading

Coakley FV, Hricak H, Filly RA, Barkovich AJ, Harrison MR (1999) Complex fetal disorders: effect of MR imaging on management – preliminary clinical experience. Radiology 213:691–696

Simon EM, Goldstein RB, Coakley FV, Filly RA, Broderick KC, Musci TJ, Barkovich AJ (2000) Fast MR imaging of fetal CNS anomalies in utero. AJNR Am J Neuroradiol 21:1688–1698

Levine D, Barnes PD, Robertson RR, Wong G, Mehta TS (2003) Fast MR imaging of fetal central nervous system abnormalities. Radiology 229:51–61

Sheth SH, Nussbaum RJ, Sanders R (1986) Sacrococcygeal teratoma: sonographic-pathologic correlation. Radiology 169:131–136

Tuladhar R, Patole SK, Whitehall JS (2000) Sacrococcygeal teratoma in perinatal period. Postgrad Med J 76:754–759

Miscellaneous

In collaboration with Sudhir Kathuria, MD

Introduction

As MR imaging technology improves and becomes more widely used, its role in patients' medical workup increases. This applies not only to the conditions in which genetics play a key role, such as phakomatoses, disorders of cortical development and inborn errors of metabolism, but also to many isolated and acquired conditions.

Malformations of cortical development are important to detect because they often cause developmental delay and seizures. Proper localization of these malformations can lead to surgical treatment of the epilepsy altering significantly the patient's life but also the life of the whole family. A particular subset of partial seizures is the complex partial seizure that has a focal onset. Approximately 70% of complex partial seizures have their origin in the temporal lobe and many of these patients become refractory to medical treatment. Because temporal lobectomy is an effective treatment, MR imaging has an important role in patients' clinical workup to guide the possible surgical treatment. Mesial temporal sclerosis is seldom discovered in a young child; it is more often seen in patients 10 years and older.

Phakomatoses are a group of disorders that are connected by a similar tendency to produce manifestations in the CNS and many other tissues. Phakomatoses belong to a group neuroectomesodermal dysplasias with characteristic malformation of tissues and neoplastic growth emanating from three germ layers. Presently none of the phakomatoses has an effective prevention, and medical treatment and management are limited to following these patients and treatment of progressive lesions. MR imaging plays a key role in the detection of CNS lesions and in the follow-up of the progression of these lesions.

Neurofibromatosis 1 (von Recklinghausen disease) is the most common neurocutaneous disorder, described as long ago as 1882. It is inherited as an autosomal dominant disorder with variable penetrance. It is caused by defects in chromosome 17. Neurofibromatosis 1 affects multiple cell types and multiple organs. The common intracranial manifestations include optic pathway tumors, astrocytomas and "neurofibromatosis spots" (myelin vacuolization), in addition to peripheral nerve involvement. Both T1 and T2 signal abnormalities in the basal ganglia typically resolve by adulthood.

Neurofibromatosis 2 was described in the 1930s. Symptomatic patients with neurofibromatosis 2 seem to be older than patients with neurofibromatosis 1. The hallmark of neurofibromatosis 2 is bilateral acoustic neuromas (vestibular schwannomas). In contrast to neurofibromatosis 1, in which glial tumors predominate, the tumors associated with neurofibromatosis 2 generally arise from Schwann meningothelial cells. Meningiomas are often multiple in patients with neurofibromatosis 2. Ependymomas are a common occurrence and usually arise within the spinal cord. Increased clinical awareness, better imaging techniques, and molecular diagnostics have made pediatric diagnosis of neurofibromatosis 2 possible, but outcomes appear to be worse than in adult patients.

Tuberous sclerosis is a congenital autosomal disorder associated with mutations in least two different chromosomes. The imaging hallmark of tuberous sclerosis is cortical tubers and subependymal nodules along the striothalamic groove. Although the calcified subependymal nodules are best visible on CT scan, MR imaging plays a major role in outlining the cortical nodules, white matter changes, radial bands and giant cell astrocytomas near the foramen of Monro. The classic clinical triad includes facial angiofibromas, mental retardation and seizures. All three symptoms are only seen in one-third of the patients. In the CT era, contrast enhancement was considered as neoplastic transformation; however, gadolinium enhancement on MR images has been seen in nongrowing lesions.

Von Hippel-Lindau syndrome (HLS), hemangioblastomatosis, is a congenital autosomal dominant disorder linked to a mutation on chromosome 3. Most lesions in HLS are infratentorial or in the spinal canal. The appearance of the hemangioblastomas varies from completely solid to cystic lesions with mural nodule. There are no cutaneous findings in HLS; however, the patients develop retinal angiomas that are hemangioblastomas. Since these patients may have multiorgan symptoms, including being at risk of renal cell carcinoma, they need life-long screening. In addition to retinal and cerebellar hemangiomas, patients may develop the same tumors in the spinal cord and nerve roots. These are not drop metastases; they are intramedullary tumors.

Sturge-Weber syndrome is a sporadic, congenital (but not inherited) syndrome of uncertain inheritance. The main feature is lack of normal development of the fetal cortical veins leading to chronic venous ischemia. Patients present also with pial angiomatosis with underlying cortical atrophy, white matter calcification and facial "port-wine nevus".

Arachnoid cysts are benign congenital intra-arachnoid collections of CSF. Although small lesions are asymptomatic and incidental findings, some cysts may expand over time. The exact mechanism for the expansion is still under discussion and several theories have been proposed.

Dermoid cysts arise from the inclusion of embryonic ectoderm into the neural tube during the 5th and 6th week of fetal life. They typically occur in the midline. Characteristically they are bright, fatty lesions in the T1-weighted image, but vary from hypo- to hyperintense in the T2-weighted image. They are rare lesions and usually not symptomatic until adulthood. They expand over the years and may rupture, resulting in chemical meningitis leading to vasospasm and infarctions, and even death.

Posterior reversible encephalopathy syndrome (PRES) is a condition long-recognized in association with hypertensive encephalopathy in pregnant patients with eclampsia. It is also seen as a consequence of chemotherapeutic agents, intrathecal methotrexate treatment and treatment of acute lymphoblastic leukemia in children. It is not uncommonly seen in transplant patients with antirejection medication. The hallmark of this condition is vasogenic edema in the posterior circulation area. DW imaging with ADC map is a useful method for recognizing the condition and guiding aggressive treatment to prevent infarction.

Suggested Reading

Ciricillo SF, Cogen PH, Harsh GR, Edwards MS (1991) Intracranial arachnoid cysts in children. A comparison of the effects of fenestration and shunting. J Neurosurg 742:230–235

Farina L, Bergqvist C, Zimmerman RA, Haselgrove J, Hunter JV, Bilaniuk LT (2004) Acute diffusion abnormalities in the hippocampus of children with new-onset seizures: the development of mesial temporal sclerosis. Neuroradiology 4:251–257

Nunes F, MacCollin M (2003) Neurofibromatosis 2 in the pediatric population. J Child Neurol 10:718–724

Otsuki T (2004) Neuroimaging and presurgical evaluation of symptomatic epilepsies. Psychiatry Clin Neurosci 3:S13–S15

Smirniotopoulos JG (2004) Neuroimaging of phakomatoses: Sturge-Weber syndrome, tuberous sclerosis, von Hippel-Lindau syndrome. Neuroimaging Clin North Am 2:171–183

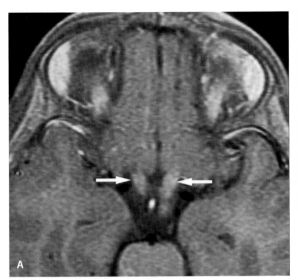 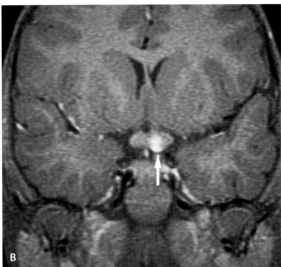

Figure 12.1

Neurofibromatosis 1 and bilateral optic nerve and chiasm glioma

Neurofibromatosis

Neurofibromatosis 1 and Bilateral Optic Nerve and Chiasm Glioma

Clinical Presentation

A 3-year-old asymptomatic female with neurofibromatosis. Previous MR image revealed an optic nerve glioma.

Images (Fig. 12.1)

A. The proximal optic nerves appear enlarged on the axial T1-weighted image with contrast enhancement (*arrows*)
B. Both optic nerves and also optic chiasm is thickened. An abnormal high signal nodule is seen in the undersurface of the enlarged optic chiasm and optic nerves displacing the pituitary stalk slightly towards the right. This lesion enhances with contrast (*arrow*)

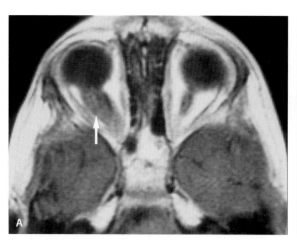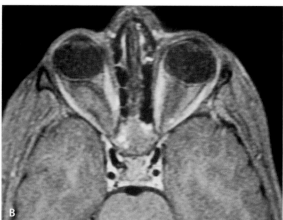

Figure 12.2

Neurofibromatosis 1 and unilateral optic nerve glioma

Neurofibromatosis 1 and Unilateral Optic Nerve Glioma

Clinical Presentation

An 8-year-old child with known optic nerve glioma on right.

Images (Fig. 12.2)

A. Axial T1-weighted image without contrast enhancement shows right optic nerve enlargement (*arrow*)
B. Contrast-enhanced image with fat suppression reveals the enlarged right optic nerve without contrast enhancement

Neurofibromatosis 1 and "Hamartomas": Myelin Vacuolization in Supratentorial Area

Clinical Presentation

A 6-year-old female with skin freckling discovered in routine examination is referred to MR imaging.

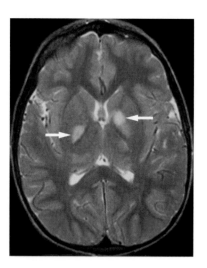

Figure 12.3

Neurofibromatosis 1 and "hamartomas": myelin vacuolization in supratentorial area

Image (Fig. 12.3)

A. Rounded foci of increased signal intensity are seen in both globi pallidi (*arrows*) and both thalami on axial T2-weighted image

Figure 12.4

Neurofibromatosis 1 and "hamartomas": myelin vacuolization in
cerebellum and pons

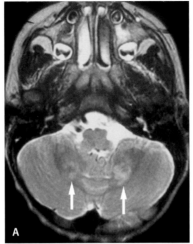 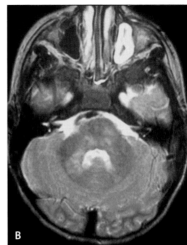

Neurofibromatosis 1 and "Hamartomas": Myelin Vacuolization in Cerebellum and Pons

Clinical Presentation

A 6-year-old asymptomatic child discovered in routine examination to have skin manifestations of neurofibromatosis 1.

Images (Fig. 12.4)

A. Axial T2-weighted image through the cerebellar white matter shows ill-defined T2 prolongation in the white matter of the dentate nuclei (*arrows*)
B. T2 prolongation is also seen in the middle cerebral peduncles and dorsal pons

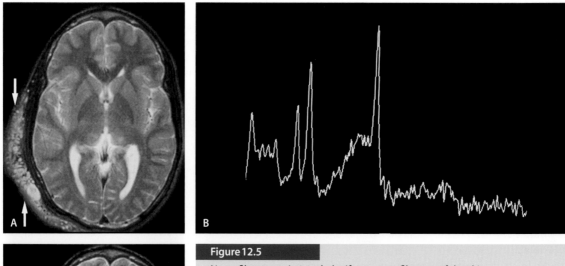

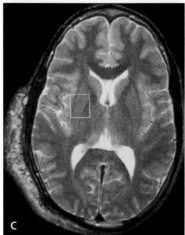

Figure 12.5

Neurofibromatosis 1 and plexiform neurofibroma of the skin

Neurofibromatosis 1 and Plexiform Neurofibroma of the Skin

Clinical Presentation

A 17-year-old male with neurofibromatosis 1 experienced new onset of dizziness and tremor on left arm and leg.

Images (Fig. 12.5)

A. A large plexiform neurofibroma is seen in the right side (*arrows*)
B. Single voxel MR spectroscopy of the basal ganglia with TE=35 ms is unremarkable
C. T2-weighted image shows voxel placement

Discussion

Neurofibromatosis type 1 is the most common neurocutaneous disorder that results from production of nonfunctional protein neurofibroma due to an abnormal gene on chromosome 17. It is mainly characterized by multiple neurofibromas along the peripheral nerves, optic nerve gliomas, sphenoid wing dysplasia, pigmented iris nodules, café-au-lait spots, and the so-called "unidentified neurofibromatosis objects" (UNOs) or hamartomas.

Neurofibromas are complex benign tumors arising in the peripheral nerves accompanied by thickened perineurium with increased size and number of Schwann cells. Cutaneous neurofibromas are confined to a single fascicle within a nerve and begin to appear in mid-childhood, while diffuse plexiform neurofibromas involve multiple fascicles and are almost always congenital. On imaging they give signal similar or slightly greater than muscle in T1 images with homogeneous hyperintense or characteristic "target sign" on T2-weighted images. Typically, the lesion can form a "dumbbell" appearance and often is associated with displacement of the spinal cord by the mass.

Optic pathway gliomas and brainstem gliomas are the most common intracranial neoplasms found in this disorder. Optic pathway gliomas can arise anywhere from the globe to the occipital cortex. The majority of these intracranial neoplasms are benign pilocytic astrocytomas that behave in a less-aggressive manner than histologically identical tumors in a non-neurofibromatosis type 1 patient.

On brain MR imaging, areas of T2 hyperintensity (neurofibromatosis spots or hamartomas) are seen in the pons, cerebellar white matter, internal capsule and splenium of the corpus callosum. Histologically, these represent myelin vacuolization and separation of myelin layers around the axons. These lesions typically start appearing at about 3 years of age and increase in number and size until 10 to 12 years, and then again decrease in number and size. They are rarely seen in adults.

Other intracranial manifestations of this disorder include bone dysplasia, macrocephaly, a larger midsagittal surface area of the corpus callosum, and vascular dysplasia. Sphenoid wing dysplasia is of clinical importance as it may sometime result in herniation of the temporal lobe into the orbit causing pulsating exophthalmos. It can be associated with orbital or periorbital plexiform neurofibromatosis.

Suggested Reading

Palmer C, Szudek J, Joe H, et al (2004) Analysis of neurofibromatosis 1 (NF1) lesions by body segment. Am J Med Genet 125:157–161

Visrutaratna P, Oranratanachai K, Singhavejsakul J (2004) Clinics in diagnostic imaging (96). Plexiform neurofibromatosis. Singapore Med J 45:188–192

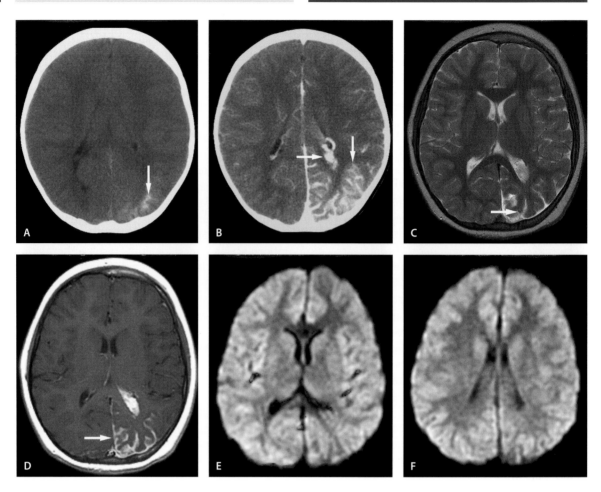

Figure 12.6

Classic Sturge-Weber syndrome

Sturge-Weber Syndrome

Classic Sturge-Weber Syndrome

Clinical Presentation

An 8-year-old female with seizures and history of Sturge-Weber syndrome. Patient has glaucoma. MR imaging is done to evaluate extent of the disease.

Images (Fig. 12.6)

A. Noncontrast CT scan at the age of 17 months following seizures shows abnormal calcification in the left posterior parietal cortex (*arrow*)

B. Contrast-enhanced CT scan shows extensive enhancement in the angiomatosis area and in the left choroid plexus (*arrows*)

C. On T2-weighted image there is evidence of pial-leptomeningeal enhancement consistent with angiomatosis. There are calcifications identified as areas of low signal intensity on T2-weighted images in the adjacent cortex (*arrow*). The occipital horn of the left lateral ventricle is prominent and is related to an enlarged choroid plexus. There is a

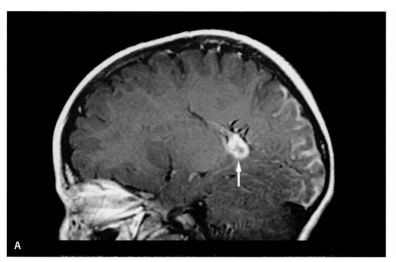

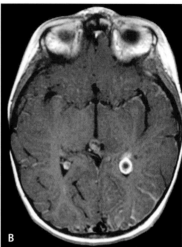

Figure 12.7

Leptomeningeal angioma and prominent choroid plexus

dilated periventricular vein. Cortical atrophy is present on the area. There is thickening of the diploic space over the involved cortex

D. Contrast-enhanced image shows marked enhancement in the area of angiomatosis (*arrow*)

E. No area of restricted diffusion is seen on DW image

F. DW image at the higher cortical level is also normal

Leptomeningeal Angioma and Prominent Choroid Plexus

Clinical Presentation

A 2-year-old boy with Sturge-Weber syndrome and a seizure disorder now presents with behavioral changes.

Images (Fig. 12.7)

A. Sagittal contrast-enhanced T1-weighted image reveals enlarged choroid plexus (*arrow*). Extensive leptomeningeal enhancement is also seen over the surface of the left cerebral hemisphere posteriorly

B. Axial contrast-enhanced image confirms the findings seen in A

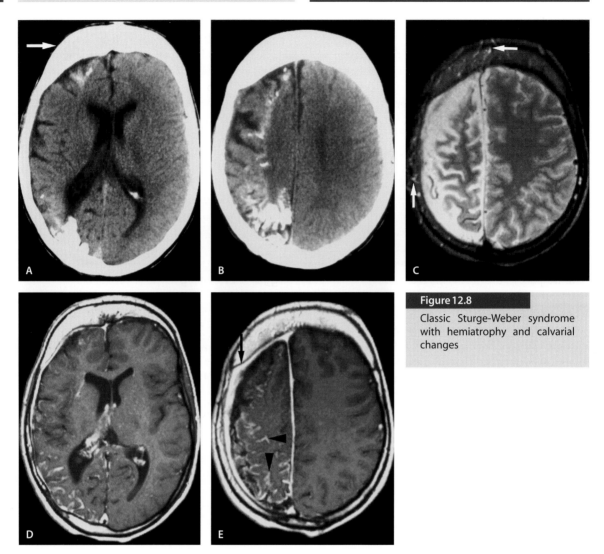

Figure 12.8

Classic Sturge-Weber syndrome with hemiatrophy and calvarial changes

Classic Sturge-Weber Syndrome with Hemiatrophy and Calvarial Changes

Clinical Presentation

A 12-year-old girl with long history of seizures has a port-wine nevus on the right side of her face.

Images (Fig. 12.8)

A. Axial noncontrast CT scan shows abnormal calcification in the cortex of the right frontal and occipital lobes. Note also the frontal calvarial thickening (*arrow*)

B. Axial noncontrast CT scan in this patient shows more extensive cortical calcification also in the parietal region

C. The cortical calcification is difficult to appreciate on T2-weighted image. The right hemisphere is smaller with cortical atrophy. Note the multiple transcalvarial vascular channels (*arrows*)

D. Contrast-enhanced T1-weighted image shows extensive leptomeningeal enhancement. The right choroid plexus is enlarged and shows significant enhancement

E. Contrast-enhanced T1-weighted image also shows leptomeningeal (*arrowheads*) and pachymeningeal (*arrow*) enhancement in the atrophic right hemisphere. Note the enlarged right hemicranium with prominent vascular channels

Discussion

Sturge-Weber syndrome, encephalotrigeminal angiomatosis, is a sporadically occurring phakomatosis characterized by a port-wine vascular nevus in the territory of the trigeminal nerve, particularly of the first division. The clinical features include seizures, mental retardation and hemiplegia or paresis. The primary lesion is abnormality in the circulation for the brain and skin that is mainly postcapillary with dilated veins. The abnormal circulation involves skin of the face, brain, eye and leptomeninges. The facial nevus is often described "port-wine stain". Some children are born with an enlarged globe (buthalmos, ox eye). Intracranially an abnormal venous drainage is seen, with angiomatous change in the choroid plexus. Chronic ischemia in the cortex leads to progressive cortical atrophy and calcification.

Although diagnosis can be made on clinical features, imaging is important to confirm the diagnosis as well as to exclude unsuspected bilateral Sturge-Weber syndrome. Intracranial gyral calcification in the form of a "tram-track " pattern located in the occipital and posterior parietal lobes ipsilateral to facial angioma is the common radiological manifestation of Sturge-Weber syndrome.

Calcification is unusual before the age of 2 years. CT scan is the ideal modality for detection of cortical calcifications and determining their extent. MR imaging is better than CT imaging in showing the extent and degree of brain parenchymal atrophy, the presumed ischemic changes affecting the gray and white matter, and the cranial diploetic prominence on the affected side. Contrast-enhanced MR image shows the extent and patency of the leptomeningeal angiomatous malformation and the parenchymal venous anomalies. ^{99m}Tc HMPAO (^{99m}technetium hexamethylpropyleneamine oxime) imaging serves as a useful adjunct for preoperative road map of the lesions.

Suggested Reading

Griffiths PD, Boodram MB, Blasre S, Armstrong D, Gilday DL, Harwood-Nash D (1997) 99m Technetium HMPAO imaging in children with the Sturge-Weber syndrome: a study of nine cases with CT and MRI correlation. Neuroradiology 39:219–224

Marti-Bonmati L, Menor F, Poyatos C, Cortina H (1992) Diagnosis of Sturge-Weber syndrome: comparison of the efficacy of CT and MR imaging in 14 cases. AJR Am J Roentgenol 158:867–871

Sperner J, Schmauser I, Bittner R, et al (1990) MR imaging findings in children with Struge-Weber syndrome. Neuropediatrics 21:146–152

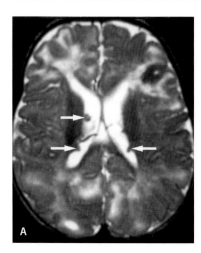 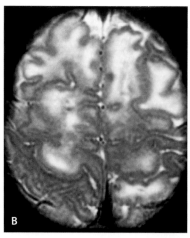

Tuberous Sclerosis

Tuberous Sclerosis and Subependymal Nodules and Cortical Tubers

Clinical Presentation

A 7-month-old child with seizures since infancy.

Images (Fig. 12.9)

A. Axial T2-weighted image shows multiple areas of subcortical white matter hyperintensities. Subependymal nodules are well seen (*arrows*)
B. Cortical tubers are seen as marked hyperintensities with associated expansion of the overlying gyri

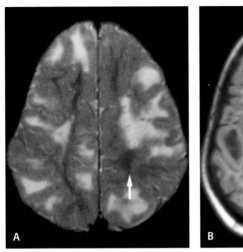
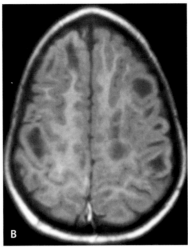
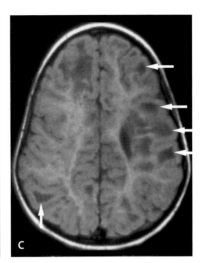

Figure 12.10

Tuberous sclerosis and radial bands and cortical tubers

Tuberous Sclerosis and Radial Bands and Cortical Tubers

Clinical Presentation

A 3-year-old with seizures and mental retardation.

Images (Fig. 12.10)

A. Axial T2-weighted image shows tubers of marked hyperintensities with associated expansion of the overlying gyri. Hypointense radial bands are seen on left (*arrow*)

B. The radial bands can be seen as hypointense on the T1-weighted image. Cortical tubers are also hypointense

C. T1-weighted image shows numerous hypointense tubers (*arrows*)

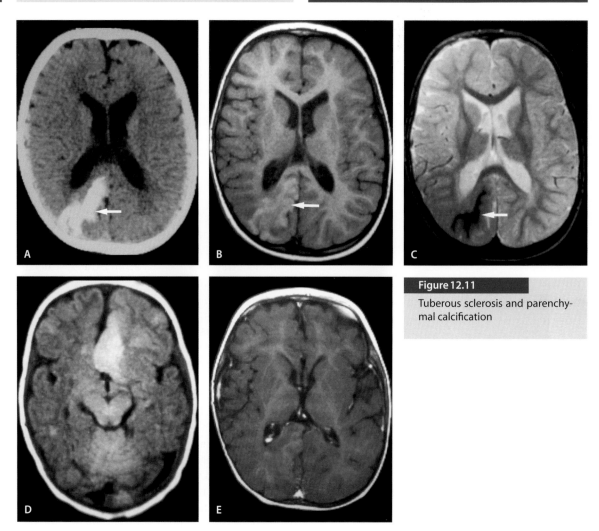

Figure 12.11

Tuberous sclerosis and parenchymal calcification

Tuberous Sclerosis and Parenchymal Calcification

Clinical Presentation

A 10-year-old with seizures and developmental delay.

Images (Fig. 12.11)

A. CT scan shows a large parenchymal calcification (*arrow*)
B. The right occipital calcification is slightly hyperintense on T1-weighted image (*arrow*)
C. Calcified tuber is hypointense on T2-weighted image (*arrow*)
D. Left frontal lobe tuber is hyperintense on T1-weighted image
E. Contrast-enhanced image through the calcified lesion; no enhancement is present

Tuberous sclerosis and cortical dysplasia-mimicking lesion

Tuberous Sclerosis and Cortical Dysplasia-Mimicking Lesion

Clinical Presentation

A 12-year-old girl with tuberous sclerosis and seizures.

Image (Fig. 12.12)

A. Axial FLAIR image shows wedge-shaped cortical lesion tapering towards the ventricle and simulating focal cortical dysplasia of Taylor type

Tuberous Sclerosis and Giant Cell Astrocytoma, Subependymal and Subcortical Tubers

Clinical Presentation

A 12-year-old girl with tuberous sclerosis. She has had recent clinical deterioration with difficulty ambulating and new behavioral changes.

Images (Fig. 12.13)

A. Noncontrast CT shows parenchymal (*arrow*) calcification and subependymal calcification at the foramen of Monro and the right trigone
B. Noncontrast CT scan demonstrates calcified subependymal nodules. The ventricles are mildly enlarged
C. T2-weighted image at the ventricle level shows a heterogeneous subependymal giant cell astrocytoma (SEGA) at the foramen of Monro (*arrow*). A calcified tuber is vaguely seen adjacent left trigone (*arrowhead*)
D. FLAIR image shows cortical and subcortical tubers
E. Calcified subependymal nodule is seen at the right trigone (*arrow*) on T2-weighted image
F. The SEGA is isointense to the gray matter on T1-weighted image (*arrow*)
G. Contrast-enhanced T1-weighted image shows robustly enhancing SEGA on right side. Mild hydrocephalus is present

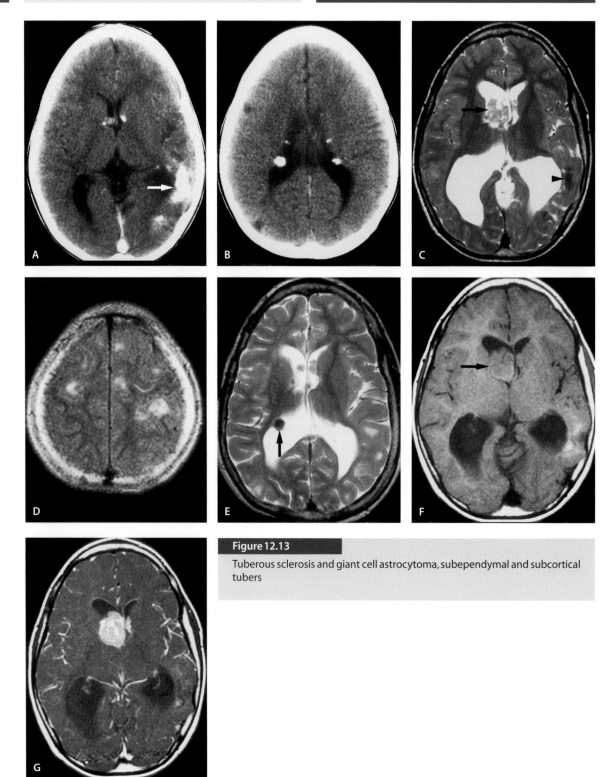

Figure 12.13

Tuberous sclerosis and giant cell astrocytoma, subependymal and subcortical tubers

Tuberous Sclerosis and Low-Grade Glioma

Clinical Presentation

A 9-year-old male with symptomatic tuberous sclerosis since childhood. He presents with seizures and increasing behavioral changes.

Images (Fig. 12.14)

A. Axial T2-weighted image reveals multiple cortical and subcortical tubers. There is a cystic lesion with a solid component in the cyst wall which shows enhancement and reveals low-grade glioma. This left frontal lesion has increased in size and has now a mild mass effect to the lateral ventricle (*arrow*). Other cortical/subcortical lesions are unchanged in size

B. The cystic lesion shows low signal on FLAIR image. The smaller lesions are surrounded by vasogenic edema

C. None of the lesions shows high signal on DW image

D. The cystic lesion shows no restricted diffusion

E. A large right cerebellar lesion is of low signal on T2-weighted image; it probably contains calcification

F. Coronal T2-weighted image shows the full extent of the cerebellar lesion

G. The cerebellar lesion is also hypointense on FLAIR image

Discussion

Tuberous sclerosis is an autosomal dominant neurocutaneous syndrome with multisystem involvement including the brain, kidney, skin, retina, heart, lung, and bone. Two separate genes have been identified that are mutated or deleted in patients with tuberous sclerosis. The brain is the most frequently affected organ. The hallmark of tuberous sclerosis is calcified subependymal nodules, best seen on CT scan. The classical clinical triad of adenoma sebaceum, seizures, and mental retardation is found in fewer than half of the patients. The cerebral lesions in tuberous sclerosis are of three kinds: cortical tubers, white matter abnormalities, and subependymal nodules; they are almost always benign hamartomas. Not all kinds of lesions are seen in the same patient. Clinically 80% of patients present with myoclonic seizures beginning in infancy.

Cortical Tubers. Cortical hamartomas ("tubers") can be seen in both brain and cerebellum. They may vary from a few millimeters to several centimeters in size. On MR imaging, tubers show somewhat thick cortical gray matter and a less distinctive gray/white matter junction compared with normal cortex. The peripheral component of tubers is isointense to mildly hyperintense to normal gray matter on both T1- and T2-weighted images. Calcification may be seen in more than 50% of cortical tubers. The cortical tuber may show central depression.

Subependymal Nodules. Subependymal nodules are the most characteristic lesions of tuberous sclerosis. They are found in 95% of patients with tuberous sclerosis. Subependymal nodules may occur in the third and fourth ventricular walls, but most are found in the lateral ventricular walls near the sulcus terminalis. CT scan shows higher sensitivity in detection of subependymal nodules because of calcification. Calcification may be globular, partial, or ring-like in appearance. Giant cell astrocytoma may be seen in 10–15% of patients. This is always seen near or at the foramen of Monro (see Chapter 6).

White Matter Lesions. White matter lesions are composed of bizarre, heterotopic giant cells ("balloon cells") and associated hypomyelination. MR imaging shows four distinct patterns of white matter lesions: straight or curvilinear bands ("radial bands"), wedge-shaped lesions, nonspecific "tumefactive" or conglomerate foci; and cerebellar radial bands. Straight or curvilinear bands extend from the ventricular wall through the cerebrum toward the cortex. Most white matter lesions are seen as isointense to hypointense on T1-weighted images and hyperintense on T2-weighted images in older children and adults. In infants these bands are hypointense to unmyelinated white matter on T2-weighted image.

Balloon cell focal cortical dysplasia of Taylor type resembles tuberous sclerosis in terms of its histological and imaging findings. In the absence of systemic or cutaneous symptoms it is difficult to distinguish them apart from forme fruste tuberous sclerosis. Many authors believe that these disorders may represent a spectrum of the same entity.

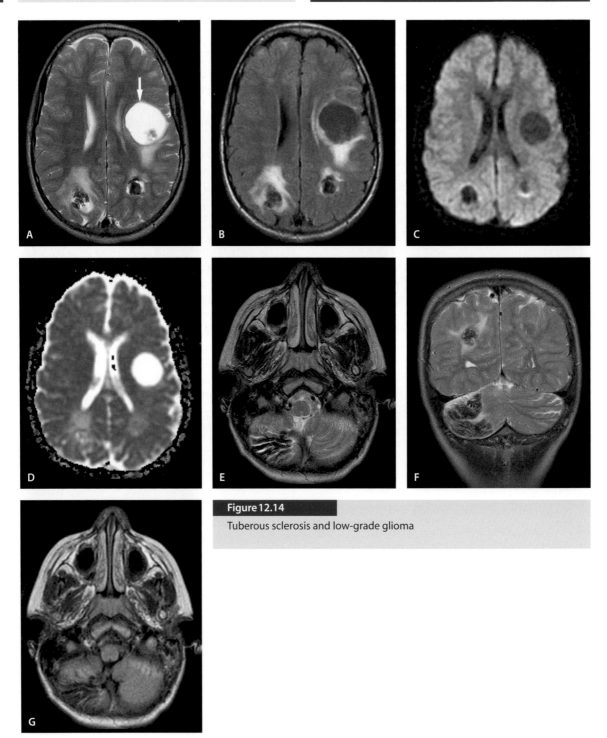

Figure 12.14
Tuberous sclerosis and low-grade glioma

Suggested Reading

Baron Y, Barkovich AJ (1999) MR imaging of tuberous sclerosis in neonates and young infants. AJNR Am J Neuroradiol 20:907–916

Griffiths PD, Martland TR (1997) Tuberous sclerosis complex: the role of neuroradiology. Neuropediatrics 28:244–252

Inoue Y, Nemoto Y, Murata R, et al (1998) CT and MR imaging of cerebral tuberous sclerosis. Brain Dev 20:209–221

Mesial Temporal Sclerosis

Bilateral Mesial Temporal Sclerosis

Clinical Presentation

A 15-year-old male with seizure disorder presents after a small head trauma.

Image (Fig. 12.15)

A. Coronal T2-weighted image shows hyperintensity and atrophy of both hippocampi (*arrows*)

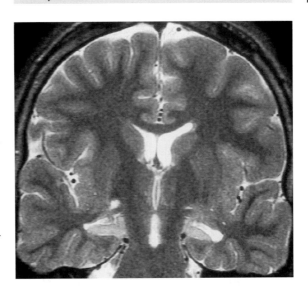

Figure 12.15

Bilateral mesial temporal sclerosis

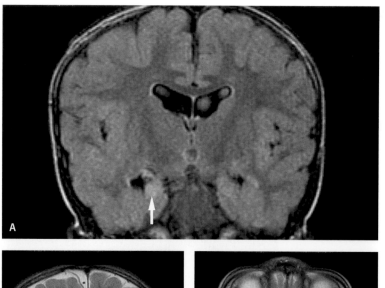

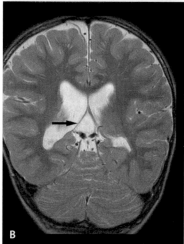
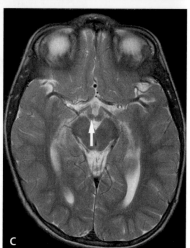

Hippocampus, Fornix and Mamillary Body Involvement in a Patient with Mesial Temporal Sclerosis

Clinical Presentation

A 3-year-old male with developmental delay and seizures.

Images (Fig. 12.16)

A. Coronal FLAIR reveals bilateral round hippocampi with disturbed internal architecture. The right hippocampus is smaller with increased signal (*arrow*)

B. High signal is noted also in the right atrophic fornix (*arrow*). This is best seen on T2-weighted image

C. The right mamillary body is smaller than the left (*arrow*). These features are suggestive of mesial temporal sclerosis on the right side

Unilateral Mesial Temporal Sclerosis

Clinical Presentation

A 14-year-old male with partial complex seizures.

Image (Fig. 12.17)

A. Left atrophic hippocampus with T2-hyperintensity (*arrow*) is seen

Discussion

Mesial temporal sclerosis, also known as hippocampal sclerosis or Ammon horn sclerosis, is the most common entity associated with medically intractable temporal lobe epilepsy. It is pathologically characterized by neuronal loss and gliosis that is also considered as the focus of such seizures. Although more commonly seen in adults, this disease is more prevalent in children than realized, and has been found in up to 12% of all brain MR imaging studies for seizures in children.

It is difficult to detect this entity on routine brain MR imaging, and visualization if the hippocampus requires a specific epilepsy protocol with thin coronal sections through the anterior hippocampi angled perpendicular to the long axis of the hippocampus. No contrast is needed unless a focal lesion is seen. The hallmark of this disease on MR imaging is an atrophic hippocampus associated with increased hippocampal signal on T2-weighted images, and decreased hippocampal signal on T1-weighted images. Other supporting findings include disruption of the internal hippocampal structure, and atrophy of other ipsilateral structures including temporal lobe, fornix, mamillary body and collateral white matter (white matter between the hippocampus and gray matter overlying the collateral sulcus), with increased temporal horn size. MR spectroscopy is often helpful: it shows decreased NAA in the hippocampus and/or temporal lobe. NAA/Cho ≤0.8 also suggests mesial temporal sclerosis. Quantitative hippocampal volumetry may increase sensitivity of mesial temporal sclerosis detection in doubtful cases. One has to be careful with MR images obtained soon after a seizure or status epilepticus, because T2 hyperintensity or gyriform enhancement in the hippocampus may be a misleading finding.

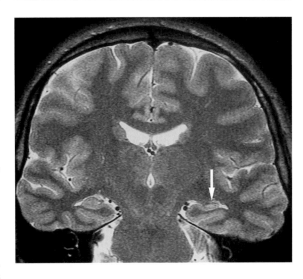

Figure 12.17

Unilateral mesial temporal sclerosis

MR imaging has a critical role in accurate identification and lateralization of this pathology before considering surgery to potentially cure such patients with medically intractable seizures. The Wada test with intraarterial sodium amytal injection into the carotid artery is a useful test to lateralize memory and language function.

Suggested Reading

Bronen R (1998) MR of mesial temporal sclerosis: how much is enough? AJNR Am J Neuroradiol 19:15–18

Ng YT, McGregor AL, Wheless JW (2004) Magnetic resonance imaging detection of mesial temporal sclerosis in children. Pediatr Neurol 30:81–85

Wasenko JJ, Gharagozloo AM, Smith MV, Thomas D (1997) High resolution MR technique in the diagnosis of mesial temporal sclerosis. Correlative MRI and pathological features. Clin Imaging 21:319–322

Figure 12.18

Absent pituitary gland

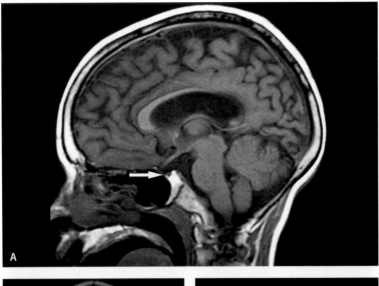

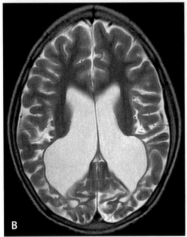

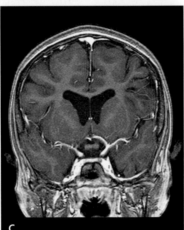

Pituitary-Hypothalamic Axis Anomalies

Absent Pituitary Gland

Clinical Presentation

A 16-year-old male with global developmental delay, multiple congenital anomalies as well as panhypopituitarism.

Images (Fig. 12.18)

A. Sagittal T1-weighted image reveals absent or markedly hypoplastic pituitary gland (*arrow*)
B. Axial T2-weighted image shows bilateral occipital atrophy with shrinkage of the cerebral cortices as well as significant loss of posterior white matter and consequent ex-vacuo dilatation of the lateral ventricles
C. Coronal contrast-enhanced T1-weighted image through the pituitary region reveals no visible gland

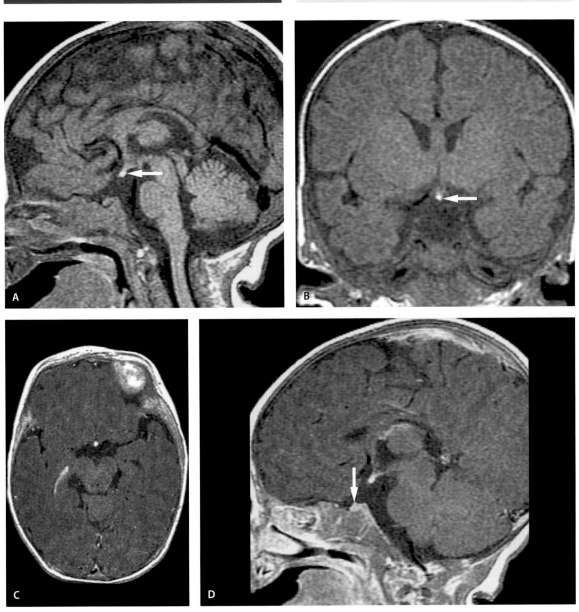

Figure 12.19

Ectopic posterior pituitary gland

Ectopic Posterior Pituitary Gland

Clinical Presentation

An 8-week-old infant with abnormal eye movement.

Images (Fig. 12.19)

A. Sagittal T1-weighted image without contrast shows focal increased signal intensity just inferior to the hypothalamic region in the midline (*arrow*). Normal pituitary stalk extending from the hypothalamus to the pituitary gland is not identified. The normal pituitary bright spot anterior to the dorsum is missing

B. Coronal T1-weighted image showing high intensity in an ectopic posterior pituitary gland (*arrow*)

C. Axial T1-weighted image confirms the location of the ectopic pituitary gland

D. Sagittal T1-weighted image with contrast enhancement shows enhancement of the normal (*arrow*) and ectopic gland

Thickening of the Pituitary Stalk

Clinical Presentation

A 6-year-old female with known Langerhans cell histiocytosis who recently developed headaches of increasing severity and diabetes insipidus.

Images (Fig. 12.20)

A. Sagittal T1-weighted image shows thickening of the pituitary stalk (*arrow*). Note the absence of the posterior pituitary bright spot

B. On coronal T1-weighted image the lesion appears isointense to surrounding brain parenchyma

C. On coronal T2-weighted image the thickened stalk is also isointense to the brain parenchyma (*arrow*)

D. On axial FLAIR the lesion is bright (*arrow*)

E. On DW image the lesion is slightly hyperintense (*arrow*)

F. The focal mass in the hypothalamus enhances with contrast more than the pituitary gland or thickened stalk (*arrow*)

G. The difference in contrast enhancement is seen also on coronal image: the hypothalamic mass enhances more than the stalk or gland

Discussion

Pituitary-hypothalamic axis anomalies can be due to the stalk, the neurohypophysis, or the adenohypophysis. The neurohypophysis comprises the posterior pituitary lobe, the infundibulum, and the median eminence of the hypothalamus. The posterior lobe of the pituitary gland normally gives high signal on T1 image presumably because of neurosecretory granules. During the first 2 months, the anterior lobe also gives bright signal on T1 images due to marked endocrine activity of the gland during the neonatal period.

Absent Pituitary Gland and Hypoplasia. The pituitary gland may be very small, and sometimes absent. It is important to correlate the hormonal profile and clinical symptoms with imaging findings before making the diagnosis of absent pituitary. A small gland in the presence of normal endocrine profile is usually of no concern. The pituitary gland may shrink following trauma, irradiation, resection, infarction, hemorrhage, or infection.

Ectopic Pituitary Gland, Stalk or Median Eminence. The ectopic pituitary may be seen with absent gland, with prior transection of the stalk due to trauma or birth-related injuries, or following destruction of the glands by adenoma. It is unusual to find ectopic posterior lobe in the presence of a normal-appearing stalk and gland. Various midline brain malformations have been associated with ectopic posterior pituitary lobe, including Chiari 1 malformation, optic nerve hypoplasia, septo-optic dysplasia, agenesis of the corpus callosum, Kallman syndrome, basilar impression, cerebellar atrophy, and vermian dysplasia. Ectopic pituitary appears as a focal, rounded area of increased signal intensity on noncontrast T1 images. It is usually seen in the region of the hypothalamus or along the superior aspect of the stalk. Translocation of the posterior pituitary lobe can be seen following tumor invasion into the gland, as hormones then cannot descend to its normal location.

Pituitary Stalk Thickening. Pituitary stalk thickening may be seen due to germinoma, Langerhans histiocytosis and putative antivasopressin cell antibody-induced central diabetes insipidus. A thickened pituitary stalk can also be seen in self-limiting lymphocytic infundibuloneurohypophysitis that has usually resolved on follow-up examination.

Suggested Reading

Castillo M (2002) Neuroradiology. Lippincott Williams and Wilkins, Philadelphia, pp 177–192

Mitchell LA, Thomas PQ, Zacharin MR, Scheffer IE (2002) Ectopic posterior pituitary lobe and periventricular heterotopia: cerebral malformations with the same underlying mechanism? AJNR Am J Neuroradiol 23:1475–1481

Mootha SL, Barkovich AJ, Grumbach MM, et al (1997) Idiopathic hypothalamic diabetes insipidus, pituitary stalk thickening, and the occult intracranial germinoma in children and adolescents. J Clin Endocrinol Metab 82:1362–1367

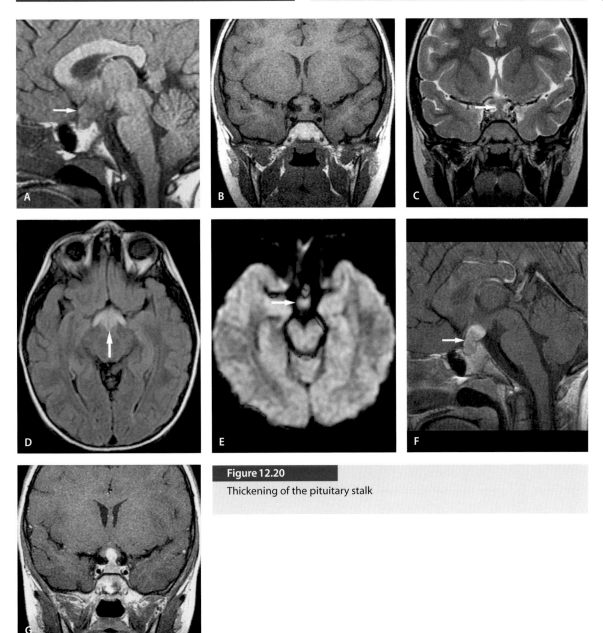

Figure 12.20

Thickening of the pituitary stalk

Posterior Reversible Encephalopathy Syndrome (PRES)

Clinical Presentation

A 12-year-old female with leukemia. Following intrathecal methotrexate treatment she had headache, altered mental status, seizure, tremors and nystagmus. She also experienced temporary renal failure with increased blood pressure. After the blood pressure was under control, her mental status normalized and headache disappeared.

Images (Fig. 12.21)

A. Noncontrast CT scan shows bilateral, diffuse white matter low density involving both frontal and occipital white matter

B. Axial FLAIR image reveals widespread bilateral white matter hyperintensities involving the occipital, parietal and frontal lobes. It predominantly affects the subcortical white matter. There is some mass effect on the adjacent sulci

C. Contrast enhanced T1-weighted image shows vague leptomeningeal enhancement or slow flow in meningeal vessels

D. DW image shows slight increase in signal

E. ADC map does not show restricted diffusion; the white matter lesions are hyperintense

F. Follow-up FLAIR image obtained 10 days after B shows resolution of white matter edema. She was asymptomatic at this time

Discussion

PRES is a heterogeneous group of disorders that share common clinical symptomatology and imaging findings. It presents clinically with headache, seizures, visual changes and altered mental status. CT and MR imaging typically show vasogenic edema in the posterior circulation; however it can also be seen more anteriorly and in the posterior fossa and brainstem. The edema mainly involves the white matter but also the cortex can be involved. When detected early enough, the imaging abnormalities can be completely reversed. Endothelial cell damage is the pathological hallmark of PRES. This allows breakdown in the cerebral autoregulation resulting in leakage of fluid into the interstitium seen as vasogenic edema on DW images. The findings are best seen in the T2 and FLAIR images. DW images and ADC map can reliably distinguish vasogenic edema seen in PRES from cytotoxic edema seen in the setting of brain ischemia.

The etiology of PRES is broad: it has been seen following a subacute elevation in the blood pressure in hypertensive patients and it has long been recognized in pregnant patients with eclampsia. In transplant patients PRES is a well-known complication of antirejection therapy with cyclosporin A and tacrolimus. In children it is seen following intrathecal methotrexate therapy and multidrug treatment of acute lymphoblastic leukemia. If a patient's condition remains unrecognized, it can progress to ischemia, infarctions and even to death. DW imaging with ADC map is a fast and efficient way of recognizing the condition and DW imaging may help recognize those patients at risk of having nonreversible edema leading to infarctions.

Suggested Reading

Covarrubias DJ, Luetmer PH, Campeau NG (2002) Posterior reversible encephalopathy syndrome: prognostic utility of quantitative diffusion-weighted MR images. AJNR Am J Neuroradiol 6:1038–1048

Kinoshita T, Moritani T, Shrier DA, et al (2003) Diffusion-weighted MR imaging of posterior reversible leukoencephalopathy syndrome: a pictorial essay. Clin Imaging 5:307–315

Lamy C, Oppenheim C, Meder JF, Mas JL (2004) Neuroimaging in posterior reversible encephalopathy syndrome (review). J Neuroimaging 2:89–96

Vazquez E, Lucaya J, Castellote A, et al (2002) Neuroimaging in pediatric leukemia and lymphoma: differential diagnosis. Radiographics 6:1411–1428

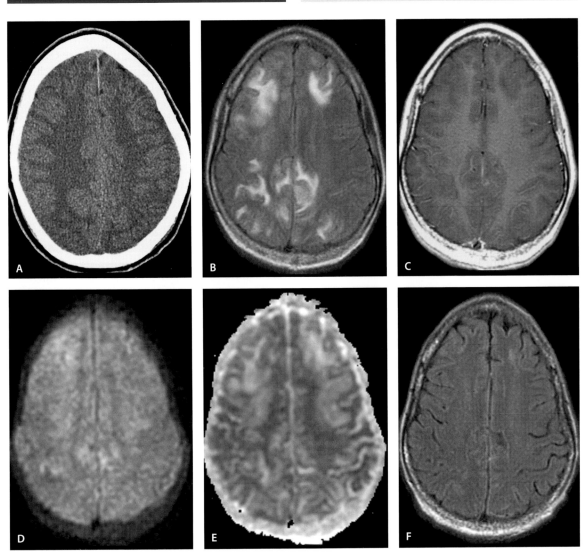

Figure 12.21

Posterior reversible encephalopathy syndrome

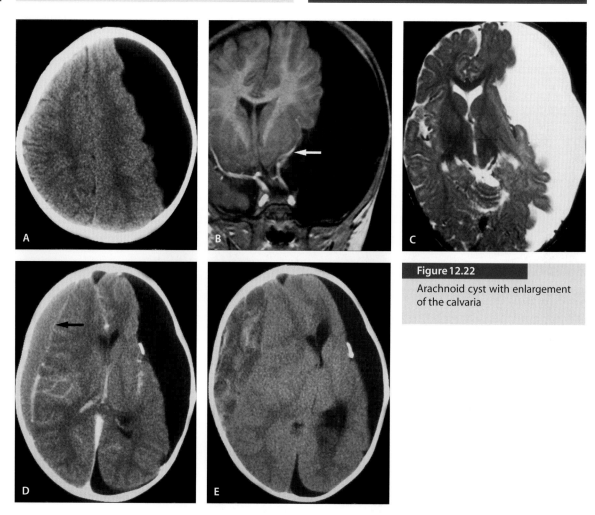

Figure 12.22

Arachnoid cyst with enlargement of the calvaria

Arachnoid Cyst

Arachnoid Cyst with Enlargement of the Calvaria

Clinical Presentation

A 10-month-old male with large head circumference. Patient presents after a fall to evaluate for a hematoma.

Images (Fig. 12.22)

A. Noncontrast CT scan demonstrates a large hypodense arachnoid cyst with enlarged left hemicranium and displacement of the white matter

B. Coronal T1-weighted image shows enlarged middle cranial fossa with an arachnoid cyst that expands in the left hemicranium and causes a midline shift. The lesion displaces the left MCA medially (*arrow*)

C. Axial T2-weighted image shows displacement of the temporal lobe and midline structures by the hyperintense cyst. The cyst has a typical "box-shaped" appearance

D. Following a shunt procedure a contralateral subdural hematoma develops (*arrow*)

E. Two weeks later the SDH has increased in size with a significant midline shift

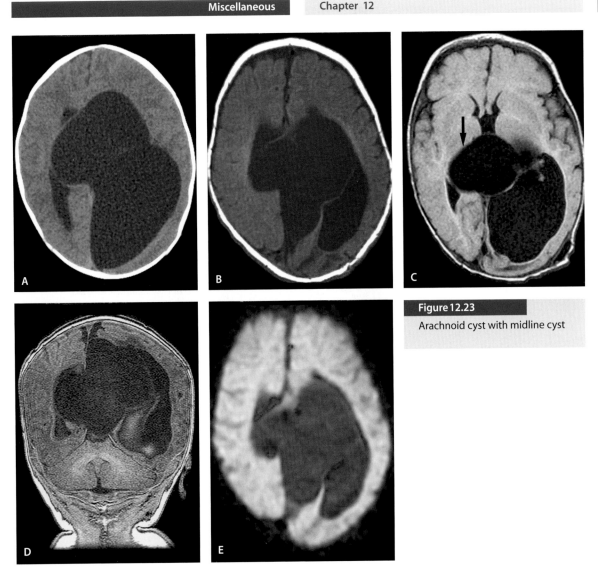

Figure 12.23

Arachnoid cyst with midline cyst

Arachnoid Cyst with Midline Cyst

Clinical Presentation

A 3-week-old baby with a cystic midline lesion obstructing the left lateral ventricle.

Images (Fig. 12.23)

A. CT scan shows a CSF density cyst in the midline causing left lateral ventricle dilatation
B. T1-weighted image. There is a large midline arachnoid cyst leading to obstructive hydrocephalus. Particularly the temporal and occipital horns of the left lateral ventricle are dilated. The corpus callosum is present, but appears markedly thinned due to the hydrocephalus
C. FLAIR image at the level of the ventricles shows again the large cyst (*arrow*) with CSF signal
D. Coronal gradient echo (SPGR) image through the cyst shows the relationship of the cyst to the ventricles. The left hemisphere is enlarged
E. DW image shows that there is no restricted diffusion in the cyst

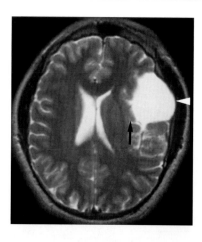

Arachnoid cyst with calvarial remodeling

Arachnoid Cyst in the Posterior Fossa

Clinical Presentation

A young adult male who was examined because of nonspecific symptoms: "pressure" feeling in the back of the head and ringing in the right ear. The diagnosis was confirmed with a cisternogram.

Images (Fig. 12.25)

A. Axial T2-weighted image shows a mass in the right cerebellopontine angle. The mass remains isointense to CSF. The fourth ventricle is displaced to left (*arrow*)
B. Axial T1-weighted image. The mass follows the CSF signal
C. Coronal T1-weighted image shows the stretched seventh/eighth nerve complex (*arrow*)
D. The fifth cranial nerve (*arrow*) is stretched on the sagittal T1-weighted image

Arachnoid Cyst with Calvarial Remodeling

Clinical Presentation

A young man, examined for increasing headaches.

Image (Fig. 12.24)

A. T2-weighted image shows a mass in the right Sylvian fissure. The mass is isointense to CSF and exerts a mass effect on the temporal lobe (*arrow*) and left lateral ventricle. The calvaria are thinned at the site of the cyst (*arrowhead*)

Discussion

Arachnoid cysts are congenital lesions of the arachnoid membrane that expand by CSF secretion. The true arachnoid cysts are intra-arachnoid in location and their inner and outer walls consist of arachnoid cells. Cells lining the arachnoid cysts contain specialized membranes and enzymes for secretory activity. When the cyst forms, the mechanism appears to be accumulation of CSF secreted by the cells in the cyst wall rather than a ball-valve mechanism or infiltration of CSF. The middle cranial fossa is the most common location followed by suprasellar, quadrigeminal, cerebellopontine angle and posterior retrocerebellar cistern. Arachnoid cysts can also be seen in the interhemispheric fissure and in the cerebral convexity. Small cysts are usually asymptomatic and are discovered incidentally. Large supratentorial cysts may cause hydrocephalus. Large suprasellar cysts may cause visual symptoms, hypothalamic dysfunction and craniomegaly.

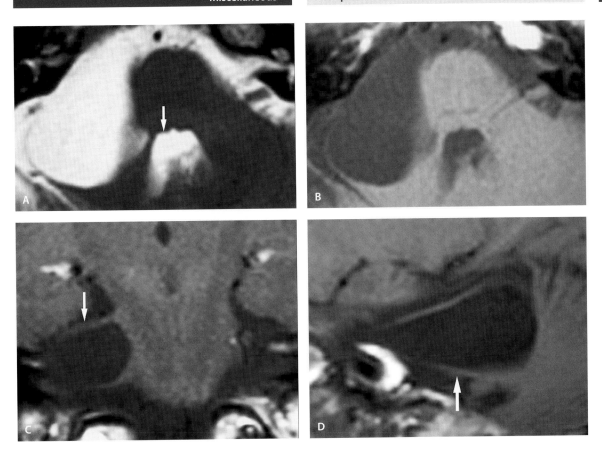

Figure 12.25

Arachnoid cyst in the posterior fossa

The CT and MR imaging appearance is that of a homogeneous, well-defined CSF mass without enhancement. Suprasellar arachnoid cysts can expand in all directions. They may extend into the sella turcica, laterally in the middle cranial fossa and posteriorly to the prepontine cistern. The differential diagnosis includes epidermoid tumors and cystic astrocytomas. In the posterior fossa the differential diagnosis includes the spectrum of Dandy-Walker malformation. Large retrocerebellar cysts may be associated with anomalies of the dural venous sinuses.

Suggested Reading

Ciricillo SF, Cogen PH, Harsh GR, Edwards MS (1991) Intracranial arachnoid cysts in children. A comparison of the effects of fenestration and shunting. J Neurosurg 742:230–235

Piatt JH Jr (2004) Unexpected findings on brain and spine imaging in children (review). Pediatr Clin North Am 2:507–527 (review)

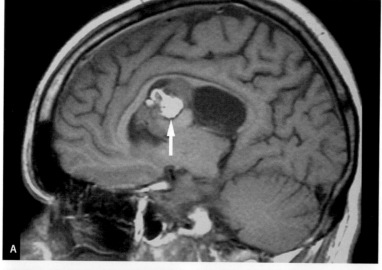

Figure 12.26

Dermoid cyst (ectodermal inclusion cyst)

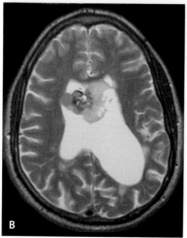

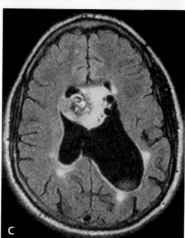

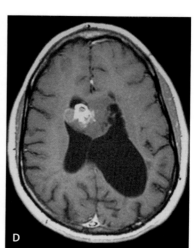

Dermoid Cyst (Ectodermal Inclusion Cyst)

Clinical Presentation

A young male was referred for MR imaging because of headaches.

Images (Fig. 12.26)

A. Sagittal T1-weighted image shows a fat-containing, well-circumscribed dermoid cyst near the midline. T1 shortening (*arrow*) is related to the fatty component of the lesion

B. Axial T2-weighted image shows a mixed signal intraventricular mass causing hydrocephalus; especially the left lateral ventricle is enlarged

C. FLAIR image shows again a heterogeneously hyperintense lesion near the midline

D. Axial postcontrast image reveals minimal enhancement on the right side of the lesion

Discussion

Dermoid cysts are considered to be in the category of congenital ectodermal inclusion cysts. They are felt to result from inclusion of ectodermal elements during neural tube closure. They are rare lesions, and less common than epidermoid tumors that they resemble in many respects. Dermoids contain hair, sebaceous and sweat glands, and squamous epithelium, in contrast to epidermoids that have only squamous epithelium. Both arise from trapped pouches of ectoderm. Both dermoids and epidermoids share the same symptomatology. These slowly expanding, cystic masses may produce only mild symptoms. They may be complicated by rupture leading to chemical meningitis. Dermoids are most commonly seen in the midline. Both types of lesions share a tendency to cause chemical meningitis secondary to leakage of the cyst elements into the CSF space. Such an event is typically devastating for the patient. These lesions may also occur as a result of trauma where skin elements can be driven into the subarachnoid space. The spinal lumbar puncture may give rise to such a lesion as skin cells desquamate and enlarge inside a canal. If the lesion ruptures, the best imaging clue to the nature of the lesion is the fat signal or droplets in the cisterns, sulci or ventricles.

The lesion is hyperintense to isointense on T1-weighted image and mixed signal intensity in the T2-weighted image. The nature of the lesion can easily be confirmed by using fat-suppressed sequence to confirm the presence of fat. On MR spectroscopy there is a strong and broad resonance peak from mobile lipids at 0.9 and 1.3 ppm. Differential diagnosis of dermoid cysts includes epidermoids, craniopharyngioma and teratoma.

Suggested Reading

Jacqueline Y, Brown AP, Morokoff P, Mitchell J, Gonzales MF (2001) Unusual imaging appearance of an intracranial dermoid cyst. AJNR Am J Neuroradiol 22:1970–1972

Smirniotopoulos JG, Chiechi MV (1995) Teratomas, dermoids, and epidermoids of the head and neck. Radiographics 15:1437–1455

Neuroepithelial (Ependymal) Cyst

Clinical Presentation

A 5-year-old male with developmental abnormalities and left-hand shaking. Patient was referred for MR imaging because a structural lesion was suspected.

Images (Fig. 12.27)

A. Axial T2-weighted image shows a cyst within the right lateral ventricle with signal intensity isointense to CSF in all pulse sequences
B. On coronal T2-weighted image a thin wall is seen
C. The lesion crosses the midline but does not cause significant dilatation of the left lateral ventricle. There is some effacement of the cortical sulci on the right side
D. Axial CT scan shows a large cyst with mass effect. Contrast was injected through the ventriculostomy tube that was placed within the body of the cyst. Air and high density contrast material is seen within this cyst as well as dependent layering in the posterior horn of the right lateral ventricle. The cyst communicates with the ventricle

Discussion

Neuroepithelial cysts (ependymal cysts, glioependymal cysts) are rare congenital, benign ependymal-lined cysts. They are usually clinically asymptomatic, but can present with headaches, seizures and gait disturbance. There is a male predominance. The symptoms can be related to obstruction to the CSF flow and a mass effect. The best diagnostic clue is their imaging appearance: they are thin-walled with CSF signal intensity in all pulse sequences. They typically locate in the lateral ventricle, but can be seen in the brain parenchyma, and in the central white matter of the temporoparietal and frontal lobes. They are less common in the subarachnoid space. They are typically thin-walled cysts from 2–3 mm up to 9 cm in diameter. These lesions may be indistinguishable from arachnoid and choroid plexus cysts.

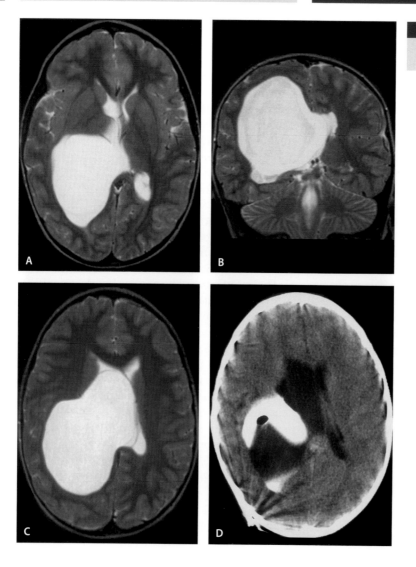

Figure 12.27

Neuroepithelial (ependymal) cyst

Suggested Reading

Boockvar JA, Shafa R, Forman MS, O'Rourke DM (2000) Symptomatic lateral ventricular ependymal cysts: criteria for distinguishing these rare cysts from other symptomatic cysts of the ventricles: case report. Neurosurgery 5:1229–1232

Heran NS, Berk C, Constantoyannis C, Honey CR (2003) Neuroepithelial cysts presenting with movement disorders: two cases. Can J Neurol Sci 30:393–396

Temporal Lobe Cysts and Fetal Alcohol Syndrome

Clinical Presentation

A 2-year-old female born to a young mother who abused alcohol and marijuana during her pregnancy. She was born after a 36-week pregnancy and had very low birth weight. The patient has no speech, but she is deaf. She understands visual clues. Head size is on 25th percentile. A previous MR image showed delayed myelination.

Images (Fig. 12.28)

A. Parasagittal T1-weighted image shows cystic intraparenchymal lesion (*arrows*) in the temporal tip. The cysts are limited to the white matter and outlined by normal-appearing gray matter
B. T2-weighted image shows bitemporal intraparenchymal cysts (*arrows*). The cysts do not communicate with the ventricular system and there is no visible gliosis around them. They are most likely consistent with neuroglial cysts
C. T2-weighted image shows that myelination has progressed centrally with large hyperintense areas behind the occipital horns and spotty nonmyelinated areas in the subcortical areas (*arrows*). The corpus callosum is present but hypoplastic. She has also a small cavum septum pellucidum (in a lower cut). At the age of 2 years the myelination is normally seen in the peripheral white matter already. The white matter volume is low
D. The temporal lobe cysts follow the CSF signal on FLAIR image
E. Proton MR spectroscopy of the white matter is normal
F. Localizer to demonstrate the sample collection

Discussion

Prenatal alcohol exposure has long been associated with alterations in behavioral and brain structural changes. The corpus callosum can be affected by heavy prenatal alcohol exposure, and agenesis of this structure occurs more often in children with fetal alcohol syndrome than in the general population. Although the majority of children with fetal alcohol syndrome do not have agenesis of the corpus callosum, the callosal area is reduced in this population. The following morphological anomalies have been also reported: cortical atrophy, dilated ventricles, corpus callosum hypoplasia, and cerebellar atrophy. Delayed myelination of the white matter is not uncommonly seen in these patients. More recent MR imaging studies, particularly when combined with quantitative analysis, have indicated that specific brain areas in addition to the corpus callosum – such as the basal ganglia and diencephalon and parts of the cerebellum – might be especially susceptible to the teratogenic effects of alcohol.

Temporal lobe intraparenchymal cystic lesions are also seen in the megaloencephalic leukoencephalopathy (MLC, van der Knaap leukoencephalopathy) that is an inborn genetic error disease. Other temporal lobe cystic lesions include arachnoid cysts (extraaxial in location), porencephalic cysts (rarely symmetric) and infectious cysts.

Suggested Reading

Riikonen R, Salonen I, Partanen K, Verho S (1999) Brain perfusion SPECT and MRI in fetal alcohol syndrome. Dev Med Child Neurol 10:652–659

Roebuck TM, Mattson SN, Riley EP (2002) Interhemispheric transfer in children with heavy prenatal alcohol exposure. Alcohol Clin Exp Res 12:1863–1871

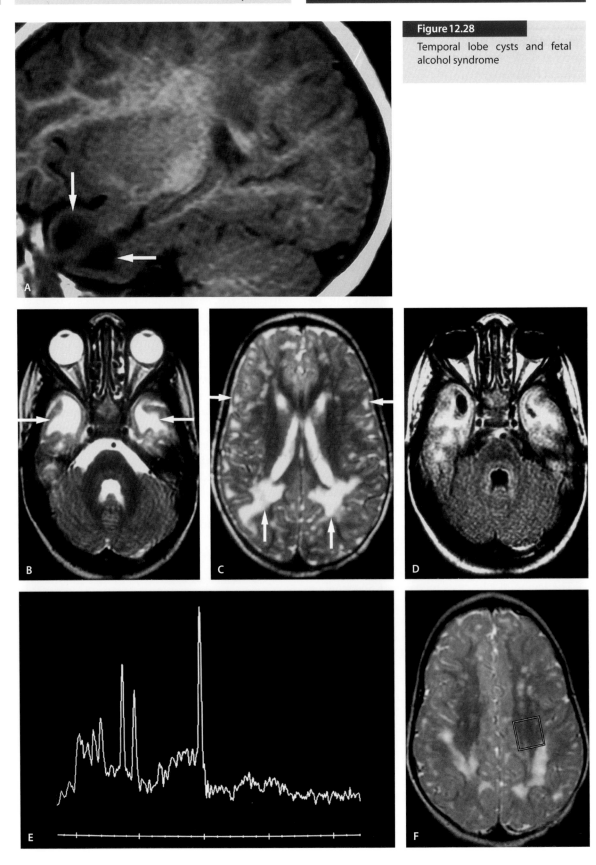

Figure 12.28

Temporal lobe cysts and fetal alcohol syndrome

Lenticulostriate Vasculopathy

Clinical Presentation

A 3-year-old female with macrocephaly, hypotonia, and developmental delay. Mother has a history of intake of multiple medications during early pregnancy.

Images (Fig. 12.29)

A. On coronal contrast-enhanced SPGR image, the lenticulostriate vessels are prominent within the basal ganglia (*arrows*)
B. On axial T2-weighted image the basal ganglia are normal
C. The cross sections of prominent lenticulostriate vessels are seen on axial T1-weighted image (*arrows*)
D. DW image is normal
E. Basal ganglia MR spectroscopy (TE=144 ms) fails to demonstrate abnormal metabolites
F. No abnormal metabolites are seen with short echo (TE=35 ms) MR spectroscopy

Discussion

The lenticulostriate arteries with diameters less than 0.5 mm that supply the basal ganglia are distinct from the brain parenchyma in normal infants on high-resolution US, CT and MR imaging studies. Radiating ramified echogenic stripes in these regions suggest lenticulostriate vasculopathy. This finding is nonspecific and may be seen in congenital infections, fetal alcohol syndrome, certain trisomies and neonatal hypoxia, besides others, and in some asymptomatic patients. Lenticulostriate vasculopathy is merely an indicator of nonspecific early insults to the developing brain.

Suggested Reading

El Ayoubi M, de Bethmann O, Monset-Couchard M (2003) Lenticulostriate echogenic vessels: clinical and sonographic study of 70 neonatal cases. Pediatr Radiol 33:697–703

Wang HS, Kuo MF, Chang TC (1995) Sonographic lenticulostriate vasculopathy in infants: some associations and a hypothesis. AJNR Am J Neuroradiol 16:97–102

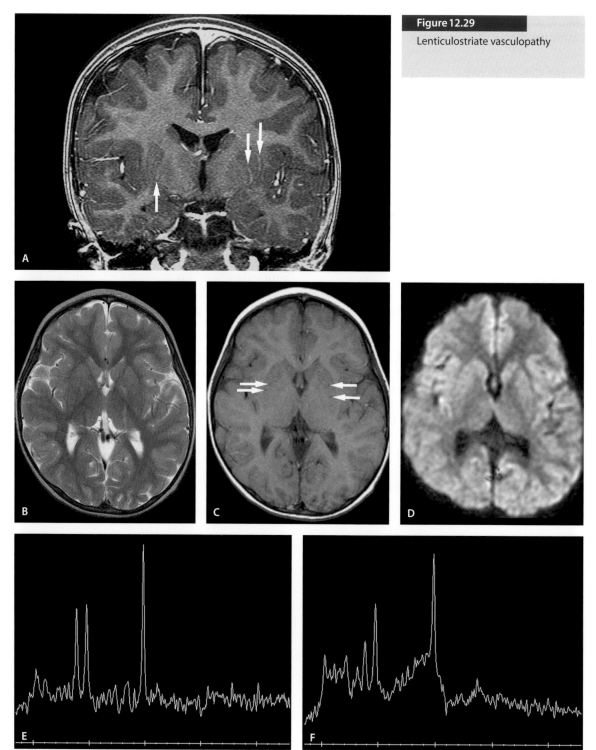

Figure 12.29
Lenticulostriate vasculopathy

Craniosynostosis

Clinical Presentation

A 5-month-old child with calvarial asymmetry is referred for CT and MR imaging with clinical suspicion of craniosynostosis.

Images (Fig. 12.30)

A. Bone window of axial CT scan shows synostosis of the right coronal suture with resulting calvarial asymmetry. The metopic suture is closed as well
B. The 3D reconstruction shows asymmetric calvaria with closed right coronal suture (*arrow*)
C. Right side of the calvaria of the 3D reconstruction shows again the closed coronal suture
D. MIP image clearly shows the premature fusion of the right coronal suture (*arrow*)
E. Noncontrast CT scan shows agenesis of the corpus callosum
F. Agenesis of the corpus callosum is better seen on coronal FLAIR image
G. Axial FLAIR image also reveals the corpus callosum aplasia without parenchymal pathology
H. No parenchymal abnormality is seen on DW image
I. No restricted diffusion is seen on ADC map

Discussion

Craniosynostosis results from premature closure of the sutures thereby leading to growth retardation of the skull. Craniosynostosis is classified as either simple synostosis, involving fusion of a single suture, or compound synostoses, involving fusion of two or more sutures. The majority of cranial synostoses involves single suture and is non-syndromic. The single suture synostosis involves the sagittal, coronal, lambdoid or metopic suture. The multiple suture synostoses are more often associated with an underlying syndrome such as Apert syndrome, Crouzon syndrome, Pfeiffer syndrome and Carpenter syndrome.

CT gives the precise spatial depiction of pediatric craniofacial malformations. 3-D CT and MIP (maximum intensity projection) reconstruction have been shown to be an important tool to assist spatial orientation in planning the surgery.

Suggested Reading

Binaghi S, Gudinchet F, Rilliet B (2000) Three-dimensional spiral CT of craniofacial malformations in children. Pediatr Radiol 30:856–860

Levi D, Rampa F, Barbieri C, Pricca P, Franzini A, Pezzotta S (2002) True 3D reconstruction for planning of surgery on malformed skulls. Childs Nerv Syst 18:705–706

Figure 3.30 ▼

Craniosynostosis

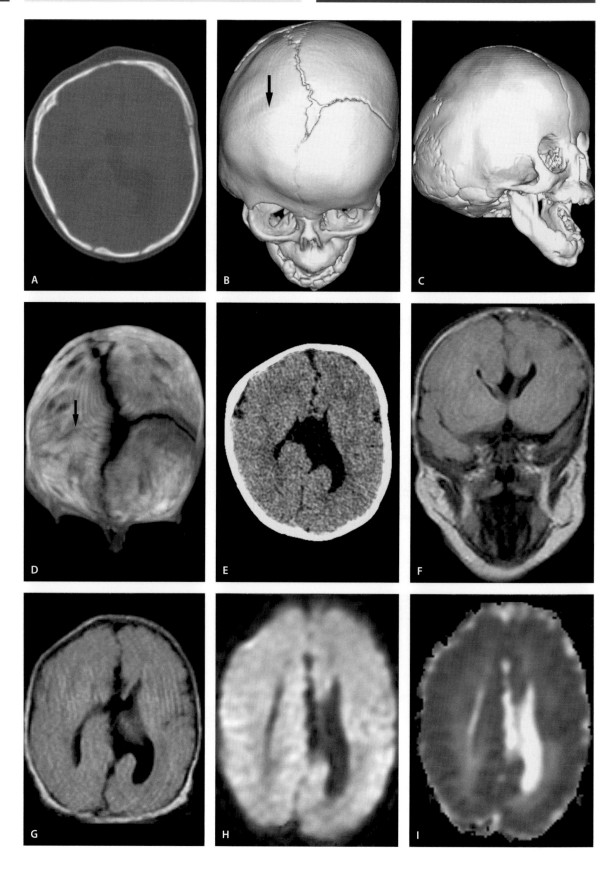

Subject Index

A

abscess
- brain 133, 134
- - tuberculous 161, 162
- epidural, spine 434
acinic cell carcinoma,
    parotid gland 352, 353
acyclovir treatment 143
ADC map 188
ADEM (acute disseminated
    encephalomyelitis) 110–112, 165
- cervical cord 433
- thoracic cord 432
adenoma
- pituitary
- - macroadenoma 222, 223
- - microadenoma 224, 225
- pleomorphic, nose 349, 350
adrenoleukodystrophy 79, 80
Aicadi's syndrome 20, 60
AIDS 155
alcohol syndrome, fetal 483
amino acid/organic acid metabolism,
    disorders
- galactosemia 102, 103
- maple syrup urine disease
    (MSUD) 101, 102
- ornithine transcarbamylase
    (OTCD) deficiency 104
- phenylketonuria (PKU) 98, 99
- propionic acidemia 100
amino acid peaks 126
anal duct, cyst 448
anemia, macrocytic 435
anencephaly 17, 27, 34, 440
anesthesia, epidural 425
aneurysm 24
- berry 322, 324
- fusiform 323
angioma
- leptomeningeal 457
- venous 312
angiomatosis,
    encephalotrigeminal 459
angiopathy,
    post-varicella 287
anisotropy, fractional 102
anophtalmos 354, 355
anosmia 217

arachnoid cyst 18, 181, 203, 450,
    476–479
Arnold-Chiari malformation 20, 53, 54
artery, choroideal 13
arteriovenous malformation
    (AVM) 287, 302–305
arthrogryposis
    (*Larsen's* syndrome) 388
astrocytoma 167, 398
- cerebellar 175
- fibrillary 179
- giant cell 463, 464
- juvenile pilocytic (JPA) 191, 192
- - optic nerve 230, 231
- low-grade 203
- pilocytic 173–176
- spinal cord 391–393
- subependymal giant cell
    (SEGA) 225, 226
- xanthoastrocytoma,
    pleomorphic (PXA) 192–194, 203
ataxia 56, 89
- truncal 87
atrophy 82, 244, 483
AVF (dural arteriovenous fistula) 287
axonal injury,
    diffuse (DAI) 241, 251–257

B

B12 deficiency 435
balloon cells 465
Balò's disease 109
Blake's pouch 18
blood-CSF barrier 126
brachial plexus trauma
- blunt trauma 423, 424
- nerve root avulsion 421
- obstetric injury 422
brain malformations,
    congenital 17–67
- cephalocele 28–34
- *Chiari* malformation 20, 51–57
- classification 17
- cloverleaf skull syndrome
    ("Kleeblattschädel" anomaly) 64,
    65
- corpus callosum, agenesis/
    dysgenesis 19, 20, 61

- cortical dysplasia 35–37
- *Dandy-Walker* malformation 18, 20,
    58–61, 445, 479
- hemimegalencephaly 66, 67
- heterotopia, gray matter 40–45
- holoprosencephaly 45–50
- hydranencephaly 25–27
- *Joubert's* syndrome 18, 61
- lipoma 20–24
- lissencephaly 34, 35, 39, 149,
    439
- meningocele 28–34
- micrencephaly 18, 34, 35
- rhombencephalosynapsis 18, 63,
    64
- schizencephaly 37, 38
brain stem glioma 178, 179

C

café-au-lait spots 455
calcification, dystrophic
    parenchymal 260
callosal dysgenesis 14, 20, 61, 444,
    483
candida 132
caudal regression syndrome 383
cavernous malformation 287
- with developmental venous
    anomaly 308
- exophytic 307
- intrinsic parenchymal lesion 306
- multiple 309
- simulating neoplasm 311, 312
cavum
- c. septi pellucidi 11
- c. velum interpositum 12, 13
- c. vergae 13
centrum semiovale 96
cephalhematoma
- CT scan 280
- with hypoxic-ischemic
    insult 283–286
- MR imaging 281, 282
cerebellar degeneration,
    associated with coenzyme Q10
    deficiency 90, 91
cerebellitis 164, 165
cerebritis, citrobacter 142, 143

Chiari malformations
- *Chiari* I 51, 52, 372
- *Chiari* II (*Arnold-Chiari* malformation) 20, 53, 54
- Chiari III 55–57
choline, peak 104, 168, 188, 206
chordoma 185
choroid plexus
- papilloma 199–201
- tumor 403
chromosome Xq22 94, 398
cingulate gyrus 20, 84
citrobacter
- cerebritis 142, 143
- meningitis 141
cleft lip, midline 444
cloverleaf skull syndrome ("Kleeblattschädel" anomaly) 64, 65
coenzyme Q10 deficiency 90, 91
coloboma, chorioretinal 61
colpocephaly 57, 444
combined degeneration, subacute (SCD) 435
contusion 251
conus medullaris 15
cord compression 74
cord sign 318
corpus callosum
- agenesis/dysgenesis 19, 20, 61, 483
- aplasia 444
cortical tubes 465
CPM (central pontine myelinolysis) 278
craniopharyngioma 220–222
craniorachischisis 34
craniosynostosis 487
CSF hernia 29
CT scanning 125, 126
cyclosporin-induced encephalopathy 277, 278
cyst
- anal duct 448
- arachnoid 18, 181, 203, 450, 476–479
- dental radicular 367
- dermoid 450, 480, 481
- epidermoid 18, 448
- glioependymal 481
- hemispheric 444
- neuroepithelial 18, 481, 482
- porencephalic 203, 483
- subcortical 117
- temporal lobe 483
- thyroglossal duct 337, 338
- *Tornwald* 339
cysticercosis 126
- calcified 59
- intraventricular 157
- parenchymal 158
- subarachnoid 157
cytomegalovirus infection 125
- congenital 149, 150
- encephalitis 151

D

DAI (diffuse axonal injury) 241, 251
- corpus callosum and parenchyma 252, 253
- excitotoxic mechanism 256
- hemorrhagic contusion 254
- multiple areas, corpus callosum 255
Dandy-Walker malformation 18, 20, 58–61, 445, 479
De Morsier syndrome 49
degeneration, myxoid 401
delayed myelination 483
dementia 81
dental radicular cyst 367
dermal sinus
- sacral 61
- tract 378, 379
dermoid 346, 347, 413
- cyst 450, 480, 481
developmental delay 18, 39, 485
developmental venous anomalies (DVA) 287, 312, 313
Devic's disease 109
diabetes insipidus 472
diastematomyelia 376–378
diploic space 165
diseases (*see* syndromes)
dissection
- common carotid 290, 291
- internal carotid artery 288, 289
Duchenne-Erb's syndrome 423
DW imaging 126, 167, 188
dysarthria 92
dysembryoplastic neuroepithelial tumor (DNET) 208
dysmorphy 17, 79
dysplasia
- cortical, generalized 35–37
- dural 396
- fibrous 364, 365
- mesodermal 57
- septo-optic 20, 45, 46, 443, 472
- vermian 472
dysraphism 376

E

eclampsia 425, 450
edema
- brain 263
- cord 418
emboli, septic 138, 139
embryonic cell carcinoma 212–214
empyema
- epidural 137
- subdural 135, 136
encephalitis
- cytomegalovirus 151
- herpes simplex virus 143–149

- influenza 152, 153
- limbic (paraneoplastic) 162
- *Rasmussen's* encephalitis 165, 166
encephalocele
- occipital 28, 55
- parietal 29, 30
- skull base 31
encephalomalacia, multicystic 268–270
encephalomyelitis, acute disseminated (ADEM) 110–112, 165, 432, 433
encephalopathy
- anoxic ischemic (AIE) 235
- cyclosporin-induced 277, 278
- hypertensive 450
- hypoxic 267, 268
- hypoxic ischemic (HIE) 235, 263–266
- – preterm 260
- influenza 152, 153
- with lactic acidemia 287
eosinophilic granuloma 220
ependymoblastoma 407, 408
ependymoma 167, 176–178, 197, 398, 403
- conus 395
- holocord 394
- myxopapillary 395
epidermoid 413
- cyst 18, 448
- tumor 180, 181
epilepsy 112
- status epilepticus 270–275
EPM (extra pontine myelinolysis) 278
Epstein-Barr virus 165
Erb's palsy 423
esthesioneuroblastoma 217, 218

F

facial dysmorphism, with hypotelorism 47
Fahr's syndrome 122
fetal hydrops 446, 447
fetus, normal 438–440
fibrous dysplasia 364, 365
filum terminale 391
fistula, arteriovenous (AVF)
- dural 287
- vertebral artery 369, 370
folic acid deficiency 440
fornix 468
fracture
- burst 426, 427
- compression 428, 429
- skull 237
- spine 426–429
Fukuyama congenital muscular dystrophy 39

G

galactosemia 102, 103
Galen, vein malformation 332–334
ganglioglioma 192, 203, 204
ganglioneuroblastoma 406
ganglioneuroma 406, 407
germinal matrix 18
germinoma 208, 209, 403
glaucoma 456
glial fiber, radial 18
glioblastoma multiforme
  (GBM) 189–191, 403
– congenital 230
glioependymal cyst 481
glioma
– brain stem 178, 179
– hypothalamic 232
– intraspinal 395
– low-grade 465
– optic nerve 230–233
– optic pathway 232, 233
gliomatosis cerebri 202, 203
globus pallidus 93
globoid cell leukodystrophy 70
glutamine/glutamate peaks 104, 266,
  257
glycosaminoglycans 390
goiter, multilobulated 335, 336

H

Hallervorden-Spatz disease 91–93
hamartoma 453, 455
– hypothalamic 233, 234
– subependymal 44
Hansen's node 415
Hashimoto's thyreoiditis 121
helmet sign 446
hemangioblastoma 182
hemangioblastomatosis 449
hemangioma
– face/orbit 359, 360
– parotid gland 358
– spine 417
hematoma
– cephalhematoma 280–286
– epidural 247, 248, 425
– intracerebral 327
– subdural 249–251
hemicord 376
hemimegalencephaly 18, 66, 67
hemiparesis 130
hemivertebra
– lumbar 384, 385
– thoracic 386
hemoglobinopathy,
  sickle cell 292–294
hemolytic anemia,
  antibody-mediated 446

hemolytic uremic
  syndrome (HUS) 326, 327
hemorrhage
– parenchymal 240
– subarachnoid 239
– subdural 238
– subgaleal 236
herpes simplex virus 125
– encephalitis
– – type 1 147–149
– – type 2 (neonatal) 143–147
– vasculopathy 296, 297
heterotopia
– band (double cortex) 44
– subcortical 41–43
– subependymal nodular 40, 44
HIE (hypoxic ischemic encephalopathy)
  235, 263–266
– brain edema 263
– infarcts 263
– post-surgery 264
– seizures 265
hippocampal sclerosis 469
histiocytosis, *Langerhans* cells 220,
  360, 361, 472
HIV 125
– congenital infection 153–156
– primary brain lymphoma 156
– progressive multifocal
  leukoencephalopathy 155, 156
– toxoplasmosis 155, 156
holocord 394
holoprosencephaly 441, 442
– alobar 18, 47
– semilobar 18, 48–50
– septo-optic dysplasia 20, 45, 46
Hunter's syndrome 77, 391
Hurler syndrome 77
Hurler-Scheie syndrome 77
– with atrophy 74
– with prominent *Virchow-Robin*
  spaces 73, 74
– spinal cord 388, 389
hydranencephaly
– with increasing head size 25–27
– with microcephaly 27
hydrocephalus 47, 179
– congenital 149
– meningitis 128
– X-linked 444
hydromyelia 56
hydrops fetalis 446, 447
hygroma
– cystic 340
– subdural 251
hyperacusis 70
hyperpnea, episodic 61
hypomyelination 98
hyponatriemia 124, 278
hypoosmolality 278
hypotelorism 47
hypotonia 78, 79, 94, 485

I

infarct 243
– meningitis 130, 131
– multiple bilateral 293
– traumatic dissection of internal
  carotid artery 288, 289
infection
– brain abscess 133, 134
– citrobacter 141–143
– cysticercosis 157–159
– cytomegalovirus infection,
  congenital 149–151
– diagnosis 125, 126
– empyema 135–137
– herpes simplex virus
  encephalitis 143–149
– HIV 125, 153–156
– meningitis 127–132
– mycoplasma 433
– nocardiosis 139
– septic emboli 138, 139
– tuberculosis 160, 161
influenza
– A 152
– encephalopathy 152, 153
intramedullary tumor, cystic 394
ischemia 240
ischemic injury, hypoxic 242
isoleucine 102

J

Joubert's syndrome 18, 61

K

Kearns-Sayre syndrome 85, 89
keratinaceous debris 181
ketoacid, oxidative
  decarboxylation 102
kidney disease, cystic 61
Kikuchi disease 344, 345
"Kleeblattschädel" anomaly 64, 65
Krabbe's disease 70–72
kyphoscoliosis 384–387
kyphosis 384–387

L

lactate 266
lactic acidosis 83, 104
laminin 115
Langerhans cell histiocytosis 220, 360,
  361, 472
Larsen's syndrome 388
Leigh's disease 86–89
lenticulostriate vasculopathy 485, 486
leucine 102

leukemia, lymphoblastic   184, 185
leukencephalopathy
- megalencephalic
  with subcortical cysts   117–119
- progressive multifocal
  (PML)   155, 156
leukodystrophy   69
- globoid cell (*Krabbe's* disease)
  70–72
leukomalacia   1
- periventricular (PVL)   235,
  258–262, 270
ligament injury   418
limbic system   13
lipofuscinosis, neuronal ceroid
  (NCL)   80, 81
lipoma
- intradural   381
- midline (callosal)   20, 23
- pericallosal   22, 444
- simple   382
- spinal   380–382
- tethered cord   373, 374
lipomeningocele, spinal   33
lipopigment   81
lissencephaly   34, 35, 39, 149, 439
- cobblestone form   39
liver disease   124
Luschka, foramina   178
lymphadenitis, histiocytic
  necrotizing   344
lymphadenopathy,
  Kikuchi-Fujimoto   344
lymphangioma   340, 448
lymphoma   155, 156, 403

M

macrencephaly   18
macroadenoma,
  pituitary   222, 223
macrocephaly   17, 117
macroencephaly   485
mamillary body   468
mandible, coronoid
  hyperplasia   365, 366
maple syrup urine disease
  (MSUD)   101, 102
Marfan syndrome   290
Markowski, vein   332
massa, m. intermedia   20, 39, 57
mastoiditis   368, 369
measles   165
medulloblastoma   167, 403
- CSF seeding   172, 173
- hemorrhagic/necrotic   170, 171
- solid   169
mega cisterna magna   18, 60
membrane oxygenation,
  extracorporal (ECMO)   320, 321

meningioma
- atypical   226–228
- spinal cord   408
meningitis
- acute pyogenic   127
- candida   132
- citrobacter   141
- subacute pyogenic,
  with hydrocephalus   128
- suppurative
- - and brain infarct   130, 131
- - with subdural effusions   128–130
meningocele   396
- lipomeningocele, spinal   33
- parietal   32
- pseudomeningocele   421, 422
- traumatic   421
meningoencephalocele, occipital   61
meningomyelocele   53, 54
mental retardation   61, 98
mental status change, acute   121
merosin   115
mesial temporal sclerosis
- bilateral   467, 468
- unilateral   469
metastases
- extramedullary
  (drop metastases)   402
- intramedullary   403
metastatic seeding, subarachnoid   167
methotrexate, intrathecal   450
micrencephaly   18
- with lissencephaly   34, 35
microadenoma, pituitary   224, 225
midbrain tectum, unsegmented   61
Miller-Dieker syndrome   39
mitochondrial disorders   83, 84, 89, 433
Monro, foramen, choroid plexus
  papilloma   201
Morquio's syndrome   390, 391
Moyamoya disease   329–332
- bilateral   329, 330
- sickle cell disease   330, 331
- unilateral   330
MR imaging   126
MR spectroscopy   126, 167, 168, 188
mucopolysaccharidoses (MPS)   73–77
- *Hunter's* syndrome (MPS II)   77, 391
- *Hurler* syndrome (MPS I)   77
- *Hurler-Scheie* syndrome
  (MPS I)   73, 74, 388, 389
- *Morquio's* syndrome
  (MPS IV)   390, 391
- *Sanfilippo* syndrome
  (MPS III)   76, 77
- *Sly* disease (MPS VII)   77
multiple sclerosis (MS)   106, 433
- acute, with ring-enhancing
  lesions   108
- classic   107
mumps   165
muscle-eye-brain disease   39

muscular dystrophy
- *Fukuyama* congenital   39
- merosin-deficient
  congenital   114, 115
mycoplasma   433
myelin disorders, hereditary
- adrenoleukodystrophy   79, 80
- cerebellar degeneration,
  associated with coenzyme Q10
  deficiency   90, 91
- *Hallervorden-Spatz* disease   91–93
- *Kearns-Sayre* syndrome   85, 89
- *Krabbe's* disease   70–72
- *Leigh's* disease   86–89
- mitochondrial disorders   83, 84, 89
- mucopolysaccharidoses
  (MPS)   73–77
- NCL (neuronal ceroid
  lipofuscinosis)   80, 81
- *Zellweger* syndrome   78, 79
myelin vacuolization   452
myelination
- delayed   119, 120
- normal brain   1–15
- - chronological imaging atlas   2 ff
myelinolysis
- osmotic   123, 124
- pontine/extrapontine   278, 279
myelogram, MR   424
myelomalacia   419, 420
myelomeningocele   34
myoinositol   104
myxoid stroma   406

N

N-acetyl aspartate (NAA)   188, 203
NCL (neuronal ceroid
  lipofuscinosis)   80, 81
near-drowning   267, 268
necrosis, cortical laminar   130, 275, 276
neocerebellum   18
neural tube defect   440, 448
neuritis, optic   107, 108
neuroblastoma   404, 405
neurocutaneous melanosis   60
neurocytoma, central   206
neurodegenerative disorders   81
neuroectodermal tumor, primitive
  (PNET)   167, 214, 215, 403, 408
neuroepithelial cyst   18, 481, 482
neurofibroma
- plexiform   398, 454
- spinal cord   400, 401
- trigeminal   218, 219
neurofibromatosis
- orbit   343, 344
- plexiform   342
- spots   449
- type 1 (NF-1)   396–398, 449, 451–455
- type 2 (NF-2)   398, 399, 449
neuropathy, cranial nerve   179

nocardiosis 139
Noonan syndrome 52
nose, pleomorphic adenoma 349, 350
notochordal region 185
numbness, extremity 107
nystagmus 46, 87, 94

O

ocular anomaly 20
oligodendroglioma 194–197, 203
optic disc hypoplasia 46
optic nerve glioma 230–233
optic neuritis 107, 108
ornithine transcarbamylase
  (OTCD) deficiency 104
osteochondroma 415, 416
osteosarcoma, cranium 362, 363

P

p10p9 translocation 95–97
paleocerebellum 18
Pallister-Hal syndrome 233
pantothenate kinase 2 gene 92
papilloma, choroid plexus 199–201
parotid gland
 – acinic cell carcinoma 352, 353
 – hemangioma 358
Pelizaeus-Merzbacher disease 93–95
perisylvian syndrome 112–114
peritrigonal area 1
peroxisomes 79
pertussis 165
pes cavus 376
phakomatoses 449
phenylketonuria (PKU) 98, 99
Pierre-Robin syndrome 49, 50
pineal embryonal carcinoma 212–214
pineal tumor 167
pineoblastoma 211, 212, 403
pineocytoma 211
pituitary gland
 – absent 470, 472
 – ectopic posterior 471, 472
pituitary stalk,
  thickening 472, 473, 472
planar bone scintigraphy (PBS) 431
plaque, multiple sclerosis 107
pleomorphic adenoma, nose 349, 350
PNET (primitive neuroectodermal
  tumor) 167, 214, 215, 403, 408
polydactyly 61
polyglandular syndrome,
  autoimmune (APS) 121, 122
polyhydramnion 440, 448
polymicrogyria 149, 439
 – parietal (BPPP) 112
 – perisylvian syndrome 112
pontomedullary corticospinal tract 80
porencephalic cyst 203, 483

porencephaly 18
port-vine stain 459
PRES (posterior reversible leukoencephalopathy syndrome) 315,
  450, 474
Probst bundles 20
propionic acidemia 100
pseudomeningocele 421, 422
pugilist 13
PVL (periventricular
  leukomalacia) 235, 270
 – dystrophic parenchymal
  calcification 260
 – thin corpus callosum 259
 – unilateral 260
 – white matter aplasia 258

Q

18q syndrome 97, 98

R

Rasmussen's encephalitis 165, 166
Recklinghausen disease 449
Rendu-Osler-Weber syndrome 303
retinopathy, prematurity 357
rhabdoid tumor 167
 – atypical teratoid 215, 216
rhabdomyosarcoma 350, 351
 – metastatic 412
 – primary 411
rhombencephalosynapsis 18, 63, 64
rubella 125

S

Sanfilippo syndrome (MPS III) 76, 77
sarcoma
 – granulocytic 185
 – meningeal 410
 – neurogenic 401
 – osteosarcoma, cranium 362, 363
 – rhabdomyosarcoma 350, 351,
  411, 412
scalp injury 236
Schilder's disease 106, 109
schizencephaly
 – closed lip 38
 – open lip 37, 38
schizophrenia 13
Schwann cells 115
schwannoma 218
 – spinal cord 401, 413
 – tongue 348
scoliosis 384–387
SEGA (subependymal giant cell
  astrocytoma) 225, 226
seizures 78, 90, 92, 100, 106, 159, 265,
  327, 456

septo-optic dysplasia 20, 45, 46,
  443, 472
septum pellucidum 13
shaken infant syndrome 245, 246
sickle cell hemoglobinopathy 292–294
 – *Moyamoya* disease 330, 331
sinus thrombosis 245, 315–318
 – extracorporal membrane
  oxygenation (ECMO) 320, 321
Sjögren's syndrome 300
skull fracture 237
Sly disease 77
SPECT (single-photon emission
  computed tomography) 431
Spielmeyer-Vogt disease 80
spina bifida 56, 57, 373
 – occulta 376
spinal dysgenesis 383
spondylolisthesis 430, 431
squamous epithelium 181
SSFSE (single-shot fast spin-echo) 437
Staphylococcus aureus 130, 434
status epilepticus 270–275
 – permanent tissue damage 272–275
stridor 112
stroke 287
stroke-like episode 89
Sturge-Weber syndrome 318, 319, 450
 – classic 456
subependymal nodules 465
substantia nigra 93
syndactylism 376
syndromes/diseases (names only)
 – *Aicadi's* syndrome 20, 60
 – *Arnold-Chiari* malformation 53, 54
 – *Balò's* disease 109
 – *Chiari* malformation 20, 51–57
 – *Dandy-Walker* malformation 18, 20,
  58–61, 445, 479
 – *De Morsier* syndrome 49
 – *Devic's* disease 109
 – *Duchenne-Erb's* syndrome 423
 – *Fahr's* syndrome 122
 – *Fukuyama* congenital muscular
  dystrophy 39
 – *Hallervorden-Spatz* disease 91–93
 – *Hashimoto's* thyreoiditis 121
 – *Hunter's* syndrome 77, 391
 – *Hurler* syndrome 77
 – *Hurler-Scheie* syndrome 73, 74, 77,
  388, 389
 – *Joubert's* syndrome 18, 61
 – *Kearns-Sayre* syndrome 85, 89
 – *Kikuchi* disease 344, 345
 – *Krabbe's* disease 70–72
 – *Larsen's* syndrome 388
 – *Leigh's* disease 86–89
 – *Marfan* syndrome 290
 – *Miller-Dieker* syndrome 39
 – *Morquio's* syndrome 390, 391
 – *Moyamoya* disease 329–332
 – *Noonan* syndrome 52
 – *Pallister-Hal* syndrome 233

- *Pelizaeus-Merzbacher* disease 93–95
- *Pierre-Robin* syndrome 49, 50
- *Rasmussen's* encephalitis 165, 166
- *Recklinghausen* disease 449
- *Rendu-Osler-Weber* syndrome 303
- *Sanfilippo* syndrome 76, 77
- *Schilder's* disease 106, 109
- *Sjögren's* syndrome 300
- *Sly* disease 77
- *Spielmeyer-Vogt* disease 80
- *Sturge-Weber* syndrome 318, 319, 450, 456–459
- *Turner*-like syndrome 52
- *von Hippel-Lindau* disease 182, 183, 449
- *Walker-Warburg* syndrome 39, 60
- *Wiskott-Aldrich* syndrome 301, 302
- *Wolf-Hirschhorn* syndrome 356
- *Wyburn-Mason* syndrome 303
- *Zellweger* syndrome 78, 79
syphillis 125
syringohydromyelia 376, 394

T

T2-shine through 153, 181
talipes equinovarus 388
Tc HMPAO 459
teleangiectasia, capillary 287, 314, 315
temporal lobe cyst 483
teratoid rhabdoid tumor, atypical 215, 216
teratoid tumor 167
teratoma
- congenital 229
- pineal 210, 211
- sacrococcygeal 414, 415, 448
- spinal cord 413, 414
tethered cord 15, 33, 376
- lipoma 373, 374
thecal sacs, separate 376
third ventricle, rudimentary 48
thrive, failure 103

thrombosis
- herpes virus infection 296, 297
- venous sinus 245, 315–318, 368, 369
thyroglossal duct cyst 337, 338
tongue, schwannoma 348
TORCH 125
Tornwald cyst 339
toxoplasmosis 125
- HIV-infection 155, 156
trauma
- brachial plexus 421–424
- nonaccidental 236–247
- spinal 418–420
tuber cinereum, hamartoma 233, 234
tuberculoma, intracranial 160
tuberculosis 160, 161
- brain abscess 161, 162
tuberous sclerosis 225, 226, 449
- giant cell astrocytoma 463, 464
- low-grade glioma 465
- parenchymal calcification 462
- radial bands 461
- subependymal nodules 460
Turner-like syndrome 52
Turner's phenotype 52

U

ultrasonography 437
- head 125
UNO (unidentified neurofibromatosis objects) 455
urea cycle 104
urinary retention 383

V

valine 102
vanishing white matter disease 115–117
varicella-zoster virus, vasculopathy 297

vasculitis, CNS
- basal ganglia infarct 298
- posterior circulation infarct 300
vasculopathy
- herpes simplex virus 296, 297
- lenticulostriate 485, 486
- varicella-zoster virus 297
vasospasm 324
vein of *Galen* malformation 332–334
ventral induction 18
ventriculus terminalis 14, 376
vermian
- aplasia-hypoplasia 18
- dysplasia 472
vertebral body, scalloping 396
"viking helmet" configuration 20
Virchow-Robin spaces 73, 74
von Hippel-Lindau disease 182, 183, 449

W

Wada test 469
Walker-Warburg syndrome 39, 60
white matter
- aplasia 258
- lesions 465
Wiskott-Aldrich syndrome 301, 302
Wolf-Hirschhorn syndrome 356
Wyburn-Mason syndrome 303

X

xanthoastrocytoma, pleomorphic (PXA) 192–194, 203

Z

Zellweger syndrome 78, 79